1001909066

SO-EEK-994

CENTRE
GRANT MacEWAN
COMMUNITY COLLEGE

City Centre
RG
133.5
.P73

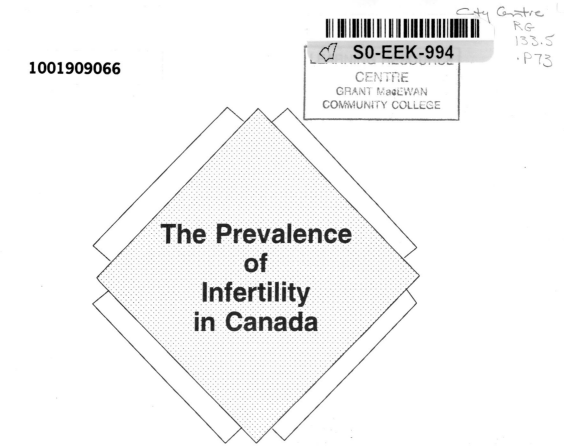

The Prevalence of Infertility in Canada

Volume 6 of the Research Studies

Royal Commission on
New Reproductive Technologies

© Minister of Supply and Services Canada, 1993
Printed and bound in Canada

This volume is available in both official languages. Each volume is individually priced, but is also available as part of a complete set containing all 15 volumes.

Available in Canada through your local bookseller
or by mail from
Canada Communications Group — Publishing
Ottawa, Canada K1A 0S9

CANADIAN CATALOGUING IN PUBLICATION DATA

Main entry under title:

The Prevalence of infertility in Canada

(Research studies ; no. 6)
Issued also in French under title: La prévalence de l'infertilité au Canada.
Includes bibliographical references.
ISBN 0-662-21380-7
Cat. no. Z1-1989/3-41-19E

1. Infertility — Canada — Statistics. 2. Health surveys — Canada. I. Canada. Royal Commission on New Reproductive Technologies. II. Series: Research studies (Canada. Royal Commission on New Reproductive Technologies) ; 6.

RG133.5P73 1993   616.6'92'00971   C94-980062-7

The Royal Commission on New Reproductive Technologies and the publishers wish to acknowledge with gratitude the following:

- Canada Communications Group, Printing Services
- Canada Communications Group, Graphics

Consistent with the Commission's commitment to full equality between men and women, care has been taken throughout this volume to use gender-neutral language wherever possible.

Contents

LEARNING RESOURCE
CENTRE
GRANT MacEWAN
COMMUNITY COLLEGE

1. Historical Overview of Medical Perceptions of Infertility in Canada, 1850-1950

Wendy L. Mitchinson

2. The Prevalence of Infertility in Canada, 1991-1992: Analysis of Three National Surveys

Corinne S. Dulberg and Thomas Stephens

Tables

Figures

⟨3⟩ Infertility Among Canadians: An Analysis of Data from the Canadian Fertility Survey (1984) and General Social Survey (1990)

T.R. Balakrishnan and Rajulton Fernando

Tables

4. Infertility, Sterilization, and Contraceptive Use in Ontario

T.R. Balakrishnan and Paul Maxim

Tables

⟨5⟩ Adoption as an Alternative for Infertile Couples: Prospects and Trends

Kerry J. Daly and Michael P. Sobol

Figures

⬦ 6 Annotated Bibliography on the Prevalence of Infertility

Michael R.P. de la Roche

Preface from the Chairperson

As Canadians living in the last decade of the twentieth century, we face unprecedented choices about procreation. Our responses to those choices — as individuals and as a society — say much about what we value and what our priorities are. Some technologies, such as those for assisted reproduction, are unlikely to become a common means of having a family — although the number of children born as a result of these techniques is greater than the number of infants placed for adoption in Canada. Others, such as ultrasound during pregnancy, are already generally accepted, and half of all pregnant women aged 35 and over undergo prenatal diagnostic procedures. Still other technologies, such as fetal tissue research, have little to do with reproduction as such, but may be of benefit to people suffering from diseases such as Parkinson's; they raise important ethical issues in the use and handling of reproductive tissues.

It is clear that opportunities for technological intervention raise issues that affect all of society; in addition, access to the technologies depends on the existence of public structures and policies to provide them. The values and priorities of society, as expressed through its institutions, laws, and funding arrangements, will affect individual options and choices.

As Canadians became more aware of these technologies throughout the 1980s, there was a growing awareness that there was an unacceptably large gap between the rapid pace of technological change and the policy development needed to guide decisions about whether and how to use such powerful technologies. There was also a realization of how little reliable information was available to make the needed policy decisions. In addition, many of the attitudes and assumptions underlying the way in which technologies were being developed and made available did not reflect the profound changes that have been transforming Canada in recent decades. Individual cases were being dealt with in isolation, and often in the absence of informed social consensus. At the same time, Canadians were looking more critically at the role of science and technology in their lives in general, becoming more aware of their limited capacity to solve society's problems.

These concerns came together in the creation of the Royal Commission on New Reproductive Technologies. The Commission was established by the federal government in October 1989, with a wide-ranging and complex mandate. It is important to understand that the Commission was asked to consider the technologies' impact not only on society, but also on specific groups in society, particularly women and children. It was asked to consider not only the technologies' scientific and medical aspects, but also their ethical, legal, social, economic, and health implications. Its mandate was extensive, as it was directed to examine not only current developments in the area of new reproductive technologies, but also potential ones; not only techniques related to assisted conception, but also those of prenatal diagnosis; not only the condition of infertility, but also its causes and prevention; not only applications of technology, but also research, particularly embryo and fetal tissue research.

The appointment of a Royal Commission provided an opportunity to collect much-needed information, to foster public awareness and public debate, and to provide a principled framework for Canadian public policy on the use or restriction of these technologies.

The Commission set three broad goals for its work: to provide direction for public policy by making sound, practical, and principled recommendations; to leave a legacy of increased knowledge to benefit Canadian and international experience with new reproductive technologies; and to enhance public awareness and understanding of the issues surrounding new reproductive technologies to facilitate public participation in determining the future of the technologies and their place in Canadian society.

To fulfil these goals, the Commission held extensive public consultations, including private sessions for people with personal experiences of the technologies that they did not want to discuss in a public forum, and it developed an interdisciplinary research program to ensure that its recommendations would be informed by rigorous and wide-ranging research. In fact, the Commission published some of that research in advance of the Final Report to assist those working in the field of reproductive health and new reproductive technologies and to help inform the public.

The results of the research program are presented in these volumes. In all, the Commission developed and gathered an enormous body of information and analysis on which to base its recommendations, much of it available in Canada for the first time. This solid base of research findings helped to clarify the issues and produce practical and useful recommendations based on reliable data about the reality of the situation, not on speculation.

The Commission sought the involvement of the most qualified researchers to help develop its research projects. In total, more than 300 scholars and academics representing more than 70 disciplines — including the social sciences, humanities, medicine, genetics, life sciences, law, ethics, philosophy, and theology — at some 21 Canadian universities and 13 hospitals, clinics, and other institutions were involved in the research program.

The Commission was committed to a research process with high standards and a protocol that included internal and external peer review for content and methodology, first at the design stage and later at the report stage. Authors were asked to respond to these reviews, and the process resulted in the achievement of a high standard of work. The protocol was completed before the publication of the studies in this series of research volumes. Researchers using human subjects were required to comply with appropriate ethical review standards.

These volumes of research studies reflect the Commission's wide mandate. We believe the findings and analysis contained in these volumes will be useful for many people, both in this country and elsewhere.

Along with the other Commissioners, I would like to take this opportunity to extend my appreciation and thanks to the researchers and external reviewers who have given tremendous amounts of time and thought to the Commission. I would also like to acknowledge the entire Commission staff for their hard work, dedication, and commitment over the life of the Commission. Finally, I would like to thank the more than 40 000 Canadians who were involved in the many facets of the Commission's work. Their contribution has been invaluable.

Patricia A. Baird

Patricia Baird, M.D., C.M., FRCPC, F.C.C.M.G.

Introduction

At the outset of the Commission's work, it was evident that a better understanding of how significant a problem infertility is for Canadians was needed. We found that very little was known in a definitive way about the overall frequency of infertility in this country. Developing accurate and valid estimates of the prevalence of infertility was, therefore, an important Commission research activity, and this volume provides, for the first time, national data on the prevalence of infertility in Canada. Estimates of the prevalence of infertility are important for policy makers who have to make decisions about what priority to attach to responses to infertility and what resources to devote to them, be they initiatives with regard to prevention or initiatives with regard to treatment of those who are already infertile.

However, in describing the findings regarding the prevalence of infertility, it should be borne in mind that "infertility" is defined differently for different purposes. It is, therefore, important to define clearly what is being measured in any population study that is carried out and to make clear that infertility may be viewed and defined differently for different purposes.

This volume examines infertility from several perspectives. First, to provide some context, it presents a historical overview of how infertility has been perceived by the medical profession in Canada. It then sets out the methods used and the findings from the three national surveys that were commissioned on the prevalence of infertility in Canada. In addition, researchers analyzed some data from past surveys, although the usefulness of findings from these other surveys is limited, as their goals were not to measure infertility per se but, rather, to focus on fertility. However, results from these surveys are presented, as well as an annotated bibliography that provides results from various published studies in the world literature on the prevalence of infertility in different groups and populations. To put the statistics that are presented into a human context, and because it is often suggested as a way of dealing with the inability to have children, the volume also contains a study of adoption in Canada. The findings of that study underscore that adoption is no longer an available option for many of those who are unable to conceive and bear children.

The Studies

In the century between 1850 and 1950, as Wendy Mitchinson describes, the medical establishment took a less than active interest in infertility. When it finally became a topic of interest, the focus was primarily on female factor infertility and on treatment rather than prevention. There was a strong propensity to "blame the patient" for her infertility, and relationships between physicians and their patients who were infertile were structured within the context of the physician as the authority figure. There are many still-relevant implications for understanding the way infertility is viewed, prevented, and treated in the portrait of the past that Dr. Mitchinson paints. For instance, the strong belief in the power of medical technology that she outlines is still very much with us, and the relative lack of resources devoted to prevention is still very much an issue. The "blind spot" with respect to male infertility is being addressed, but it is clear that there is still much to be done to rebalance the focus of research on women. Efforts to ensure informed consent and informed choice, and new efforts toward a more equal relationship between practitioners and patients, based on mutual respect with an exchange of information about technical aspects and personal priorities, are what is needed to deal with the still-applicable situations Dr. Mitchinson describes.

In the past, almost all estimates of infertility have been the by-product of broader studies focussing on fertility. From these efforts emerged the realization that infertility must be addressed and measured in its own right, and Corinne Dulberg and Thomas Stephens have done exactly that. Three different national surveys put the same questions to respondents to find out what percentage of couples who had been married or cohabiting for a given period of time had not been using contraception throughout that time and had not had a pregnancy. Two measures were taken — the percentage without a pregnancy after one year and the percentage in that situation after two years.

As is noted in their paper on the prevalence of infertility in Canada, the results of all three surveys are very close: 8.5 percent of couples who had been married or cohabiting for one year and not using contraception had not had a pregnancy in that time period, and 7 percent of couples who had been married or cohabiting for two years and not using contraception had not had a pregnancy. This two-year figure is the more useful one, as a significant percentage of those who have not had a pregnancy in the first year will have one in the second 12 months. These results are very similar to those of the series of National Surveys on Family Growth that have been carried out in the United States over the past 20 years, and they indicate that infertility is a problem for a significant minority of Canadians of childbearing age. The fact that 250 000 couples are experiencing infertility is an important finding that puts questions of the prevention and treatment of infertility into a broader perspective.

Although necessarily limited in usefulness because of their primary focus on fertility, data from major fertility- or health-related surveys carried out in Canada over the past decade were subjected to secondary analyses by T.R. Balakrishnan. In the first of these studies, Dr. Balakrishnan and his colleague, Rajulton Fernando, examined infertility-related results from the Canadian Fertility Survey of 1984 and the General Social Survey of 1990. In the second study, Dr. Balakrishnan and Paul Maxim examined infertility, sterilization, and contraceptive use in Ontario, using results derived from a study of general health in Ontario carried out in 1990. The results of these secondary analyses demonstrate the problems inherent in attempting to extrapolate data to reach conclusions about infertility from data collected on fertility; they underscore the necessity of using tools designed to directly measure infertility in any attempt to assess prevalence. It is simply not possible to extrapolate accurately data from surveys designed for other purposes, and the findings of somewhat lower infertility figures cannot be considered as reliable as the figures reported by Drs. Dulberg and Stephens. The additional information on sterilization and contraceptive use, however, is valuable for the perspective it provides on infertility. What emerges is the reality that the preoccupation of the vast majority of Canadians of childbearing age is limiting fertility rather than overcoming infertility.

Half of the Canadians surveyed by the Commission in two different surveys said they would explore adoption if they could not have children. In this context, the results of Kerry Daly's and Michael Sobol's national study of adoption are sobering. Put succinctly, adoption is no longer a viable option for most infertile couples. There are various reasons for the sharp drop in the number of infants available for public adoption over the past 20 years, but a significant reason is that many young women are now choosing to keep their children rather than putting them up for adoption. Drs. Daly and Sobol also note that adoption raises many of the same issues for parents as infertility treatment, particularly donor insemination, because of the lack of a biological link between at least one parent and the child. The points they raise about the importance of an adopted child's knowing about his or her genetic origins are also applicable to the needs of children born through the use of donated sperm or eggs.

Finally, Michael de la Roche has examined published information on the prevalence of infertility in some groups that have been studied in Canada and other industrialized countries. His findings demonstrate how little data are available in this area, but data that are available indicate that the frequency of infertility is fairly similar in developed countries.

Conclusions

The studies in this volume lead to the conclusion that there are a significant number of Canadian couples who would like, but are unable, to have children, and that the options open to them are limited. It is of significance and concern that currently, at any given time, 250 000 couples in this country are experiencing infertility, defined as not having had a pregnancy despite two years without using contraception. It indicates the need both for more research and action in preventing infertility and for effective and safe infertility treatments. The study of Drs. Dulberg and Stephens has provided the first point in what should be an ongoing tracking of the prevalence of infertility in Canada. It is apparent that trends in prevalence must be tracked over time if we are to gauge whether infertility is increasing or decreasing — essential information for sound public policy regarding infertility.

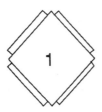

Historical Overview of Medical Perceptions of Infertility in Canada, 1850-1950

Wendy L. Mitchinson

Executive Summary

This paper examines the medical perceptions and treatment of infertility in Canada from 1850 to 1950. It begins with a study of the medical profession itself, followed by an examination of the importance of bearing and raising children during this period, and concludes that the focus was on motherhood, not fatherhood or parenthood. In the late nineteenth century, physicians did not focus specifically on infertility. This seemed to await the inter-war years — perhaps because accurate information on the female cycle became available. Doctors were vague about the way in which they defined sterility (which is the term they used), and their growing interest in the field does not seem to have been the result of increasing infertility within society. The paper examines attitudes toward male and female infertility and concludes that doctors perceived many of the causes of infertility to be the "fault" of lifestyle, that is, the way in which people lived their lives. In addition, they blamed colleagues for some of the difficulties faced by women. The paper ends with a brief look at some of the infertility treatment provided during this period and concludes that physicians focussed on hormonal therapy and on surgery. Of less interest to them were preventive measures.

This paper was completed for the Royal Commission on New Reproductive Technologies in June 1992.

Introduction

This paper addresses medical attitudes toward and treatment of infertility in Canada between 1850 and 1950. It begins in the mid-nineteenth century, when the medical profession began to assert itself and to attain the prominence and prestige it now enjoys. In the decades immediately following, Canadians first became aware of the declining birth rate and initiated a discourse on fertility (and infertility) that allows for historical analysis. The study covers a hundred-year period to allow both short-term and long-term themes to emerge; these in turn can be examined to determine whether they are time-linked, that is, related to contemporary social attitudes and cultural values, and/or profession-linked, that is, integral to the way medicine is or was practised in our society. Social attitudes, cultural values, and the way medicine is practised do not change quickly, and, consequently, an extended perspective is needed if change is to be detected. By 1950, the study of infertility had become an accepted specialty. Later, the literature becomes so voluminous and engaged in technical debate as to be deserving of a separate study; however, while infertility treatments may have changed after 1950 and some additional causes of infertility may have been perceived, it is unlikely that the themes, which had survived within the profession for a hundred years, disappeared completely.

The focus of this study is Canada. The sources used are Canadian medical journals in which physicians from across the country described their practices and debated the issues that concerned them. These journals also contain reprints of leading foreign articles, which kept Canadian physicians abreast of what was happening elsewhere and so represented the wider medical world. Examined as well were many of the textbooks used in Canadian medical schools during this period. Most were non-Canadian in origin, only because few Canadian texts existed until well into the twentieth century. Chosen by the leading physicians in Canadian medical schools as authoritative sources for medical students, these texts were influential. Both types of sources contain a wealth of information on infertility; they reflect what Canadian practitioners were being taught, were reading, and were writing. In addition, popular health manuals and periodical literature were systematically examined to get a sense of what information was available to lay Canadians.

Does it make sense to study medical perceptions of infertility from a national perspective? Surely medicine as practised in Canada was part of Western medicine and simply reflected what was happening elsewhere? Such arguments are spurious. Physicians in Canada practised in a different social milieu from those in other countries. Because medical practice cannot be divorced from the society in which its practitioners lived, it is incumbent on us as Canadians to understand the world as those who lived here in the past understood it.[1]

The Canadian Medical Profession

To understand and assess medical perceptions and treatment of infertility over one hundred years, it is necessary to be aware of the development of the Canadian medical profession. The status and position of physicians influenced what they thought and did. They could not divorce themselves from their own time and social context, and it would be expecting the impossible to assume that they could. Although a general overview of the profession is presented, training in obstetrics and gynaecology is examined in more detail because traditionally the two went hand in hand and were the medical specialties that focussed most on infertility during the period under review. Urology emerged in a major way only in the twentieth century; even then its focus on infertility was minor compared to that of gynaecology.

For much of the nineteenth century, general practitioners had little prestige and faced an array of competitors — irregular practitioners, midwives, patent medicine people, and so on. Only toward the end of the century were they able to achieve a medical monopoly, largely because of their efforts to control entry to the profession, through the development of professional organizations, and, most significantly, through the adoption of a single standard of education as a prerequisite for licensing. Thus physicians were a group on the rise but not one that had arrived.

In the early decades of the twentieth century, physicians built on their medical monopoly, and by the end of the 1940s they emerged as members of an esteemed profession. Aiding in this rise was the expansion of hospitals and their success in attracting paying rather than non-paying patients. Hospitals, with their emphasis on cleanliness and their ability to purchase the latest in medical technology that was beyond the means of individual practitioners, made explicit the distance that separated the patient and the physician. Medical specialization only added to that distance, as did increases in the length of study and training required to become a licensed practitioner.[2]

The morality of the time, particularly as it affected the examination of the female body, constrained the training of physicians, especially in obstetrics and gynaecology. In 1850, the *British American Journal of Medical and Physical Science* stated that demonstrative midwifery was a "violation of one of the fundamental rules of the lying-in chamber: that all *unnecessary exposure of the patient should be avoided.* The accoucheur's *eyes* should ... be at *his fingers' ends.*"[3] Viewing a birth was the exception rather than the rule. The fact that, from their beginnings, the Montreal Maternity Hospital and the Montreal Lying-In Hospital permitted students to do so placed both institutions in the forefront of North American training hospitals.[4]   A similar reticence existed about performing internal examinations on women, especially virgins.[5]

By the turn of the century, most medical texts insisted on the need to view and examine the female body in the interests of providing better medical care. This signalled a perceived separation between doctors as professional beings and as sexual beings; that is, in their professional lives they were physicians, not men. In obstetrics this can be seen in the insistence by most medical colleges that students view and attend at a certain number of births in order to graduate. For example, in 1912-13 a student had to have attended six maternity cases before graduating from the medical college of Dalhousie University.[6] The earlier reticence about men viewing the female body was difficult to overcome, however. Harold Atlee recalled his own training at Dalhousie during this period:

> Four or five of us [students] sat on a long bench against one wall of a rather large room, the bed of the patient being about 30 feet away against the opposite wall. Dr. Trenaman sat in a chair beside the bed, ... partly obstructing the view. From time to time he would run an ungloved hand in under the blankets, until finally ... he drew forth the baby and held it up for us to see ... I shall never forget the prudish solemnity with which he crossed the room and said to us: "Gentlemen, that's the proper way to deliver a child. A woman's private parts should never be exposed."[7]

The deficiencies of such training did not go unnoticed. In 1911, a study of obstetric education in one Canadian and 42 American medical schools found that more than one-third of the professors were general practitioners with little specialized training in obstetrics.[8] This resulted in poor care for pregnant women.[9] Those who specialized in obstetrics were concerned about this situation and determined to improve the obstetrical education of doctors, but they recognized that not all of their colleagues shared their enthusiasm. In 1917, Dr. S.P. Ford referred to a colleague who expressed disdain for obstetrics, stating that "he would rather clean out a garbage can than attend a confinement."[10] A similar situation, although not perhaps as extreme, existed in gynaecology.[11]

Physicians' perceptions of the deficient education provided them continued into the 1920s, 1930s, and 1940s. Training in obstetrics and gynaecology was certainly more intense than it had been, but, compared to other specialties and what could have been done, it was still inadequate. One physician noted in the 1929 *Canadian Journal of Medicine and Surgery*, for example, that more time was devoted to training for surgery than to obstetrics and gynaecology, by a factor of about two to one.[12] This occurred despite the fact that general practitioners needed obstetrical and gynaecological skills more than surgical ones.

No training can ever prepare a medical student for the reality of actual practice, but it is still worthwhile to question why doctors in the inter-war years and beyond believed that their medical education was deficient, especially in obstetrics.[13] Was there a general disdain for this specialty, as some continued to suggest?[14] If there was, it would partially account for what many physicians considered the poor childbirth practices followed by some of their colleagues. Such practices were often a major cause of gynaecological disorders and injuries, some of which resulted in sterility.

Although many physicians believed that they should have received a better medical education, the general public did not share this perspective. Indeed, between 1850 and 1950 the medical profession grew in public stature and essentially became the arbiter of health. One reason for this was the emergence of science. If Canadians had once looked to the Bible for guidance in understanding the world about them, by the end of the nineteenth century they increasingly looked to science, finding comfort in the notion that because science was objective, it reflected a divine purpose.[15] The alignment of medicine with science raised the status of physicians and gave them, in the eyes of many Canadians, the aura of expertise on a wide variety of issues that physicians had connected to the body — birth control, sexuality, education, and exercise, to name only a few. Medicine became the mediator between medical science and lay people, and the trend only intensified as science increased its sway throughout the twentieth century.

Given the significance of this role, it becomes important to examine in whose hands this mediation lay. Who were the doctors? For the period under study it is easy to generalize. Doctors tended to be white, middle-class males, and they saw the world through these filters. This means that members of the profession seldom challenged established social norms, but rather reflected those norms and provided a scientific rationale for them. Norms often influenced the way doctors interpreted and applied their medical "knowledge." For example, in the late nineteenth century, Canadians were concerned that women were restricting the number of children they bore. Doctors in turn criticized birth control as unhealthy, even though they were aware that non-harmful methods were available.[16] Their opinions on birth control were largely based on moral and social considerations. Similarly, they shared accepted social views as they applied to issues such as fertility, infertility, and the respective "blame" assigned to men and women for childlessness. By supporting the norms of society, practitioners maintained their control.

Motherhood

In a historical study of infertility, it is important to examine attitudes toward parenthood. Only if parenthood is deemed socially valuable is a couple's infertility a problem. In the period under review, however, there is little discussion of this issue; instead, the focus is on motherhood. The continuing perception of doctors and other Canadians over the entire period was that motherhood was central to woman's existence. Fatherhood was not central to man's.

The emotional concept of motherhood, as we know it, is a relatively new phenomenon. As Jesse Bernard points out, it is a product of affluence, for "in most parts of the world ... adult, able-bodied women have been, and still are, too valuable in their productive capacity to be spared for the exclusive care of children."[17] The word itself first appeared in the *Oxford English Dictionary* in 1597 and referred to the fact of being a mother; only in the Victorian era did the word "emerge as a concept rather than a mere statement of fact."[18] Although there were complex reasons to account for this change, the influence of science cannot be overlooked. The concept of motherhood gained support when it was understood that the woman was more than simply a receptacle for "active seminal matter." This was proven without a doubt in 1854, when scientists first saw the fusion of sperm and egg.[19] The emphasis on women as mothers was also partly a result of the Victorian penchant for distinguishing between men and women. Before the nineteenth century, lay and medical people alike had seen woman as an inferior version of man (for example, the vagina was considered an internal penis); in the nineteenth century, they saw her as something other than man.[20] Man was the norm, and the emphasis was on how woman differed from him, a perspective that persists to this day. What changed over the period was the differences perceived, not the emphasis on differences.

In the late nineteenth and early twentieth centuries, Canadians viewed women as physically weaker than and intellectually inferior to men.[21] Doctors explained the latter using scientific or medical terminology. As a physician explained in the 1905 *Canada Lancet*, puberty was the culprit. "During this time, brain weight is actually lost by the lessening of the usual blood supply to the brain, which is diverted to nourish rapidly growing organs. The child's brain is now easily fatigued, and what is acquired by a tired brain is soon lost."[22] These themes of difference continued into the 1920s and beyond. The feminist Emily Murphy argued that it is "natural for a girl to be good, also easier."[23] Again, doctors attempted to explain this and other psychological differences:

> A grand difference between plant and animal life lies in the fact that the plant is concerned chiefly with the storing of energy, and the animal with consuming it. The plant by a very slow process converts lifeless matter into living matter, expending little energy and living at a profit. The animal lives upon the plant world and in contrast to plants lives at a loss of energy.

Thus, in biological terms "the habit of the plant is predominantly anabolic, that of the animal predominantly katabolic." The conclusion: "that woman comes nearer to the metabolism of the plant than does man."[24]

Not all physicians believed differences between the sexes were biologically immutable. A very few argued that environmental factors were a cause of many of the differences.[25] But even when old stereotypes weakened, acknowledgment of their shortcomings was at times grudging. When large numbers of women entered paid employment during the Second World War, an article by Dr. Lydia Giberson in the 1944 *Canadian Medical Association Journal* still focussed on the differences between the male and female worker:

> The healthy, mature woman, if given a chance to adjust herself to the new demands, can expend without harm as much energy as the male worker, though at a slower rate and with more frequent rest periods. The energy potentials of both are not dissimilar. The male is more explosive; he can summon greater strength for a short period. But the healthy female has great reserves of endurance and recovers rapidly from fatigue; the fact that she is more subject to worry and other emotional drains on her energy obscures but does not alter these physiological generalizations.[26]

The emphasis on differences throughout this period stems partly from Canadians' perception of the proper role of men and women in society. Men were to be the breadwinners and women the nurturers; it seemed "natural" to assume that these different roles required different characteristics.[27]

Perceptions of difference would not be problematic except that they led to different treatment of the two sexes in all spheres. An examination of one sphere (in part because it is linked to the discussion of disease in women resulting in infertility) should be sufficient to make the point. Of particular concern for doctors and Canadians alike was the education girls received. An author in the *Canadian Magazine* at the turn of the century made it clear that, although girls' education should be just as thorough as that for boys, it should be different.[28] Providing as thorough an education for girls was difficult, however, because some doctors, focussing on girls' "weakness" during puberty, advocated removing girls from school for three or four days a month.[29] Even if young women were not made physical wrecks through the pressures of education, doctors argued that training girls and boys in a similar way was unnatural — that is, it did not maintain the proper role division between the sexes.[30] And certainly education was expected to maintain differences — a belief made explicit by educators as late as the 1940s.[31]

Canadians' anxiety about education for girls was linked to their perception of the roles they believed men and women should play. Sexual and gender differences existed so women and men could marry and have children; it was natural to do so. This theme dominates popular and professional literature during the period. Potential and imperative became one — that is, because women could bear children they should bear children, an idea that dates from time immemorial.[32] In the nineteenth century, this emphasis intensified as a shift occurred from the concept of parenting (or even fathering) to mothering. In a mid-century popular health manual, Eugene Becklard made it very clear that "there is no such thing as natural barrenness in natural women."[33] Thus only unnatural women were childless. The assumption underlying the Victorian view was that it was woman's responsibility to have children and her fault if a marriage remained childless.[34] As one doctor claimed, women could see this failure to produce only "as a reproach to [their] womanhood."[35]   This view deepened toward the end of the century. In his popular handbook, Pye Henry Chavasse maintained that for a wife, children were "as necessary to her happiness as the food she eats and the air she breathes." He even went so far as to argue that health was necessary for a woman, not for her own sake but so that she could bear healthy children.[36]   Doctors seldom differentiated between motherhood as a social phenomenon and as a biological one; they collapsed both into the biological.

This emphasis on the importance of maternity continued into the twentieth century. Dr. Winfield Scott Hall argued that children had the power "to keep hearts young."[37]   John Martin claimed in the 1916 *Public Health Journal* that even feminists acknowledged that a child was necessary for the "complete self-realization" of women.[38] Perhaps no one expressed this view more blatantly than Dr. Eugene St. Jacques, Professor of Clinical Surgery at the University of Montreal, when he concluded in 1923 that "the heart and soul of a woman lie in her pelvis."[39] The prospect of having children, then, controlled a woman's entire life. Dr. H.B. Atlee, head of gynaecology at Dalhousie Medical College in 1931, made this clear in an article for the *Canadian Home Journal.*   "A woman's physical upbringing from her earliest years must have childbearing as its aim and end ... It means that woman must carve out a feminine way of life, a way that differs from the male as her destiny differs from his."[40] Two of the most popular sex manuals in the 1940s also picked up on these themes. Dr. Percy Ryberg explained to readers in *Health, Sex and Birth Control* that the goal of every girl was to marry and to procreate. Alfred Tyrer, in *Sex, Marriage and Birth Control*, maintained that "every normal woman has the maternal instinct."[41]   Childless marriages were seen as unhappy marriages.[42] The irony of these perceptions is their vehemence, as if doctors feared that, unless encouraged, women would reject the maternal role and with that rejection upset the perceived "gender balance" that stabilized society.

Although the central importance of motherhood and its naturalness for women was a constant theme over the years, there was a sense that childbirth itself was not natural. This was less so in the late nineteenth century, when the nature and scope of intervention practised by obstetricians during childbirth were limited compared to what came to be the case in the twentieth century. As the twentieth century progressed, it became clear that physicians believed that there was a very fine line between physiological and pathological. Together with the realization that Canada had one of the highest maternal mortality rates in the industrialized world, this led to a very aggressive prenatal movement in the 1920s; the goal was for doctors to provide care for the woman from the time she became pregnant to the birth of her child and after.[43] Physicians were also aware of and concerned about the fact that many women were trying to escape their maternal obligations.[44] In the nineteenth and early twentieth centuries, this concern focussed on birth control, as Canadians in general and doctors in particular became aware of the declining birth rate. By the 1920s, and continuing into the 1940s, the focus shifted to the increase in the number of women working in paid employment and the perception that these women were delaying marriage.

Physicians accepted that it was woman's role to have children. Yet some were intrigued by why this burden was placed on women, the so-called weaker sex. In the nineteenth century, a few explained it by arguing that childbearing actually improved women's health. It was especially important for the maintenance of sanity. As M.L. Holbrook made clear in *Parturition Without Pain*, "the process of child-bearing is essentially necessary to the physical health and long life, the mental happiness ... of women."[45] Others were not so optimistic. Writing in 1890 in *The Physical Life of Woman*, George Napheys saw a darker side to childbearing. "Perhaps it is a wise provision that she is thus reminded of her lowly duty, lest man should make her the sole object of his worship, or lest the pride of beauty should obscure the sense of shame."[46] Childbearing, then, kept women in their place. Less dark but equally firm in arguing that childbearing was what determined the limits on women's activities was Dr. Atlee, who argued in 1931 that "woman will always be handicapped physically by the fact that she must bear the burden of the generations; it is inescapably part of her destiny."[47] Percy Ryberg echoed this view in his popular 1942 sex manual.[48] If women tried to avoid or delay childbearing they would face increasing difficulties. Older women simply could not give birth as easily as younger women.[49]

So central was childbearing to women's established social role that some physicians believed that women who could not give birth should not marry. This was particularly true in the late nineteenth and early twentieth centuries, when sexuality was considered acceptable only within marriage and for procreative purposes.[50] Late-nineteenth-century physicians believed that there was no way for women to avoid their destiny; celibacy was actually considered dangerous. According to George Napheys, celibacy could cause chorea, painful menstruation, mania, and hallucinations. Of special concern was the development of hysteria in celibate or sterile women.[51] Women's reproductive organs had specific functions, doctors argued; if they were not used, ill health, whether mental or physical, could result. Although physicians seldom discussed how lack of childbearing and ill health were inter-related, it was not an idle belief. Because physicians were convinced of the centrality of maternity for women, they were extremely sensitive about interfering with a woman's ability to conceive. Throughout the nineteenth and early decades of the twentieth centuries, they opposed birth control, and, noteworthy at the turn of the century, they were concerned about the increasing number of ovariotomies being performed.[52]

The foregoing description of doctors' and Canadians' views on women and motherhood indicates the firm place of childbearing in people's understanding of womanhood. This concept remained constant over a hundred-year period; women were to have children, and if they did not, or could not, they were considered deficient as women and lacking as wives. Given these beliefs, it is not surprising that doctors were interested in helping women have children. But what kind of help could they provide? What information did they have at their disposal?

Knowledge of Conception

The perceived causes of infertility and their treatment depend on how much doctors and others understood about conception. From the nineteenth century until the mid-1920s, doctors' understanding of conception was such that their advice to patients was unlikely to be of much help. In 1827, scientists first identified the mammalian ovum outside the body. This was followed in 1832 by the identification of the human ovum, which made the relationship between menstruation and the reproductive process more than a matter of conjecture. The role of spermatozoa in fertility was discovered when they were found to be absent in an 1853 study of 20 childless men "who had suffered from an early double epididymitis."[53] The external fertilization of mammalian egg and sperm first occurred in 1875, although the actual viewing of a human ovum took place only in the 1930s. By the turn of the century, doctors came to accept that the sperm was not carried into the uterus by the woman's actions but rather moved on its own. More significantly, in 1924 scientists accurately identified the human fertile period. Finally, in the 1940s, a physician paired a human ovum with sperm *in vitro* but did not document any fertilization.[54]

Of particular interest to physicians in the nineteenth and early twentieth centuries was the menstrual cycle. Not understanding it, they tried to explain it through the use of animal analogies — specifically to "the heat ... of the lower animals."[55] In 1904, Dr. Jennie G. Drennan of St. Thomas, Ontario, used this analogy but went so far as to suggest that menstruation, as it was exhibited in women, was actually pathological and that if women were really healthy their bodies would behave more like those of other animals; unfortunately the "pernicious environment" of modern society prevented this.[56] Even a scientist as renowned as J.B. Collip was still using the comparison between menstruation in women and the estrous cycle in the "lower animals" as late as 1930.[57] Although he recognized that the two processes were not the same, by comparing them, as others had before him, Collip aligned women with the "lower" species and made menstruation appear strange and non-human.

Linked to concerns about menstruation was a fascination with the purpose of the ovaries. Evident in the debate about the number of ovariotomies being performed, which heated up in the late nineteenth century, was the admission that most physicians could not tell a healthy ovary from a diseased one and had little concept of what the ovary actually did.[58] In 1906, the authors of *A System of Gynaecology* even felt it necessary to assure their student readers that in the event of the removal of an ovary, a woman was still capable of giving birth to children of both sexes — that is, the ovary did not determine the sex of the child.[59] With each generation the functioning of the ovary was understood better.[60] By 1915, doctors recognized that the ovaries produced internal secretions necessary for the "function of the whole genital apparatus," but no one really understood the "nature of those secretions" or "where they [were] produced."[61] By the 1930s, the medical profession had become intrigued by the sex hormone and its source, which some suggested was the ovary. Beckwith Whitehouse, Professor of Gynaecology and Obstetrics at the University of Birmingham, acknowledged in the 1933 *Canadian Medical Association Journal* that the belief that the sex hormone was "the active principle of the ovary" made sense based on the work of earlier investigators, but that newer studies revealed that the sex hormone was present in many body fluids and organs.[62]

Considering the above, it is not surprising that, until the mid-1920s, doctors were unable to give women accurate advice about the best time for conception. Indeed, some of their advice was inaccurate and guaranteed to reduce a woman's chances of bearing a child. Until well into the twentieth century, there was virtual uniformity in physicians' advice to women — "The tendency to pregnancy is greater just before, during and immediately after the menstrual week."[63] This of course is the infertile time of the menstrual cycle. As more accurate information became available, doctors corrected their advice and became interested not in when conception was possible but when the optimum time for this was. By 1930, they were estimating that ovulation occurred from the twelfth to the fourteenth day after menstruation and that conception was most likely when intercourse took place between the tenth and eighteenth days. Estimates of the optimum time for conception were narrowed again ten years later when doctors concluded that spermatozoa could survive only three days at most after ejaculation. This was a far cry from the five weeks one physician estimated earlier in the century. Considering that the ovum too had a life of only three days, the timing had to be exact.[64] By the late 1940s, physicians had a sense that this was possible.[65]

One contentious belief in the history of fertility was that orgasm in a woman was necessary for, or at least helpful in, conception. The Greek physician Galen believed this, and the belief had been passed down from one generation of physicians to another.[66] One nineteenth-century doctor even argued that women had to be in a state of greater sexual arousal than men in order to conceive male children.[67] In the early twentieth century physicians were more ambivalent. One explained that the lack of sexual pleasure on the part of the woman was not in and of itself a cause of sterility but "significant of some pathological condition being present."[68] Similar views were expressed decades later, although not with any consistency.[69] Others such as Dr. W. Blair Bell hedged their bets. He noted in 1917 that sexual aversion did not prevent fertility but that it did lessen "the likelihood of genital turgescence and follicular dehiscence," although he was not specific about how these influenced conception.[70] In 1928, Dr. William Graves told student readers that infertility and lack of sexual arousal did go together, but for him this was a result of dyspareunia or frigidity on the part of the woman, the latter itself "characteristic of the asthenic, hysteric, infantilistic, intersexual, homosexual, and old-maid types of women."[71] Most physicians did not go that far but nevertheless continued to associate fertility and sexual arousal, albeit in a way that revealed that they did not understand the relationship between the two.[72] What they did make clear was that women themselves connected these phenomena.[73]

Linked to doctors' knowledge of fertility was their ability to diagnose a pregnancy. Doctors were concerned about this for many reasons; their professional reputation was at stake, and, once prenatal care became the norm, the idea emerged that the earlier a pregnant woman came under a doctor's care, the better were her chances of bringing a live child to term.[74] This is why physicians welcomed the Zondek-Ascheim pregnancy test, which became available in the 1930s.[75] But physicians desired even more accurate tests. In the mid-1930s R. Gottlieb, a Montreal practitioner, referred to the use of the female bitterling. Apparently the fish possessed "an ovipositor which [was] supposed to elongate when the animal [was] exposed to pregnancy urine." In the 1940s, with the acceptance of women into the military, interest was raised in the efficacy of the colostrum and histidine tests to screen out pregnant applicants.[76] By this time, physicians were confident that they had an accurate grasp of the principles of reproduction, knowledge that could help in overcoming the infertility of many couples.

Infertility

Considering the importance of having children, particularly for women, it is not surprising that doctors saw infertility as a problem or condition to be overcome.[77] Patient records almost always mentioned whether a woman had given birth, and, when a childless woman consulted a physician for a disorder, was cured, and subsequently gave birth, the physician reported the birth with satisfaction, suggesting that this "lack" had also been part of the disease, at least from the point of view of the physician. In 1930, Toronto doctor M.C. Watson described what he considered a normal situation. He believed that many women sought medical relief from certain disorders in the hope that treatment would relieve their infertility even though that was not the ostensible reason for their seeking treatment.[78]

Even if this assessment was accurate, it suggests that women were not alone in their concern; doctors, too, were worried about infertility. In the nineteenth century, the concerns were not specific except in physicians' emphasis on women having babies and infertility as a consequence of other health problems. In the early twentieth century, as the birth rate in Canada continued to decline, more detailed discussions of infertility as an issue emerged. Indeed, the 1923 *Canadian Medical Association Journal* reported with approval an English speaker who declared that "the percentage of sterility is the index of the morals of a nation."[79]

One point of interest in discussions of infertility was the evolution of opinion about how long a couple had to be childless before doctors considered it a "problem." Most physicians in the nineteenth and early twentieth centuries took three years or more as a guideline.[80] It appears, however, that as the medical profession became more interested in infertility, the definition narrowed and consensus dissipated. Although some physicians continued to adhere to the three-year guideline, by the 1930s many had adopted 12 months as the definition. In the 1940s, many shifted to a two-year rule, although some still held to the one-year definition. By 1950, there was a reference once again to three years.[81]

If there was no consensus on how long childlessness should persist before doctors diagnosed infertility, there was even less agreement about terminology. Most doctors used the term sterility rather than infertility. Some physicians used sterility as the term for a situation where an egg was never fertilized,[82] but most did not, allowing them to include habitual spontaneous abortion, stillbirths, and other conditions that prevented a live birth. But these generalizations do not convey the variations. Some doctors referred to the inability to conceive as absolute sterility or primary sterility. Others referred to the inability to bring forth a living child as sterility, secondary sterility, or relative sterility. Some also referred to acquired sterility, where a woman had given birth but was unable to conceive again.[83] Acquired sterility, sometimes referred to as one-child sterility, was also mentioned under the broader category of secondary sterility. For statistical purposes, however, acquired sterility was not considered, because it was impossible to determine whether or not one-child families were a result of choice.

Defined as the number of childless couples, infertility appears to have affected not more than 10 to 15 percent of the population between 1848 and 1981. Indeed, Ellen Gee has pointed out that between 1922 and 1936 there was a significant decrease in childlessness to less than 10 percent.[84] Medical interest in infertility, then, was not linked to any perceptible increase in the degree of infertility in the population. Little discussion of the actual rates, or how physicians came to determine the rates, occurred. It would appear that most doctors based their figures on the percentage of childless couples in society — not a very accurate test, since some couples may have chosen to prevent conception. In addition, the tendency was to quote non-Canadian statistics.

Some change in the way physicians accounted for the statistics suggests the reasons for concern about infertility. Dr. Ashton Fletcher, of the Toronto Western Hospital, pointed out in 1906 that infertility was higher in the peerage of Britain than in the general community. He believed that the rate in Canada would be even lower.[85] This may have reflected a general Canadian perception that the New World was a healthier place in which to live than the Old. W. Pelton Tew, Professor of Obstetrics and Gynaecology at the University of Western Ontario, saw no class dimension to infertility in 1939; neither did E.L. Chicanot writing in reference to Britain in 1945. Tew, however, did blame modern civilization.[86]

Not until the twentieth century did Canadian doctors specifically address the issue of female fertility and infertility. For example, in a study of medical examinations given at Queen's University between 1900 and 1942, the first question concerning sterility did not appear until 1919. This was followed by increasing interest over the next two decades; questions on sterility were asked again in 1924, 1929, 1931, 1932, 1936, and 1937.[87] In 1930, Dr. M.C. Watson of Toronto confirmed this growing awareness of infertility when he noted that "During the past decade more than 500 articles have appeared in the literature on the diagnosis and treatment of sterility."[88] Seven years later Montreal physician Henry A. Baron observed that such literature a generation earlier would have covered only one printed page, but "following the pioneering work of Frank in endocrinology, of Rubin in the development of the test for tubal patency, simplified methods of basal metabolism determination, the work of Huhner and Moench in semen studies and the investigation of ovulation by means of the suction-curette, the study of sterility has made rapid strides, culminating in an excellent monograph by Meaker, only three years ago."[89]

By the 1920s, then, doctors were convinced that sterility was a "fascinating subject" on the rise.[90] This increased interest seems to have followed medical advances. Until the mid-1920s, doctors' knowledge of conception was such that their efforts to assist patients were largely ineffective. Once physicians had pinpointed women's fertile period, the situation changed, and this was reflected in the new interest in infertility. Tests such as Rubin's were also crucial, as will be seen. In the medical literature little evidence exists that interest rose in response to patients' demands other than physicians' assumption that all married couples wanted children. In the popular literature as well there was little discussion of infertility. The medical interest appears to have been self-propelling, albeit in the context of a society that was essentially pro-natalist.

Over the hundred-year period under review, the emphasis in medical and popular literature was on the importance of having children. The declining birth rate (from 1871 to the mid-1940s) did not necessarily suggest that Canadians disagreed with the prescriptive literature, except in the number of children they felt they could afford to raise. One trend that did emerge was a normative family size. In the late nineteenth century, family size varied from those with no children to those with many. No particular family size dominated. As the birth rate declined, family size became increasingly homogeneous; that is, more families were becoming similar in size through the elimination of large families, not the increase in childless families. The variety of the earlier period disappeared and conformity replaced it. Conformity has its own authority and may have made couples without children feel that they were deficient and somehow out of step with the societal norm.

Infertility in Men

What emerges in the general literature of the nineteenth century and the more specific literature of the twentieth century is that physicians saw infertility as a problem largely of women, acknowledgment of male infertility notwithstanding. In the nineteenth century, doctors generally believed that as long as a man was not impotent he could impregnate his wife.[91] From the turn of the century onward, however, physicians began to estimate the percentage of childless marriages that were the "fault" of the male partner. There was no consistency in the estimates, but one trend was visible — physicians came to see male sterility as increasingly more important. For example, in the first 20 years of the century, physicians' estimates of the incidence of childless families caused by the husband's sterility went from a low of 7 percent to a high of 40 percent.[92] In the 1920s and 1930s, estimates ranged from 20 percent to 50 percent.[93] In the 1940s, estimates ranged from 25 percent to 50 percent.[94]

Ironically, this gradual recognition of the significance of male sterility was not accompanied by changes in attitudes. Many doctors in the first half of the twentieth century made the same point — that in cases of infertility the male partner had to be examined as well as the female and that too much emphasis was being placed on the woman to her detriment.[95] That physicians expressed this view repeatedly suggests that although they recognized male sterility, many had difficulty translating intellectual recognition into medical practice. Certainly recognition of male sterility and the need to focus both on it and on female sterility was not reflected in extended discussions even by those physicians who felt male sterility was being overlooked. The reluctance of male physicians to accept that male sterility might be as significant an issue as female sterility was one that they shared with other men. When some physicians tried to account for the overwhelming emphasis on female infertility, they concluded that men ignored the possibility of their own sterility as long as they were not impotent. As a Winnipeg physician put it in 1934, "The faith of the average man in his own procreative ability and his willingness to place the blame of an unproductive union on his wife are remarkable."[96]

The medical literature reveals the perceived causes of male sterility and how the emphasis on those causes changed. The causes can be categorized under three general headings — moral-sexual, lifestyle, and physiological. The first had its greatest acceptability in the late nineteenth and early twentieth centuries. The second gained currency in the twentieth century, as did the third. Also clear is the decline in the judgmental quality of discussions of male infertility over time, particularly with reference to the first two categories.

Moral-Sexual Causes

Since physicians in nineteenth-century Canada generally assumed that a man could impregnate a woman unless he was impotent, discussions of male sterility were not explicit. Only occasionally did doctors make references to health problems that could be linked to sterility (although doctors did not always phrase it that way). For example, in his 1867 medical manual, William Buchanan warned readers that spermatorrhoea was a result of "excessive venery" and masturbation, both of which were considered morally reprehensible because they were evidence of lack of control.[97] In 1883, the *Canada Medical Record* also emphasized the connection between spermatorrhoea and masturbation, as did Hamilton Ayers in *Everyman His Own Physician*.[98] Ayers went further, in fact, linking masturbation to eventual impotency. Equally damaging, according to nineteenth-century sources, was withdrawal as a form of birth control.[99] Thus when physicians addressed male fertility problems, they connected the cause to moral failings. This reflected the nineteenth-century abhorrence of sexual activity outside a legitimate heterosexual relationship and of sexuality that was not controlled and controlled naturally. One of the few references in the nineteenth century to a non-moral cause was in an article in *The Canada Lancet* in 1894. The author argued that civilization in general had led to an inability to reproduce, stating bluntly, "Wild animals in confinement seldom propagate their own kind."[100]

The focus on immoral sexual behaviour never disappeared entirely from the medical literature during the period under review. Indeed, its link with infertility became more explicit. What did alter in the twentieth century were attitudes; moral indignation about masturbation, over-indulgence in sexual activity, and birth control declined. Of the three, masturbation seemed to be the least important. In an eccentric 1916 medical manual entitled *Tokology*, Alice Stockham declared masturbation a cause of impotency and sterility.[101] Little mention in the medical literature is made after that except in passing. For example, Dr. F.S. Patch,

Clinical Professor of Urology at McGill University in 1924, listed masturbation as a cause of male sterility but made it clear that "masturbation to
excess" was the problem. Indeed, the discussion emphasized the medicalization of masturbation. The act itself was not the difficulty (as was true
in the nineteenth century); the issue was the possible physiological
consequences of masturbation, in particular azoospermia.[102]

Something similar occurred with respect to the perception of birth
control. In 1907, J. Clifton Edgar connected the use of birth control (most
likely withdrawal) with male sterility. He also claimed that it caused
"dissatisfaction with imperfect coitus with [the] wife, which often foments
dislike, unfaithfulness, marital infelicity and divorce."[103] Alice Stockham,
too, drew a link between withdrawal and sterility.[104] By 1927, however, the
medical interest in birth control had declined, perhaps because it had
become clear that Canadians were going to practise birth control with or
without doctors' approval, and whether birth control was legal or not. In
that year, Dr. Little and Dr. Percival of Montreal mentioned the use of
chemical contraceptives in a general discussion of factors that could affect
the vitality of sperm.[105] But there was no suggestion that birth control
generally was a problem, simply this particular form of birth control. Only
in non-mainstream medical publications did the moral overtones persevere
in discussions of birth control and masturbation.[106]

More significant in the twentieth century was physicians' concern
about the effects on men of excessive sexual activity. Throughout the first
50 years of the twentieth century, doctors referred to it regularly as a cause
of sterility, believing that it weakened the vitality of the sperm.[107] In 1903,
Dr. J.J. Ross explained that, although it was not a primary cause of
infertility, "debauchery" on the part of the man was a factor.[108] Ross may
not have been referring directly to sexual intercourse but to venereal
disease, the most significant cause of male sterility recognized by the
medical profession. Three years later in *A System of Gynaecology*, Thomas
Allbutt, W.S. Playfair, and Thomas Watts Eden mentioned too-frequent
intercourse in marriage as a cause of male sterility.[109] Concern about
sexual "excesses" continued to be expressed; as with masturbation and
birth control, practitioners saw sexual excess as medically problematic,
because they thought it temporarily reduced the vitality of the sperm.[110]
Sexuality was no longer socially problematic, largely because psychologists
were seeing sexuality as positive and acceptable even when not associated
with procreation.

Lifestyle Causes

Although twentieth-century doctors did not express moral indignation
about sexual activities to the same extent as their nineteenth-century
colleagues, there were concerns about what could be called lifestyle factors,
some of which certainly contained the germ of moral judgment. Perhaps
the mildest reproach was that modern society was not conducive to

reproduction. As noted above, this was expressed as early as the late
nineteenth century, coinciding with the declining birth rate in Canada.[111]
It was only decades later, however, that this theme re-emerged in
discussions of infertility. In a 1939 study of human sterility, W. Pelton Tew
expressed the belief that "[i]ntensive living in the modern world may lead
in time to unhealthy sex cells. This is exemplified by the modern business
or professional man who carries heavy responsibilities with their
accompanying worries and improper hours of rest."[112] Others, too, believed
that exhaustion, a sedentary life, and overwork were factors in sterility
(including impotence).[113] Physicians, who were predominantly middle-class,
did not pay close attention to the work hazards to which many
working-class men were exposed. They acknowledged the danger of chronic
poisoning from lead, mercury, and exposure to "heavy metals" and other
occupational hazards, but gave little detail.[114]

Of more interest after 1930 was diet, perhaps because the Depression
concentrated attention on the problems associated with inadequate
nutrition and also because of the growing knowledge of vitamins. "Errors
in diet" were seen to result in fewer spermatozoa, as well as weak or
immature sperm.[115] Doctors focussed specifically on the effects of obesity
and the lack of vitamin E on sterility, the latter concern emerging in the
late 1930s.[116] Also linked to diet, and certainly an aspect of lifestyle, was
the attention paid to alcohol and its effect on spermatozoa.[117]

More significant than any of these factors in both male and female
sterility — and a factor on which doctors focussed more than any other —
was venereal disease (VD). VD was recognized as a cause of male sterility
early in the century.[118] To appreciate the significance of this perception,
one needs to realize the perceived incidence of VD in the male population.
One physician argued in 1906 that 75 percent of men had had gonorrhoea
once in their lives, while 30 percent carried the "latent germ to the nuptial
couch." For this physician the solution was to apply to men the same
moral standards as applied to women, an argument that gained currency
in the first two decades of the century among reformers working in the
purity movement.[119] Within the movement, physicians were prominent in
arguing that prostitution and the double standard had to be eliminated.
Purity reformers saw prostitutes as temptresses of innocent middle-class
young men and the existence of a double standard of morality as a
reflection of the new wave of immigrants coming to Canada from Europe
and Asia, immigrants unfamiliar with the norms of Canadian society.
Enmeshed in this was also middle-class distrust of working people.[120]

The purity movement had declined by the early 1920s, but medical
concern about VD in men did not, partly as a result of soldiers returning
infected after the First World War and the government's involvement in
establishing VD clinics. In 1923, Dr. Alan Brown made clear the urgency
of the problem: "Gonorrhoea affects the future of the race by making men
and women childless. Syphilis affects the race by destroying outright
75 percent of the children of syphilitic parents before they are born or

during the first year of life, and by crippling or weakening a considerable proportion of those who survive."[121] Brown may have been vague about the connection between VD and male sterility, but others were not. F.S. Patch pointed to the link between generalized syphilis and azoospermia in 1924, and a decade later S.C. Peterson made clear the connection between gonorrhoea and male sterility in the majority of cases.[122] In the 1930s and 1940s, physicians still attended to both gonorrhoea and syphilis, although they gave gonorrhoea pride of place along with its treatment with penicillin.[123]

The focus on lifestyle choices as a cause of male sterility gave the medical profession hope for a cure, given that adjustments in lifestyle did not appear to be outside the realm of possibility. With respect to VD, of course, damage could be so extensive as to eliminate the possibility of cure, but generally the damage could be contained if doctors diagnosed the condition early enough. Focussing on lifestyle also permitted an expansion of medical expertise into areas not traditionally considered part of the medical world. Poor employment conditions and inadequate diet began to receive attention from the medical community, although physicians were never too specific about how to overcome them. Similarly, factors such as exercise (or lack of it), hygiene, indeed anything that contributed to general ill health, were potential causes of sterility and thus came under the scrutiny of doctors.[124]

Physiological Reasons

More directly linked to sterility and more problematic for the individual man were, for want of a better word, physiological causes. Impotence was one such factor. In the nineteenth and early twentieth centuries, doctors often saw impotence as a consequence of immoral acts and were not therefore particularly sympathetic. Impotence could be caused by factors over which an individual had little control, however, and in those cases physicians acknowledged the problem in a straightforward manner.[125] Of particular note were problems in the development of the reproductive organs. In a 1924 article entitled "Sterility in the Male," F.S. Patch pointed to the need for thorough examination "of all organs concerned in the formation and conveyance of spermatozoa ... of the urethra and its glandular apparatus and of the prostate and seminal vesicles." Certainly when doctors mentioned the need to consider male sterility in treating infertile couples they assumed that such an examination would follow.[126] At various times doctors also remarked on diseases such as tuberculosis, diabetes, mumps, and others as factors in male sterility.[127] Over time, the list of causes became longer as new ones were added by each generation of physicians. Interestingly, considering the emphasis placed on endocrinal causes in women, doctors did not focus on this as a significant cause of male sterility.[128]

The twentieth-century literature conveys the sense that most physicians believed that impotence, developmental problems, and various illnesses, although causes of sterility, were relatively minor compared to the problem of inadequate or unhealthy sperm. Many of these factors, as well as the other causes of male sterility that have been examined, had adverse effects on the sperm. For example, VD, excessive sexual intercourse, and masturbation were all identified as potentially problematic, as were poor hygiene, inadequate diet, overwork, and lack of exercise. By themselves they did not cause sterility, but through their effects on the sperm they did. Physicians linked aspermia, too, with VD and masturbation in the 1920s. H.G. Osborne acknowledged in 1950 that the prognosis for treatment of this condition was poor.[129] In some cases doctors viewed the physiological processes of aging as a factor in inadequate sperm production, although they certainly did not emphasize it and referred to it as a problem only of very elderly men.[130] Rarely did physicians mention problems in sperm production being the result of specific medical practices such as the treatment of other conditions using X-rays.[131] As the twentieth century progressed, the reasons for the lack of sperm, inadequate sperm, and unhealthy sperm did not receive particular attention.[132] What seemed to be of concern was the problem as diagnosed through sperm samples, not its origins. Doctors treated the problem but did not develop strategies for preventing the condition or alleviating its causes.

While not exhaustive, this examination of male sterility as discussed in the medical literature reveals the main focus of physicians' concerns. What emerges is a gradual shift in emphasis, from blaming men's behaviour for their sterility to a more value-neutral approach. This shift should not be exaggerated, however. Although much of the discussion of VD in the 1930s and 1940s did not have the moral tone of the earlier period, underlying it was the conviction that if men behaved better they would not have contracted VD in the first place.

Causes of Sterility in Women

As in the case of male sterility, doctors blamed women's lifestyles for their inability to conceive or carry a child to term. Sexual practices, the food they ate, the education they received, even their individual personalities — all were subjects for criticism. Discussion of a second major group of factors was virtually absent in discussions of male sterility, however: iatrogenic causes of female infertility. Doctors devoted considerable attention to how medical treatment itself could cause problems, in particular how poor obstetrical practices could lead to sterility. The third group of factors identified in the literature consisted of those related to the physiological nature of the body.

Volitional Factors

The medical literature reflects general social discomfort with the notion of female sexuality. In the nineteenth century, medical and lay people alike extolled the virtues of sexual restraint. Not until the 1920s were some Canadians prepared to accept that sexuality and reproduction did not have to go together. Nonetheless, throughout the entire period under review, the female sexual drive was always perceived to be weaker than the male's and somehow more dangerous for women. In the late nineteenth century, doctors acknowledged that women's sexual feelings were natural, but only within a heterosexual, marital relationship; unease occurred when women expressed sexual feelings in ways society did not approve of. In 1882, for example, writing in *The People's Common Sense Medical Adviser*, R. Pierce described the symptoms that could accompany female masturbation — deafness, decline in strength, loss of memory, and leucorrhoea.[133] In his authoritative 1894 text, Henry Garrigues reasserted what Pierce had written — that masturbation could lead to gynaecological disorders.[134] The link to infertility was that physicians believed that gynaecological diseases of all types, including leucorrhoea, contributed to and sometimes caused sterility. The 1910 *English Herbal Dispensary* made the link explicit, stating that "self-abuse" was a cause of sterility.[135] By the second decade of the twentieth century, however, doctors no longer saw masturbation in women as morally reprehensible, wasteful of energy, or dangerous, or connected it to sterility.

Masturbation was a specific case, but physicians had long considered sexual excess (solitary or otherwise) problematic. Doctors in the late nineteenth century discussed in general terms the debilitating effects on women of long engagements, sexual activity during menstruation, reading prurient novels, and engaging in too violent coitus.[136] Some physicians argued that violation of the "laws" of sexual congress was a cause of miscarriages.[137] As in other areas, the tendency to moralize dissipated in the 1920s, and doctors often stated in non-judgmental terms that sexual excess, "faulty" sexual habits, or even lack of sexual enjoyment could lead to sterility or to problems that could cause sterility.[138] Notable in discussions where female sexuality is mentioned is the inability of physicians to explain the precise connection between sexual habits and sterility. For men the connection was clear — depletion of sperm; for women it was less clear, which suggests that doctors' unease with female sexuality was cultural.

Linked to sexuality was concern about birth control in general and abortion in particular. Birth control was very much a moral issue in the late nineteenth and early twentieth centuries. In addition, doctors were convinced that birth control was unnatural and anything unnatural was bound to be detrimental to health. Besides this indirect connection, some physicians directly linked birth control to sterility.[139] Although birth control was not legalized in Canada until 1969, the medical literature does not focus on it much after 1920; the moral indignation characteristic of the earlier period was no longer a factor.

Abortion, however, continued to be a concern. From the mid-nineteenth century onward, physicians saw non-therapeutic abortion as a cause of ill health and gynaecological disorders.[140] The lengths to which women went to obtain an abortion appalled physicians. One physician in the 1916 *Public Health Journal* expressed concern about the use of harmful abortifacients, claiming that he had seen "young women run the gauntlet of losing their lives ... paralyzed in hands and feet, lose their eyesight, pass through a long and trying illness, and for months afterwards be nothing but a drag upon the financial resources of a husband with slender wages."[141] Perhaps not surprisingly, given the economic pressures on families, doctors detected an increase in self-induced abortions during the 1930s. Dr. W.A. Dafoe estimated that 40 percent of the incomplete abortion cases in the Toronto General Hospital wards were self-induced; the health of patients was sometimes destroyed by the use of quinine, castor oil, ergot, tinet, cantharidis, quaiacum, salts, lead pills, and a variety of patent preparations.[142] Similar concerns were evident during the war years that followed.[143] Although doctors believed that ill health in general could contribute to a woman's sterility, at times they made the link explicit between abortion, along with its attendant consequences, and sterility.[144]

In discussing female sexuality physicians assumed that such activity was harmful because they accepted the prevailing view that it was socially unacceptable. This connection between medical and social opinion is even more evident in discussions of female education and how it contributed to weakening women's health, which in turn reduced their ability to conceive. Physicians feared that education was physically harmful to both sexes, but especially to women. Of special note was their belief that women needed all their energy in the years after puberty to develop their reproductive systems; if this was prevented by educational and other pressures, the reproductive system would not develop properly. William Goodell was more honest than most practitioners about what bothered him about educating women — "Too much brain-work, too little housework."[145] The link between education and ill health did not disappear until early in the twentieth century; after that, the debate on education was not medical so much as social — the concern was not that it weakened the female body but that it encouraged women to reject their "natural" roles of wife and mother. By that time, however, physicians were not a significant group participating in the debate.

Nor were doctors comfortable with the increasing participation of women in paid employment. In 1887, a noted physician drew a link between women who habitually miscarried and physical activity, specifically running a sewing machine.[146] This was a serious charge, because the garment industry was a major employer of women at the time. Early in the new century doctors also noted such employment hazards as carbolic acid gas and lead poisoning.[147] In 1916, *The Public Health Journal* — perhaps in response to the increased number of women in the workforce as a result of the war — published an article suggesting that working conditions were often "a peril to womankind and a menace to the race."[148] These conditions were also dangerous to men, but there was a sense that women's reproductive responsibility made them particularly susceptible to industrial poisons, especially lead, mercury, arsenic, and phosphorus.

This direct connection between workplace hazards and female sterility was also acknowledged in the 1930s and beyond.[149] Physicians argued that hard work in factories delayed puberty and the employment of mothers was a factor in infant mortality.[150] Some doctors equated paid employment with "emancipation," which, according to one physician writing in the 1936 *Canadian Medical Association Journal*, resulted in increased spontaneous abortions.[151] The fact that thousands of women were flocking to industrial jobs during the Second World War raised concerns about the potential effects on their capacity to bear children and how exposure to poisonous substances such as mercury, manganese, lead, and petroleum would affect their health.[152] Other than pointing out the problem, however, physicians appear to have done little to follow up on their concerns.

One aspect of women's lives and health about which physicians had long written was the way women dressed. Of particular concern was the use of corsets in the late nineteenth century and other tight clothing around the waist and abdomen in the twentieth. In the earlier period, doctors believed that tight corsets caused "falling of the womb," miscarriage, headache, bad temper, local inflammation of the liver, gall-stones, enteroptosis, flexions of the womb, anaemia, chlorosis, weak eyes, and Bright's disease.[153] As an American doctor explained in the 1902 *Canadian Practitioner and Review*, "Tight lacing ... predisposes to pelvic disorders by interfering with circulation and exciting uterine displacements."[154] Uterine displacements were considered a possible cause of sterility. Although hostility toward women's fashions as a cause of disease declined as fashions changed and allowed the body more freedom, concern about them never disappeared. In 1930, doctors expressed anxiety about the idealization of the "boyish figure," whose achievement often entailed dieting and drug-taking, as well as the pursuit of "extraordinary physical exercises and mechanical appliances to prevent the normal development of the hips and bust."[155]

The mainstream medical literature of the nineteenth century did not reveal any particular sensitivity to problems of women's diet or the connection between diet and ill health. The concern about the link between poor diet and the ability to conceive and bear children became more common in the twentieth century.[156] In 1917, for example, physicians reported that nutrition affected fertility in animals "in a marked degree" and noted that "girls in factories, who are badly fed and live in unhygienic surroundings, may be late in arriving at maturity, and consequently relatively sterile."[157] In the first three decades of the century physicians linked obesity and sterility,[158] and occasionally sterility and vitamin E deficiency.[159] Particularly disturbing were studies conducted on Canadians' diets during the 1930s, which concluded that in poorer families it was women's diets that were most likely to be deficient.[160] By the early 1930s, doctors viewed alcohol as a contributing factor in sterility; before then they had seen it as a factor in spontaneous abortions.[161]

The literature also shows that when physicians could not attribute sterility to any particular cause they looked to the more general aspects of women's lives. In 1882, Henry Chavasse, author of *Advice to a Wife*, made clear his belief that it was not poor women who had trouble conceiving but the pampered rich. In the 1902 *Canadian Practitioner and Review*, Dr. Charles Shepard was concerned not so much about the wealthy as about the emergence at the turn of the century of the "new woman," whose "new ideas and practices" had retarded the growth of her natural menstrual processes and who had descended into ill health as a result.[162] Physicians continued to be concerned about lifestyle, whether because certain choices or practices caused sterility in women or because they led to health problems that could be linked to sterility.[163]

Underlying some of this concern was a feeling that women who lived without regard to the consequences for their reproductive capacity were selfish. Dr. W. Pelton Tew made this clear in 1939, explaining that "human energy is expended in two ways, for individuation and genesis. The more used for individuation, the less remains for genesis. It seems therefore, that the manifold strains of a complex and artificial mode of life have operated slowly over centuries to reduce the energies available for reproduction."[164] Women clearly had to decide between their own needs and those of the species.

Lifestyle choices such as diet, exercise, and sleeping habits could be changed by the individual. But physicians' criticisms also alluded to vague factors that individuals had little hope of changing. The result was that doctors had great latitude for intervention and an almost endless range of causes to blame for sterility.[165] Nowhere was this more evident than in the occasional references to the personality of women as a source of infertility. In 1870, the *Canada Medical Journal and Monthly Record* linked infertility in women to hysteria.[166] During this period most physicians believed hysteria to be a feigned disease and one of self-centredness; not surprisingly, then, the sympathy expended on these women was limited. Eighty years later Dr. Jessie McGeachy was even more vehement about the blame individual women should accept:

> In assessing a case of sterility from the emotional standpoint, it is important to judge the personality type ... For example, is she vain and egocentric, able to give love and attention only to herself in the way of clothes and personal adornments and elaborate housing equipment? If this is so, she has not developed beyond the narcissistic stage of childhood and she is emotionally unable to love anyone else but herself. Does she desire a child, not with the aim of being a good parent, but to be one of a group of women with social prestige because they can gossip

about formulas and training?   Is it too visionary to venture the suggestion that this type of egocentricity and emotional maldevelopment may be accompanied by altered physiology such as faulty ovulation?[167]

Less judgmental was the recognition that the older the woman the less her chances of conceiving. While in the early years doctors emphasized both youth and age, acknowledging that if a woman married too young she too would have difficulty conceiving,[168] the emphasis was generally on the "older" woman, who was defined most often as over age 35, although sometimes even 30 was seen as problematic.[169] Women simply should not delay childbearing, was physicians' message; they should accept their role in society and the constraints it imposed.

Medical Intervention

Despite the considerable attention paid to the role of lifestyle factors in infertility, some physicians did acknowledge that often doctors, not women, were responsible for problems affecting fertility. A strong theme emerges from the medical literature concerning excessive interventions practised by many physicians; such treatment could have dire consequences for patients. Ironically, nineteenth-century practitioners admitted this more readily than twentieth-century ones, despite the expanding scope and nature of intervention in the present century.

Of particular concern was the increasing number of gynaecological interventions that accompanied the rise of gynaecology as a specialty. For example, in 1882 R. Pierce criticized the frequency with which physicians examined women's uteri, arguing that this often resulted in lasting injury. Certainly the introduction of carbolic acid or nitric acid into the uterus was not without harmful effects, nor was the constant probing of the uterine cavity with various surgical tools. As one physician noted, a great deal of time and effort was spent on an organ just three inches long, two inches wide, an inch thick, and weighing only an ounce and a half at most.[170] In his textbook, Henry Garrigues warned students about physician-induced gynaecological problems associated with the use of sounds, curettes, tents, dilators, and pessaries, all of which could absorb septic material.[171] In a few instances in the twentieth century as well, doctors explicitly connected specific treatments with infection causing sterility.[172] Similar concerns were expressed about frequent gynaecological surgery interfering with a woman's ability to conceive.[173]

This was not a major focus for most physicians writing in the twentieth century, but there was the occasional acknowledgment that surgery intended to cure sterility at times actually caused it.[174] Equally problematic were childbirth practices, which many saw as increasingly interventionist in the nineteenth century and which gynaecologists in both centuries blamed for many of women's gynaecological problems. In 1882, Dr. Tye observed that "after seeing all the forceps and scoops and other iron instruments, he really congratulated himself that he was not a woman," and noted that in his own practice he seldom felt the need to resort to them but trusted in nature.[175] Not all followed his lead; physicians and patients alike complained that the ill health of many women stemmed from poor obstetrical practices.[176]

Many twentieth-century doctors deemed childbirth, or the medical practices surrounding it, a cause of disease and ill health and a factor in fertility problems. As one physician described his obstetrical colleagues in 1911, "The dictum, that forceps is only to be applied when the cervix is fully dilated, is unknown to the majority of practitioners who have little or no compunction about dragging a head through a cervix but half dilated."[177] Similar concerns about obstetrical practices continued to appear in the literature, as did the view that childbirth itself was a factor in subsequent difficulties, including sterility.[178] Of particular note was concern about the increasing number of Caesarian sections and their relationship to subsequent sterility.[179]

Like the Caesarian section, the use of X-rays and radium treatment became a tool in the hands of practitioners in the twentieth century. Effective in combatting various conditions, their connection to sterility was not always appreciated. In the early decades, radiologists emphasized consistently that only those trained in the field should attempt to use the new technology. That these warnings had to be repeated suggests that this did not always occur. In 1928, the use of "weak therapeutic doses of x-ray" for sterility was mentioned in the literature, a situation of understandable concern.[180] In the 1931 *Canadian Medical Association Journal*, Dr. L.J. Carter expressed reservations about X-raying women who could still bear children, fearing the effect it would have on the children they bore. D. Kearns made it clear in 1943 that radium therapy could cause sterility.[181] Doctors could be part of the problem rather than part of the solution.

Physiological Reasons

Rather than focus on physician-induced fertility problems, doctors were more inclined to blame the female body for "failing" to reproduce. They explored every possible aspect of a woman's health experience in attempting to explain her infertility. Did she, or had she, suffered from tuberculosis, rheumatism, cholera, enteric fever, scarlatina, or myxedema?[182] How healthy were her various reproductive organs? Disease of the ovaries was one potential source of problems,[183] but disease of "the vagina, the vaginal canal itself, the external os uteri, the cervical canal, the internal os uteri, the cavity of the uterus, its cornua, the fallopian tubes, [and] the peritoneal opening of these tubes" also had to be taken into account.[184] Given this vast terrain, it would be impossible even to survey all the perceived medical causes of sterility in women over a hundred-year period; only the more prominent perceptions are examined here.

First among causes was VD, specifically gonorrhoea. This was the factor mentioned most often and consistently during the entire period under study. Physician after physician acknowledged that women most often contracted gonorrhoea from their husbands. Women were innocent victims. As a result, physicians urged their colleagues through the medical journals to be very careful about advising a man who had or had had gonorrhoea that it was safe for him to marry.[185] The importance physicians attached to this problem is suggested by a 1906 report by Dr. Fletcher of the Toronto Western Hospital who estimated that 40 percent of one-child sterility was caused by gonorrhoeal infection and that it accounted for about 30 percent of primary sterility. In 1908, E.C. Dudley pointed to what he saw as a perilous practice, in *The Principles and Practice of Gynaecology for Students and Practitioners*: "Young men sometimes are advised to marry in order to improve their sexual hygiene, and so to cure an intractable chronic but 'innocent gleet.' Such advice may result in the destruction of the reproductive organs of an innocent woman."[186] As late as 1951 physicians were pointing out that

> gonorrhoea should still be accorded great emphasis; for it produces sterilizing lesions in both sexes — inflammatory lesions in the cervix and occlusion of the fallopian tubes of the wife, as well as devastating chronic infection of the prostate and obstructions of the passageways for spermatozoa in the male genital tract.[187]

Doctors also saw syphilis as a problem but perceived it slightly differently. It did not cause sterility by itself, but it often resulted in miscarriage or stillbirth with the same result — childless homes.[188] One early estimate was that 30 to 40 percent of syphilitic women aborted spontaneously. This compares with a 1923 estimate that syphilis destroyed 78 percent of the children of syphilitic parents either before they were born or within a year of birth.[189] Some physicians believed that the incidence of syphilis varied depending "upon the class of patients with which one has to deal," while others argued that it had been overestimated as a cause of stillbirth.[190]

The real significance of VD is the damage it causes in the reproductive system. For example, gonorrhoeal infection can cause blocked fallopian tubes, which physicians in the present century determined a major cause of sterility. They did not always discuss the original cause of the blockage (if there was one), so that their expressed concerns about the patency of the fallopian tubes could in part be added to the problems arising from VD.

Physicians perceived closed tubes as a significant problem very early in the literature. Some physicians blamed nature for the design of the female reproductive organs. Dr. R.E. Cutts explained in the 1900 *Canada Lancet*, for example, that "notwithstanding the wonderful make-up of the female generative system it does seem as if nature had complicated conditions unnecessarily in its connecting link between the ovary and uterus. The fallopian tube is, no doubt, the weakest part of the entire system. The smallness, length and tortuosity of its canal all favour its occlusion with the slightest pathological change."[191] A further problem arose from the belief, expressed early in the century, that if one fallopian tube was diseased sufficiently to cause removal, the other tube, even if apparently healthy, would soon follow; thus efficiency demanded its removal at the same time. Such beliefs, of course, imposed sterility on the woman.[192]

The focus on the fallopian tubes remained constant throughout the twentieth-century literature examined.[193] One reason was Rubin's 1920 introduction of a test for the patency of the tubes "by allowing carbon dioxide gas under pressure to escape into the abdominal cavity by means of a cannula introduced into the uterine cavity." Successful escape proved the patency of the tubes; non-escape suggested blockage.[194] The test was taken up quickly as diagnostic procedure that was easier and less intrusive for the woman than the exploratory surgery used previously to determine the condition of the tubes.

The perceived advantage of the Rubin test was that it could lead to a cure by confirming the cause of sterility and thus suggesting treatment, that is, removal of the blockage through surgery. For other factors the situation was not as bright. Malformation of any of the reproductive organs was recognized as problematic, but doctors offered few straightforward solutions. They comforted themselves, however, that these causes of infertility were in the minority; apart from noting that practitioners conducting physical examinations should check for such malformations, not a great deal of attention was devoted to them in the literature.[195]

One factor that had a chequered history was uterine displacements. From the turn of the century until the late 1930s and beyond, doctors believed that uterine displacements were linked to sterility, although the occasional voice emerged, especially in the 1940s, to suggest that this link was much exaggerated.[196] The underlying theme in discussions of uterine displacements was that women's bodies should conform to a norm and that deviation from that norm was problematic even if it appeared that the "deviation" itself was quite normal. Doctors seemed to believe that women's bodies were the problem.[197]

So much seemed to go wrong with women's bodies — menstrual disorders and to a lesser extent endocervitis, for example. One 1902 estimate was that more than half the women who suffered from "menstrual derangements" at puberty were sterile.[198] If this were true, however, the incidence of infertility would have been much higher than it was. Nonetheless, many physicians writing in the journals continued to focus on these disorders for at least the first two decades of the century.[199] After that period, an appreciation emerged that menstrual disorders were symptomatic of other conditions rather than being primary causes of infertility. This never seemed true of what doctors referred to as "abnormal secretions"; although they were not harmful to the woman producing them, they were harmful to sperm. Thus their "abnormality" was judged on the basis of whether sperm could survive them. At times, physicians referred to such secretions in volitional terms, making references to the "incorrigible hostility" of such secretions to the sperm as if it was the woman who was incorrigibly hostile.[200]

Also intriguing was the discussion of endometriosis, which first emerged in the 1930s.[201] Seen as a cause of sterility, it was portrayed in the *Canadian Medical Association Journal* of 1947 as "an antivenereal disease, being associated with sexual unfulfillment. The prophylaxis appears to be early marriage and a child every few years." It is difficult not to conclude that this was a social prescription, not a medical one. In the same year, Drs. Fallon, Bronson, and Moran claimed in *Modern Medicine of Canada* that endometriosis developed "more readily in childless or sexually dormant women."[202]

The last of the significant physiological causes in the literature were endocrinal. These causes of sterility awaited the early twentieth century for recognition. In 1915, an article in the *Canadian Medical Association Journal* linked deficiencies in the production of thyroid secretions and in the functioning of the anterior lobe of the pituitary to sterility. Physicians writing in the same journal in 1934 and 1939 agreed, pointing out how endocrine disturbances (in the pituitary, thyroid, and sex glands) were significant, and in the 1939 journal claimed that nearly 60 percent of primary sterility was connected to these disturbances.[203] Others concurred, leading to significant reliance on hormonal treatment for sterility.[204]

This review of the medical literature shows that once physicians identified a factor as a cause of sterility in women it tended to persist throughout the period, although the extent to which it was identified as a cause might ebb and flow and attitudes toward it might alter. New factors were added to older ones over time. Many of these, such as those related to disease or congenital conditions, were beyond women's control. Doctors saw many causes, however, as the fault of the woman or the way she lived. This view was similar to their perceptions of the lifestyle factors leading to male sterility; somehow blame had to be assigned. This can also be seen in attempts to apportion responsibility between the man and the woman for their childlessness. Although doctors continued to do this, they recognized that it was a fruitless exercise. For example, included in discussions of infertility was the concept of selective sterility — "when two individuals of opposite sexes are unable to procreate, although each may be potent in this respect with another partner." As Dr. W. Blair Bell wrote in 1917, the cause of selective sterility was unknown, but he speculated that "some of the biological processes of natural selection ... lie behind this so-called incompatibility."[205] Thus perhaps it was appropriate that mismatched couples remained childless; nature knew best. Dr. Pelton Tew was not as deterministic. Writing in 1939, Tew noted that "in most cases of human infertility the cause of that defect is not some single abnormality but rather the summation of several factors, there being 4.79 factors for each childless couple ... The several factors present in each case are seldom limited to one partner."[206] Doctors had long been intrigued by the fact that with different partners, individuals supposedly sterile were no longer so.[207] Selective or sterile mating was proof of the oftentimes impossibility of apportioning "blame," but physicians continued to make the attempt nonetheless.

Treatment

Encouragement of conception goes back to the ancients. In the time of Hippocrates, physicians suggested that women who wanted to conceive should eat "butter in the morning on an empty stomach and [drink] milk from a woman nursing a boy." In ancient Greece, drinking certain waters was thought to be beneficial. Alternatives to natural conception and birth were also available. Angus McLaren, for example, has described the use of both surrogacy and child exchange in the ancient world. "Formal adoptions were practised in the ancient world, disappeared in the Christian west and resurfaced in the last century."[208]

These stories from the past point to an aspect of infertility that persists to this day: in many cases individuals can take control of the problem of childlessness and deal with it themselves. Much of the advice given to men and women early in this century concerned remedies they could control. Some of this advice took the form of popular lore published in lay health manuals. In *The Physical Life of Woman*, for example, Napheys suggested that to cure sterility in a woman the breasts should be stimulated, she should rest in bed after having intercourse, or she should go horseback riding to the point of fatigue.[209] The importance of such advice lies not in its efficacy but in the fact that it allowed individuals to take charge of their condition rather than becoming totally dependent on medical treatment. Although patent medicines such as Dr. Jayne's Alternative, Dr. Pierce's Favourite Prescription, and popular tonics continued to be available and advertised as remedies for sterility well into this century, sterility treatment became increasingly medicalized.[210]

Men and women could, of course, change aspects of their lifestyle that physicians saw as problematic. Those whose diets were deficient were to alter them, taking particular care to ensure a sufficient intake of Vitamin E. In the case of obesity, the individual was to lose weight.[211] If sexual excess was a problem for either partner, restraint was recommended. If there was a difficulty associated with the method of sexual intercourse practised by the couple, it too could be adjusted. If douching was harmful, the woman could stop that practice. Both men and women were to live more healthful lives — get plenty of sleep and exercise regularly.

For some people this was easier said than done. A 1904 article in the *Canadian Practitioner and Medical Review*, for example, suggested a change in environment and climate, but how practical was this for working-class people?[212] Indeed, for the first half of the twentieth century, many

Canadians simply did not have access to adequate nutritious food. Equally problematic were environmental and workplace hazards. There was no suggestion in the medical literature that laws should be passed to protect workers from these dangers to their general and reproductive health. Nor were there suggestions that individuals should change their work situation, which would have been difficult for many to do in any case. In discussions of work-related hazards, the only direct reference to action was to suggest that women should not be involved in such jobs.

Medical therapy for sterility was extremely varied during the period under review. Since physicians believed that almost any pathological condition of the reproductive system could cause sterility, in theory whatever the current treatment for the condition was should have been a cure for sterility. Treatment ebbed and flowed. For example, early in the century some practitioners supported the benefits of divulsion and dilatation; in the 1920s, others rejected such procedures, indeed saw them as conducive to sterility rather than beneficial in curing it. The issue was still being raised in the 1940s, however, suggesting that not all practitioners were convinced,[213] and by 1950 there appeared to be a minor revival of dilation of the cervix, one text arguing that it "relieves obstruction of the canal."[214] Other therapies included the use of pessaries or curettage for a retroverted uterus, although physicians were questioning the safety and efficacy of both by the 1930s.[215]

In some cases new diagnostic tests allowed more precise pinpointing of the problem and suggested where treatment efforts were best concentrated. From the mid-1920s onward, for example, there was an emphasis on testing male sperm for quantity and quality. As some physicians pointed out, however, it was not always easy to get a semen specimen for testing since many men found it a challenge to their virility. By the 1930s, the ability of the sperm to survive within the generative tract could be determined from a post-coital examination devised by Huhner.[216] Rubin's test for tubal patency also became available in the 1920s. Although there was little supporting evidence in the literature, Rubin claimed that his test was not only diagnostic but also curative, with an estimated 10 percent cure rate.[217] Related to the Rubin test was injection of the fallopian tubes with opaque substances such as lipoidal; the resulting shadow on a radiograph would show the physician where the blockage was. The idea behind both these tests was the possibility of surgical correction of the blockage through, among other means, a salpingostomy. The success rate of such surgery was so low, however, and its consequences, in the form of high rates of spontaneous abortion and ectopic pregnancies, so worrisome that many physicians warned their colleagues about its dangers.[218]

Their better understanding of the female cycle allowed physicians to give patients more accurate advice on the most advantageous time to engage in sexual activity if conception was the goal. This knowledge and advice were not widespread until the mid-1920s, but after that time physicians had a good sense of when conception was most likely to occur. As the authors of a 1948 article reported, "Knowledge of the exact time of ovulation is of special importance for relatively infertile women since conception is favoured by intercourse on the day ova escape. The exact date of ovulation was determined by injecting patients' urine into rats."[219] In the late 1940s, specialists advised daily oral temperature readings to pinpoint ovular and anovular cycles.[220] While certainly not as invasive as Rubin's test, daily temperature readings did remind a woman of her childlessness every day.

Surgery was mentioned occasionally as a treatment for male sterility,[221] but most of the emphasis was on the female. This was related in part to the rise of gynaecology as a specialty and particularly to the tendency to equate gynaecology with surgery (although not all physicians accepted this equation). Ovariotomies had become popular in the late nineteenth century, and surgery to remove diseased ovaries for infertility or otherwise did not hold any terror for physicians.[222] Indeed, surgery seemed to be the favoured treatment, second only to endocrine therapy. The types of surgery varied, of course, but this is not the place for detailed discussion. It is more appropriate to evaluate physicians' attitudes toward such intervention.

In the late nineteenth century, one of the guiding tenets of gynae-cological surgery for various conditions was to attempt to maintain the woman's fertility. This remained true in the first half of the twentieth century as well. Removing a woman's ability to bear children was a very serious step and one doctors did not take lightly. Only for older women or women who had borne children was such surgery acceptable. Deliberate sterilization of certain groups did occur, however. For example, Angus McLaren has detailed the sterilization of "feebleminded" women in the 1930s.[223] Another strong theme in the literature is the apparent ease with which surgery was performed. Physicians acknowledged the seriousness of surgery and its potential consequences, but they had great faith in their technical abilities. This confidence came no doubt from the increasing number of operations that many doctors were performing; it was also the result of the acceptance of germ theory in the late nineteenth century and the impetus this gave all types of surgery.[224] But some commentators suggested that surgery to treat sterility was not particularly effective. Writing in the *Dominion Medical Monthly* in 1909, Dr. Cleland noted:

> From this rather extensive classification, it is readily seen that there is hardly any pathological condition affecting a woman's generative organs which may not have to do with sterility. Upon first thought, it would seem that there would naturally be many cases where operative procedure would be not only justifiable, but indicated. But this is not so, for in reality the field for surgical interference is a limited one. In the first place, all of those cases classed as absolute sterility are beyond the surgeon's help. And of the contingent class, many of the cases are either of too grave a nature, or would require too extensive an operation to

justify operative measures for sterility per se. It is, however, gratifying to know that sterility is sometimes cured by the correction of these more extensive pathological conditions by means of operation or treatment undertaken on account of the woman's ill-health alone.[225]

Thus, operate for ill health but not for sterility. Others, too, warned that abdominal surgery was likely not to be successful and could be harmful.[226] Perhaps the warning was needed. In 1924 Dr. Polak, a U.S. physician writing in the *Canadian Medical Association Journal*, remonstrated that "more unnecessary operations have been done for the relief of backache, than for any one symptom, except that of sterility."[227] Four years later Dr. William Graves asserted:

> Surgery is an important field in the treatment of sterility. This form of therapy has to a certain extent been discredited owing to the fact that until comparatively recent times operative measures have been almost the only resource, and have been undertaken in a haphazard manner, successes being more or less accidental. With the wider knowledge of the etiology of sterility and the newer methods of diagnosis, surgery is now employed with much greater intelligence, but it still remains our most important expedient.[228]

Few further warnings in this vein appeared until 1950, when the authors of a textbook repeated the assertions of Polak and Graves about the lack of surgical success in treating sterility and recommended that physicians refrain from surgery except when there was a pelvic pathology to justify it. The authors were not as vehement as their predecessors, however, for they declared that "sometimes, of course, the desire of the patient to do everything possible to bear a child may be sufficient reason for abdominal exploration even in the absence of pelvic distress."[229] The reasons for surgery had broadened.

Most surgical procedures were performed to treat "abnormal" conditions within the reproductive system, conditions physicians believed they could correct using traditional gynaecological procedures, for example, suspension of a retroverted uterus.[230] But sterility was a complex condition, stemming at times from a combination of several, often untreatable, factors. In such cases more adventuresome treatment might be tried. The oldest of these in the Canadian literature was artificial insemination. It was detailed lovingly in the 1870 *Canada Lancet*.[231] Doctors in the early decades saw problems with it, however, describing it as "revolting" and useless.[232] Physicians in the 1920s and 1930s were more optimistic, although unease had not disappeared completely.[233] In *Sex, Marriage and Birth Control*, Alfred Tyrer describes its use for sterile couples, using either the husband's sperm, if it was suitable, or that of a donor. Tyrer's matter-of-fact attitude is fascinating. By 1941, he claimed nearly 10 000 such procedures had been successful in the United States.[234]

Not all doctors were equally sanguine. A 1950 textbook by Curtis and Huffman suggested that donor insemination was fraught with "undetermined legal problems, religious restrictions, and delicate personal reactions; [yet] even those of us who have a distaste for donor insemination should accord consideration to the advantage of the theoretically better heredity in a donor conception baby in contrast with an illegitimate or foundling infant."[235] Extraordinary in this statement is the return to the age-old belief about inherited traits. The desire was not for a baby but for a certain kind of baby.[236]

The development of hormone therapy made it the new hope in infertility treatment. As early as 1915 there were references to lutein therapy to treat sterility and spontaneous abortion. Later references were to various hormonal extracts, including thyroid, pituitary, and ovarian, although there was not always the sense that physicians understood why these treatments seemed to work.[237] Some doctors also questioned the efficacy and safety of such extracts. One Toronto physician referred to the "scientifically unjustifiable prescribing of literally tons of internal gland extracts," while another pointed out the "close relationship that exists between the oestrogenic hormones and the carcinogenic factor," concluding that "hormonotherapy may not be without its dangers."[238]

Despite such concerns, endocrine therapy continued to be a favoured way of treating not only sterility (in both men and women) but also conditions that could result in sterility, such as amenorrhoea.[239] The extent of development in this field is illustrated by a physician who noted that at least 27 estrogenic hormones were available in 1940 but that only six were standardized and only six had any "appreciable oestrogenic potency." Reporting the successful treatment of male sterility, a group of physicians noted the case of a man who had been deemed sterile but whose wife became pregnant; the doctors' reaction was that "we cannot attach too much importance to this unless we carefully considered the moral habits of the wife."[240] If such an attitude was common, many marital relationships could have been jeopardized by physicians' injudicious pronouncements. A new synthetic estrogen that was causing some excitement in its varied application was diethylstilbestrol, the dangers of which were not always appreciated.[241] One physician pointed out in 1947 that in hormone therapy "Dosage is still to a large extent empirical, but modern fashions are probably fallacious in many instances. For example, stilboestrol is almost consistently used in over-doses, with the result that toxic effects are commonly experienced."[242]

Doctors writing about sterility acknowledged at times that treatment was often experimental and not very successful. This necessitated explaining very carefully to patients what was occurring, indeed at times letting the patient make the decision about therapy, especially in cases when sterility was the only complaint.[243] Such voices were few and far between, however. Said one physician in 1935, summarizing the current state of fertility treatment for women, "The wombs of childless women have been subjected to so much assault in the guise of treatment."[244]

As in most other medical specialties, infertility treatment changed greatly over time. By the 1950s, there was a sense that sterility could be overcome, although doctors also recognized that much more information was needed before a new age of therapy could claim many successes. As Drs. Harvey, Best, and Andison wrote in 1949:

> It is often noted that a couple desperately anxious for offspring and who have finally given up all hope and have adopted a child, sometimes will achieve a pregnancy. Many cases are cited where a rest, a trip, or change of employment will be rewarded with a pregnancy. It is all these factors which make one feel that we are still working on the fringe of knowledge and that the future may present many enlightening facts regarding this fascinating subject.[245]

Conclusion

Perhaps one of the differences between those who practise medicine and those who study the practice of medicine historically is that the former have traditionally seen medicine in absolute terms, as an objective science. Some aspects of medicine may meet this ideal, but most do not. This underlying theme permeates the history of medicine as a discipline. By studying medical practice in a broader framework, historians perceive the relationship between certain medical practices and their social and cultural context. A survey of medical attitudes toward and treatment of infertility in Canada between 1850 and 1950 reveals an overwhelming emphasis in the literature on female infertility, at the expense of male infertility. Despite early recognition of male sterility, the tendency of doctors was to focus on a woman's difficulty in conceiving, rather than the man's inability to impregnate her. This persisted even when physicians increased their estimates of the extent to which male infertility was responsible for childless marriages. One reason for this was the emphasis Canadian society has placed on motherhood. This led doctors and others to focus on women rather than on men in their search for infertility treatments. The rise of gynaecology also played a part. As Emil Novak stated in 1944, "It is of interest to note that the subject of sterility has become almost entirely a gynaecological problem." Urology simply did not play the same role, Novak argued, nor was it as developed or as focussed as gynaecology.[246] Moreover, underlying gynaecology was the assumption that women's bodies were often not up to their allotted task; that is, they kept breaking down. This was not simply a medical perception but a social perception as well. Finally, most doctors during this period were male and shared, or at least recognized, the difficulty men had with the concept of male sterility.

What also emerges from this study is the tendency of the medical profession to apportion blame. Despite the recognition of what doctors termed "selective mating," almost every discussion of sterility came to some conclusion about what percentage of childless marriages were the "fault" of the male or the female. This focus suggests that infertility was considered akin to deviance; one party in an infertile union was "innocent" and the other "guilty" and in need of treatment (or reform). This reflected the importance of virility to a man's sense of self and of maternity to a woman's. It also reflected the tendency of the medical profession to isolate "cause" in order to "treat." With a multitude of potential causes existing in both partners of a childless marriage, the chances of successful sterility treatment were not good.

Despite the link that doctors carefully drew between medicine and science, they were surprisingly imprecise in their explanations and use of terminology. The definition of sterility varied from one text to another, which must have caused confusion among student readers; this must also have reflected the lack of consensus within the profession itself. Despite this ambiguity and lack of consensus, physicians often gave opinions in ways that suggested pronouncements so authoritative as to need no explanation. For example, birth control practised by women caused sterility — no explanation of why. Hysterical women were generally sterile — no explanation of why.

The treatment of infertility was also subject to fads, from the folk wisdom of the earlier period, to the gynaecological operations of the turn of the century, to the various forms of endocrine therapy between the wars. This is in keeping with the nature of medicine. As Dr. Charles Shepard noted as early as 1902, "New medicines are made, achieve a short-lived success, and then pass on to obscurity. This is true, most especially in medicines for gynaecological diseases. Of the newer remedies it is hard indeed to get one that may be depended upon for long. They soon lose their reputation and potency, and are relegated to the past." Others agreed with this analysis. In a major 1928 text on gynaecology, the discussion of sterility made it clear that "the treatment must necessarily often be experimental."[247] Only after experiments on infertile couples could useful treatments be identified.

Throughout these writings on infertility, hardly any mention was made of the morality of intervention, the societal need for intervention, or the need to question the underlying assumption that couples had a "right" to have children. Doctors worked in a technological world; they were fascinated by developments in medicine and their applications. Although they recognized some of the social factors in sterility, such as work-related hazards and diet, they spent very little time advocating social change. There was no evidence in the literature that medical organizations or individual physicians were pressuring governments or employers to make work sites less hazardous for workers. Indeed, any awareness of class was absent from doctors' discussions of sterility and its causes. They left preventive medicine to their public health colleagues.

Swept up by medical advances, physicians did not always consider the side-effects of treatment or, as some of their colleagues pointed out, that some kinds of treatment may actually have caused sterility. Doctors were not alone in their faith in the efficacy of medical technology and treatment to overcome almost any health problem. Patients, too, believed in a technological fix. Although there is little evidence in the literature that many men and women consulted physicians for infertility in the nineteenth century, by the inter-war period this seemed to have changed, judging by what doctors were writing.

The voices of women and men, the childless couples, are not heard in the medical literature. They were not being heard in the popular literature either. This is not surprising considering the position of medicine in our society. As Barbara Ehrenreich has astutely observed, medicine "stands between biology and social policy, between the 'mysterious' world of the laboratory and everyday life. It makes public interpretations of biological theory; it dispenses the medical fruits of scientific advances."[248] In such a schema, patients remain relatively passive except in their ability not to accept the sick role. But once accepted, medical practitioners take charge. They determine how we look at our bodies. As seen in this study, this was particularly true with respect to the female body. At times, physicians seemed to view it as problematic.

Also lacking in the medical literature is any sense of the success rate of the various treatments, attributable no doubt in part to the complexity of factors involved in infertility and the myriad treatments available. The question that nevertheless remains is the extent to which the choices made by infertile couples during this period were informed by adequate and accurate information about the causes of infertility, the efficacy of the various treatments available, and the potential side-effects of treatment.

Abbreviations

AMB — Alberta Medical Bulletin
BAJMPS — British American Journal of Medical & Physical Science
CH — Canadian Health
CHJ — Canada Health Journal
CJMS — Canadian Journal of Medicine and Surgery
CL — The Canada Lancet
CLNH — Canada Lancet and National Hygiene
CLP — The Canada Lancet and Practitioner
CMAJ — Canadian Medical Association Journal
CMJ — The Canada Medical Journal and Monthly Record of Medical and Surgical Science
CMR — The Canada Medical Record
CMSJ — Canada Medical and Surgical Journal
CMT — The Canadian Medical Times
CP — Canadian Practitioner
CPHJ — Canadian Public Health Journal

CPMR — *Canadian Practitioner and Medical Review*
DMM — *Dominion Medical Monthly*
DMMOMJ — *Dominion Medical Monthly and Ontario Medical Journal*
MMC — *Modern Medicine of Canada*
MMJ — *The Montreal Medical Journal*
MMR — *Manitoba Medical Review*
PHJ — *The Public Health Journal*
SJ — *The Sanitary Journal*
WCMJ — *Western Canada Medical Journal*

Notes

1. In a paper that covers one hundred years, it is clearly not possible to provide a detailed social context. Where applicable, I will note how changes in the social milieu have been reflected in medical perceptions and treatment of infertility. For a more in-depth look at Canada during this period, readers are directed to A. Prentice et al., *Canadian Women: A History* (Toronto: Harcourt, Brace, Jovanovich, 1988), and R.D. Francis, R. Jones, and D.B. Smith, *Destinies: Canadian History Since Confederation,* 2d ed. (Toronto: Holt, Rinehart and Winston of Canada Ltd., 1992). Little research has been done on the history of infertility. Margarete Sandelowski has written a general overview of the American context, but her study does not really address treatment. Nor does it pay much attention to male sterility. M. Sandelowski, "Failures of Volition: Female Agency and Infertility in Historical Perspective," *Signs* 15 (1990): 475-99. Until more historical studies are completed, it will be impossible to place the Canadian experience in any comparative context.

2. For an overview of the history of the medical profession in Canada see R. Hamowy, *Canadian Medicine: A Study in Restricted Entry* (Vancouver: Fraser Institute, 1984), and more particularly C.D. Naylor, *Private Practice, Public Payment: Canadian Medicine and the Politics of Health Insurance, 1911-1966* (Montreal: McGill-Queen's University Press, 1986).

3. *BAJMPS* (November 1850), 333.

4. R. Kenneally, "The Montreal Maternity, 1843-1926: Evolution of a Hospital," M.A. thesis, McGill University, 1983, 20.

5. See W. Mitchinson, *The Nature of Their Bodies: Women and Their Doctors in Victorian Canada* (Toronto: University of Toronto Press, 1991), 240-44.

6. *Dalhousie University Medical Calendar, 1912-13,* 95.

7. H. Oxorn, *Harold Benge Atlee M.D.: A Biography* (Hantsport: Lancelot Press, 1983), 199-200.

8. N. Devitt, "The Statistical Case for Elimination of the Midwife: Fact Versus Prejudice, 1890-1935," [Part 1] *Women and Health* 4 (1)(1979), 84-85.

9. *CMAJ* 1 (2)(1911), 131.

10. *CMAJ* 7 (5)(1917), 413. Ann Oakley in her contemporary study of the English medical profession has discovered similar disdain. She found that individuals from the upper class specialize in neurology, while practitioners from lower-class

backgrounds specialize in gynaecology. A. Oakley, *Women Confined: Towards a Sociology of Childbirth* (New York: Schocken Books, 1980), 47.

11. Oxorn, *Harold Benge Atlee M.D.*, 36.

12. *CJMS* 65 (5)(1929), 132.

13. *CMAJ* 22 (4)(1930), 470; *CLP* 76 (4)(1931), 93; P. Stewart, "Infant Feeding in Canada: 1910-1940," M.A. thesis, Concordia University, 1982, 111. Even as late as 1950, the Chairman of the Committee on Maternal Welfare believed that the standard of obstetrics training in Canada was poor. *CMAJ* 62 (Suppl.)(1950), 233.

14. *CMAJ* 22 (4)(1930), 470.

15. For a description of this process in Canada see C. Berger, *Science, God and Nature in Victorian Canada* (Toronto: University of Toronto Press, 1983), and R. Cook, *The Regenerators: Social Criticism in Late Victorian English Canada* (Toronto: University of Toronto Press, 1985).

16. See Mitchinson, *The Nature of Their Bodies*, 125-51.

17. J. Bernard, *The Future of Motherhood* (New York: Penguin, 1975), 7.

18. A. Dally, *Inventing Motherhood: The Consequences of an Ideal* (New York: Schocken Books, 1983), 17.

19. R. Tannahill, *Sex in History* (London: Abacus, 1981), 330.

20. For a description of the changing way in which the female body was viewed see Thomas Laqueur, *Making Sex: Body and Gender from the Greeks to Freud* (Cambridge: Harvard University Press, 1990).

21. For a description of nineteenth-century attitudes, see Mitchinson, *The Nature of Their Bodies*, chap. 1. *Saturday Night* 17 (16 January 1914), 9.

22. *CL* 38 (5)(1905), 432.

23. *Canadian Child* 3 (7)(1923), 2.

24. *CMAJ* 17 (2)(1927), 208.

25. Oxorn, *Harold Benge Atlee M.D.*, 155.

26. *CMAJ* 50 (4)(1944), 315.

27. The focus on women as nurturers did not change over time, but attitudes toward women in the paid labour force did. In the late nineteenth century, Canadians felt uneasy about women (usually young and single) entering the workplace. By the early twentieth century, the reality of the working girl had been accepted, although concern was expressed about the impact of employment on her reproductive capacity. The change in the 1920s was the acceptance of middle-class women working *before* marriage. Only in the 1940s did Canadians accept married women in paid employment and only as part of the war effort. Throughout all these decades, Canadians saw the primary task of women as giving birth and nurturing their children. The number of children they had may have declined over time, but the importance of having them did not.

28. *Canadian Magazine* 15 (5)(1900), 473.

29. *CJMS* 11 (1)(1902), 3; W.S. Hall, *Sexual Knowledge* (Toronto: McClelland and Stewart, 1921), 203.

30. *DMMOMJ* 23 (5)(1904), 327.

31. *Saturday Night* 62 (28 September 1946), 30.

32. For example, the Israelites believed that the childless were "to be looked upon as not alive." *CMAJ* 40 (2)(1939), 116.

33. E. Becklard, *Physiological Mysteries and Revelations in Love, Courtship and Marriage* (New York, 1842), 20.

34. G.H. Napheys, *The Physical Life of Woman: Advice to the Maiden, Wife, and Mother* (Toronto: Rose Publishing, 1890), 83.

35. T.G. Thomas, *A Practical Treatise on the Diseases of Women* (Philadelphia: Henry C. Lea, 1868), 497.

36. P.H. Chavasse, *Advice to a Wife on the Management of Her Own Health and on the Treatment of Some of the Complaints Incidental to Pregnancy, Labour, and Suckling* (Toronto: Willing and Williamson, 1882), 3.

37. Hall, *Sexual Knowledge*, 207. Dr. James Sprague of Perth, Ontario, believed that a family was a woman's "crown of glory." *DMM* 38 (5)(1912), 148.

38. *PHJ* 7 (6)(1916), 306.

39. *CMAJ* 13 (11)(1923), 796.

40. *Canadian Home Journal* (November 1931), 83.

41. P.E. Ryberg, *Health, Sex and Birth Control* (Toronto: Anchor Press, 1943), 35; A.H. Tyrer, *Sex, Marriage and Birth Control*, 10th ed. (Toronto: Marriage Welfare Bureau, 1943), 48.

42. Tyrer, *Sex, Marriage and Birth Control*, 66.

43. *PHJ* 14 (6)(1923), 243. Intervention in childbirth and viewing it as pathological coincided with the rise in hospital births in the twentieth century.

44. *PHJ* 7 (3)(1916), 137; A. McLaren, *Our Own Master Race: Eugenics in Canada, 1885-1945* (Toronto: McClelland and Stewart, 1990), 80.

45. M.L. Holbrook, "Parturition Without Pain," in Napheys, *The Physical Life of Woman*, 311; see also Annual Report of the Medical Superintendent, Toronto Asylum 1859, Appendix 32, *Journals of the Legislative Assembly 1860*, 47; Annual Report of the Medical Superintendent, Toronto Asylum 1862, *Sessional Papers 66, Journals of the Legislative Assembly 1863*.

46. Napheys, *The Physical Life of Woman*, 22.

47. *Canadian Home Journal* (November 1931), 80.

48. Ryberg, *Health, Sex and Birth Control*, 33.

49. *CMAJ* 42 (3)(1940), 243; *Canadian Home Journal* (August 1943), 11; *Saturday Night* 58 (5 June 1943), 18; *AMB* 15 (2)(1950), 17.

50. B.G. Jefferis, *Search Lights on Health: Light on Dark Corners* (Toronto: Nichols, 1900), 194; *CP* 14 (1)(1885), 360; *CP* 19 (7)(1894), 495-96; Hall, *Sexual Knowledge*, 214; *CLP* 71 (4)(1928), 123.

51. Napheys, *The Physical Life of Woman*, 269. See also H. Lyman et al., *The Practical Home Physician and Encyclopedia of Medicine* (Guelph: World, 1884), 906; H. Ayers, *Ayers' Everyman His Own Doctor: Family Medical Advisor* (Montreal:

1884), 317; A. Edis, *Diseases of Women: A Manual for Students and Practitioners* (Philadelphia: Henry C. Lea's Son, 1882), 524; Chavasse, *Advice to a Wife*, 102, 105; H.J. Garrigues, *A Text-Book of the Diseases of Women* (Philadelphia: William B. Saunders, 1894), 127; A. Galabin, *The Student's Guide to the Diseases of Women* (London: 1884), 284.

52. For an overview of the history of birth control in Canada see A. McLaren and A.T. McLaren, *The Bedroom and the State: The Changing Practices and Politics of Contraception and Abortion in Canada, 1880-1980* (Toronto: McClelland and Stewart, 1986). For concern about ovariotomies see *CP* 9 (9)(1884), 272; *CP* 10 (12)(1885), 360; *CMSJ* 15 (1887), 143-44; *CP* 12 (10)(1887), 310; *CPMR* 19 (1894), 499-500; *DMMOMJ* 11 (5)(1898), 225; *DMMOMJ* 12 (6)(1899), 280; *CMAJ* 1 (6)(1911), 495.

53. W.P. Graves, *Gynecology* (Philadelphia: W.B. Saunders, 1928), 658.

54. A.L. Bonnicksen, *In Vitro Fertilization: Building Policy from Laboratories to Legislatures* (New York: Columbia University Press, 1989), 12; J.C. Edgar, *The Practice of Obstetrics Designed for the Use of Students and Practitioners of Medicine* (Philadelphia: P. Blakiston's Son & Co., 1907), 28; R.A. Leonardo, *History of Gynecology* (New York: Froben Press, 1944), 255; M. Goldman, *Gold Diggers and Silver Miners* (Ann Arbor: University of Michigan Press, 1981), 126.

55. W.B. Carpenter, *Principles of Human Physiology*, 7th ed. (London: John Churchill and Son, 1869), 834; *CP* 9 (4)(1884), 115.

56. *CJMS* 15 (2)(1904), 91.

57. *CMAJ* 22 (2)(1930), 214.

58. *CMSJ* 15 (1887), 143; *CMSJ* 14 (1886), 214; *CP* 12 (10)(1887), 308; R.V. Pierce, *The People's Common Sense Medical Adviser in Plain English* (Buffalo: 1882), 212; *CMAJ* 2 (1)(1912), 60-61. For a detailed look at ovariotomies see Mitchinson, *The Nature of Their Bodies*, 258-77.

59. C.A. Thomas, W.S. Playfair, and T.W. Eden, eds., *A System of Gynaecology* (London: MacMillan, 1906), 893.

60. *CPMR* 31 (10)(1906), 557.

61. *CMAJ* 5 (8)(1915), 667.

62. *CMAJ* 29 (6)(1933), 586.

63. Hall, *Sexual Knowledge*, 215; P.A. Cazeaux, *Theoretical and Practical Treatise on Midwifery* (Philadelphia: Lindsay and Blakiston, 1837), 123; W.T. Smith, *Parturition and the Principles and Practice of Obstetrics* (Philadelphia: Lea and Blanchard, 1849), 95; A. Flint, *The Physiology of Man* (New York: 1874), 293; Pierce, *The People's Common Sense Medical Adviser*, 739-40; A.L. Galabin, *A Manual of Midwifery* (Philadelphia: P. Blakiston and Son, 1886), 55; Jefferis, *Search Lights on Health*, 236; Napheys, *The Physical Life of Woman*, 71; Garrigues, *A Text-Book of Diseases*, 117; A.L. Galabin, *Diseases of Women* (London: J.A. Churchill, 1893), 72.

64. H.S. Crossen and R.J. Crossen, *Diseases of Women* (St. Louis: C.V. Mosby, 1930), 878; F.L. Adair, ed., *Obstetrics and Gynecology*, vol. I (Philadelphia: Lea & Febiger, 1940), 59; E.C. Dudley, *The Principles and Practice of Gynecology for Students and Practitioners* (Philadelphia: Lea & Febiger, 1908), 765.

65. *MMC* 3 (6)(1948), 44; *MMC* 4 (10)(1949), 49; *AMB* 13 (1)(1948), 64.

66. A. McLaren, *A History of Contraception: From Antiquity to the Present Day* (Oxford: Basil Blackwell, 1990), 49; Becklard, *Physiological Mysteries*, 44; Napheys, *The Physical Life of Woman*, 77; Galabin, *Diseases of Women*, 498; *CP* 19 (7)(1894), 495.

67. *CP* 11 (1)(1886), 43.

68. *DMM* 33 (3)(1909), 95; J. Bland-Sutton and A.E. Giles, *The Diseases of Women: A Handbook for Students and Practitioners* (London: Rebman, 1906), 69.

69. E. Novak, *Textbook of Gynecology* (Baltimore: Williams & Wilkins, 1944), 595.

70. T.W. Eden and C. Lockyer, *The New System of Gynaecology*, vol. I (Toronto: Macmillan, 1917), 412; Barton Cook Hirst, *A Text-Book of Obstetrics* (Philadelphia: W.B. Saunders, 1898), 91; Dudley, *The Principles and Practice of Gynecology*, 769.

71. Graves, *Gynecology*, 165, 671.

72. Crossen and Crossen, *Diseases of Women*, 869; Adair, *Obstetrics and Gynecology*, vol. I, 524; *MMR* 30 (5)(1950), 289; A.H. Curtis and J.W. Huffman, *A Textbook of Gynecology*, 6th ed. (Philadelphia: W.B. Saunders, 1950), 563.

73. J.M. Kerr et al., *Combined Textbook of Obstetrics and Gynaecology for Students and Medical Practitioners* (Edinburgh: E. & S. Livingstone, 1933), 731; Ten Teachers, *Diseases of Women*, ed. C. Berkeley et al. (London: Edward Arnold, 1935), 124; H. Flanders Dunbar, *Emotions and Bodily Changes*, 3d ed. (New York: Columbia University Press, 1947), 341.

74. Cazeaux, *Theoretical and Practical Treatise on Midwifery*, 238; *CMR* 28 (11)(1900), 475; *CPMR* 36 (10)(1911), 614; *CMAJ* 1 (12)(1911), 1131; *CMAJ* 17 (12)(1927), 1469.

75. *CMAJ* 22 (2)(1930), 253; *CMAJ* 24 (4)(1931), 491.

76. *CMAJ* 34 (4)(1936), 431; *CMAJ* 52 (4)(1945), 371.

77. Holbrook, "Parturition Without Pain," 315; Ten Teachers, *Diseases of Women*, 124; C.H. Davis, ed., *Gynecology and Obstetrics*, vol. III (Hagerstown: W.F. Prior, 1935), chap. 9, p. 3.

78. *CMAJ* 23 (1)(1930), 18.

79. *CMAJ* 13 (9)(1923), 678.

80. R.E. Frisch, "Nutrition, Fatness and Fertility: The Effect of Food Intake on Reproductive Ability," in *Nutrition and Human Reproduction*, ed. W.H. Mosley (New York: Plenum Press, 1978), 108; *CPMR* 29 (3)(1904), 141; A.W. Bourne, *Synopsis of Midwifery and Gynaecology*, 3d ed. rev. (Toronto: Macmillan of Canada, 1925), 415; H.A. Kelly et al., *Gynecology* (New York: D. Appleton, 1928), 158; T.W. Eden and C. Lockyer, *Gynecology for Students and Practitioners* (London: J. & A. Churchill, 1928), 128; Graves, *Gynecology*, 655. In 1912 B. Hirst proposed 18 months: Hirst, *A Text-Book of Obstetrics*, 89.

81. Ten Teachers, *Diseases of Women*, 125; Kerr et al., *Combined Textbook of Obstetrics*, 730; *CMAJ* 37 (3)(1937), 232; *CMAJ* 42 (3)(1940), 243; *CMAJ* 49 (3)(1943), 172; *MMR* 29 (3)(1949), 125; Novak, *Textbook of Gynecology*, 588; Curtis and Huffman, *A Textbook of Gynecology*, 567. It is difficult to know how to account for the fluctuations in definition. The medical profession is not a monolith, and in the past as now practitioners read a wide variety of literature that reflected diverse

orientations — national, medical specialization, and approach (research vs. applied). Today's profession still confuses issues. For example, medical researchers are not always clear (and one suspects deliberately so) about the degree of success in the treatment of infertility.

82. Eden and Lockyer, *The New System of Gynaecology*, vol. I, 404.

83. *MMJ* 29 (3)(1900), 182; *CL* 40 (1)(1906), 8-9; Bland-Sutton and Giles, *Diseases of Women*, 420-21; G.T. Gilliam, *A Text-Book of Practical Gynaecology* (Philadelphia: F.A. Davis, 1907), 79; *CL* 43 (9)(1910), 658; Hirst, *A Text-Book of Obstetrics*, 91; *CMAJ* 5 (1)(1915), 13; Bourne, *Synopsis of Midwifery*, 413; Kelly et al., *Gynecology*, 158; *CJMS* 78 (4)(1935), 106; *Saturday Night* 60 (10 March 1945), 12; *MMR* 29 (3)(1949), 122; *CMAJ* 62 (1)(1950), 51.

84. Kerr et al., *Combined Textbook of Obstetrics*, 728; *CL* 37 (10)(1904), 922; Dudley, *The Principles and Practice of Gynecology*, 763; *DMM* 33 (3)(1909), 90; Crossen and Crossen, *Diseases of Women*, 870; Davis, *Gynecology and Obstetrics*, vol. III, chap. 9, p. 3; E. Gee, "The Life Course of Canadian Women: An Historical and Demographic Analysis," *Social Indicators Research* 18 (1986), 267-68; McLaren, *A History of Contraception*, 260-61; *CMAJ* 40 (2)(1939), 117; Adair, *Obstetrics and Gynecology*, vol. I, 504-505; Novak, *Textbook of Gynecology*, 588; S.E. Tolnay and A.M. Guest, "Childlessness in a Transitional Population: The United States at the Turn of the Century," *Journal of Family History* 7 (1982), 201; *Saturday Night* 60 (10 March 1945), 13; *MMR* 29 (3)(1949), 121; Curtis and Huffman, *Textbook of Gynecology*, 562; *CMAJ* 63 (4)(1950), 344; R. Achilles, "Desperately Seeking Babies: New Technologies of Hope and Despair," in *Delivering Motherhood: Maternal Ideologies and Practices in the 19th and 20th Centuries*, ed. K. Arnup, A. Lévesque, and R.R. Pierson (London: Routledge, 1990), 287.

85. *CL* 40 (1)(1906), 8.

86. CMAJ 40 (2)(1939), 117; *Saturday Night* 60 (10 March 1945), 13.

87. Queen's University, Faculty of Medicine, Examination Papers 1900-1926; 1921-42.

88. *CMAJ* 23 (1)(1930), 17.

89. *CMAJ* 37 (3)(1937), 232; Graves, *Gynecology*, 5.

90. *CMAJ* 43 (4)(1940), 404; Crossen and Crossen, *Diseases of Women*, 870; *MMR* 29 (3)(1949), 125. It was also a practical subject, for awareness of previous sterility in the woman could aid in the diagnosis of ectopic pregnancy. *MMJ* 29 (9)(1900), 654; *MMJ* 30 (8)(1901), 617-18; *CPMR* 29 (8)(1904), 383; Adair, *Obstetrics and Gynecology*, vol. I, 527; *CMAJ* 62 (1)(1950), 51.

91. Jefferis, *Search Lights on Health*, 255; Pierce, *The People's Common Sense Medical Adviser*, 738-39.

92. R.W. Garrett, *Textbook of Medical and Surgical Gynaecology* (Toronto: J.A. Carveth, 1897), 127; *CL* 34 (1)(1900), 20; *CL* 33 (12)(1900), 679; *CL* 37 (10)(1904), 922; *CL* 40 (1)(1906), 7; J.C. Webster, *A Text-Book of Diseases of Women* (Philadelphia: W.B. Saunders, 1907), 700; Dudley, *The Principles and Practice of Gynecology*, 763; *DMM* 33 (3)(1909), 92; B.W. Bell, *The Principles of Gynaecology* (London: Longmans, Green, 1910), 217; Hirst, *A Text-Book of Obstetrics*, 90; J.W.T. Walker, *Surgical Diseases and Injuries of the Genito-Urinary Organs* (London: Cassell, 1914), 798; Eden and Lockyer, *The New System of Gynaecology*, vol. I, 404.

93. *CMAJ* 14 (2)(1924), 139; Bourne, *Synopsis of Midwifery*, 413; Kelly et al., *Gynecology*, 158; Graves, *Gynecology*, 658; Crossen and Crossen, *Diseases of Women*, 870; *CMAJ* 23 (1)(1930), 21; *CMAJ* 24 (5)(1931), 736; Kerr et al., *Combined Textbook of Obstetrics*, 729; *MMR* 14 (7)(1934), 8; *CMAJ* 31 (5)(1934), 526; Davis, *Gynecology and Obstetrics*, vol. III, chap. 9, p. 11, 14; *CMAJ* 37 (3)(1937), 232.

94. Adair, *Obstetrics and Gynecology*, vol. II, 673; *CMAJ* 49 (3)(1943), 167; Novak, *Textbook of Gynecology*, 589; *Saturday Night* 60 (10 March 1945), 13; *MMR* 29 (3)(1949), 124; *CMAJ* 63 (4)(1950), 344-45.

95. *CL* 33 (12)(1900), 679; Allbutt et al., *A System of Gynaecology*, 111; *CL* 40 (1)(1906), 7; *DMM* 35 (2)(1910), 48; *CL* 48 (2)(1914), 79; Eden and Lockyer, *The New System of Gynaecology*, vol. I, 124-25; *CMAJ* 14 (2)(1924), 137; *CMAJ* 23 (1)(1930), 21; *CMAJ* 30 (4)(1934), 402; *CMAJ* 31 (5)(1934), 526; *CMAJ* 30 (4)(1934), 401; *CMAJ* 40 (2)(1939), 118; Tyrer, *Sex, Marriage and Birth Control*, 50; Adair, *Obstetrics and Gynecology*, vol. II, 673; *CMAJ* 49 (3)(1943), 167; *Saturday Night* 60 (19 March 1945), 13; *AMB* 14 (4)(1949), 13; Curtis and Huffman, *A Textbook of Gynecology*, 569.

96. *CMAJ* 30 (4)(1934), 400; see also *DMM* 33 (3)(1909), 92; *MMR* 29 (3)(1949), 125.

97. J. Buchanan, *The Eclectic Practice of Medicine* (Philadelphia: 1867), 714.

98. *CMR* 11 (1883), 255; Ayers, *Ayers' Everyman His Own Doctor*, 221.

99. *CP* 18 (4)(1883), 296; Jefferis, *Search Lights on Health*, 247-48.

100. *CL* 27 (1894), 97.

101. A. Stockham, *Tokology: A Book for Every Woman* (Toronto: McClelland, Goodchild and Stewart, 1916), 325; see also H.H. Morton, *Genito-Urinary Diseases and Syphilis*, 2d ed. (Philadelphia: F.A. Davis, 1908), 467.

102. *CMAJ* 14 (2)(1924), 138-39.

103. Edgar, *The Practice of Obstetrics*, 38-39.

104. Stockham, *Tokology*, 325.

105. *CMAJ* 17 (12)(1927), 1473.

106. *Popular Sex Science* 11 (1 August 1940), 41.

107. C. Jewett, ed., *The Practice of Obstetrics* (New York: Lea Brothers, 1901), 343; Edgar, *The Practice of Obstetrics*, 28.

108. *MMJ* 32 (2)(1903), 101.

109. Allbutt et al., *System of Gynaecology*, 111.

110. *CMAJ* 14 (2)(1924), 138-39; *CMAJ* 24 (5)(1931), 660; Adair, *Obstetrics and Gynecology*, vol. I, 529; Ryberg, *Health, Sex and Birth Control*, 15; W.A. Scott and H.B. Van Wyck, *The Essentials of Obstetrics and Gynecology* (Philadelphia: Lea & Febiger, 1946), 338-39; *MMR* 29 (3)(1949), 125.

111. *CL* 27 (1894), 97.

112. *CMAJ* 40 (2)(1939), 117; Davis, *Gynecology and Obstetrics*, vol. III, chap. 9, p. 6.

113. Adair, *Obstetrics and Gynecology*, vol. I, 506; *MMR* 29 (3)(1949), 125; Novak, *Textbook of Gynecology*, 590; Curtis and Huffman, *A Textbook of Gynecology*, 563.

114. *CMAJ* 17 (12)(1927), 1473; Morton, *Genito-Urinary Diseases,* 473; Davis, *Gynecology and Obstetrics,* vol. III, chap. 9, p. 6; *CMAJ* 37 (3)(1937), 235; Adair, *Obstetrics and Gynecology,* vol. I, 513.

115. *CMAJ* 24 (5)(1931), 660; Graves, *Gynecology,* 673; Davis, *Gynecology and Obstetrics,* vol. III, chap. 9, p. 6; *CMAJ* 40 (2)(1939), 117; Adair, *Obstetrics and Gynecology,* vol. I, 506; Novak, *Textbook of Gynecology,* 590; Curtis and Huffman, *A Textbook of Gynecology,* 563.

116. For expressions of concern about obesity see *CL* 40 (1)(1906), 8; *PHJ* 18 (2)(1927), 95; *CMAJ* 40 (2)(1939), 117. What is interesting about the discussions of obesity is that it was not always clear whether physicians were referring to obesity in men or in women. For expressions of the value of vitamin E in diet see *CMAJ* 38 (6)(1938), 615; *CMAJ* 40 (2)(1939), 117; Adair, *Obstetrics and Gynecology,* vol. I, 57; *AMB* 14 (2)(1949), 28.

117. *CL* 40 (1)(1906), 8; Morton, *Genito-Urinary Diseases,* 473; Edgar, *The Practice of Obstetrics,* 28; *CMAJ* 17 (12)(1927), 1473; Graves, *Gynecology,* 658-59; Crossen and Crossen, *Diseases of Women,* 878; *CMAJ* 24 (5)(1931), 660; Davis, *Gynecology and Obstetrics,* vol. III, chap. 9, p. 6; *CMAJ* 40 (2)(1939), 117; Adair, *Obstetrics and Gynecology,* vol. I, 57; Novak, *Textbook of Gynecology,* 590; Scott and Van Wyck, *The Essentials of Obstetrics and Gynecology,* 338-39; *MMR* 29 (3)(1949), 125; Curtis and Huffman, *A Textbook of Gynecology,* 563. Occasionally in discussions of alcohol there would be mention of overuse of tobacco and drugs. Morton, *Genito-Urinary Diseases,* 473; *CMAJ* 14 (2)(1924), 139; Crossen and Crossen, *Diseases of Women,* 878; Davis, *Gynecology and Obstetrics,* vol. III, chap. 9, p. 6.

118. *MMJ* 32 (3)(1903), 101; *CL* 40 (1)(1906), 8; Morton, *Genito-Urinary Diseases,* 477; Dudley, *The Principles and Practice of Gynecology,* 765; *DMM* 33 (3)(1909), 91; *PHJ* 10 (9)(1919), 414.

119. *CL* 39 (12)(1906), 1078-79.

120. For a detailed look at the purity movement see M. Valverde, *The Age of Light, Soap, and Water: Moral Reform in English Canada, 1885-1925* (Toronto: McClelland and Stewart, 1991). At times the focus of immorality was on the upper classes, but whether on them or on workers, middle-class Canadians felt alienated and determined to impose their view of morality on society.

121. *PHJ* 14 (6)(1923), 245.

122. *CMAJ* 142 (1924), 139; *MMR* 14 (7)(1934), 8; *CMAJ* 30 (4)(1934), 400. See also Graves, *Gynecology,* 658-59, and Davis, *Gynecology and Obstetrics,* vol. III, chap. 9, p. 6.

123. Novak, *Textbook of Gynecology,* 609; Scott and Van Wyck, *The Essentials of Obstetrics and Gynecology,* 338-39; *MMR* 29 (3)(1949), 125; Curtis and Huffman, *A Textbook of Gynecology,* 577.

124. Eden and Lockyer, *Gynaecology for Students,* 129; *CMAJ* 24 (5)(1931), 660; Ten Teachers, *Diseases of Women,* 125; Davis, *Gynecology and Obstetrics,* vol. III, chap. 9, p. 1, 6; *CMAJ* 40 (2)(1939), 117; Adair, *Obstetrics and Gynecology,* vol. I, 506; Ryberg, *Health, Sex and Birth Control,* 181.

125. *CL* 33 (12)(1900), 679; Allbutt et al., *A System of Gynaecology,* 109; *CL* 40 (1)(1906), 12. Only when impotence was the result of medical conditions such as diabetes and testicular hypofunction did practitioners engage in any discussion

of treatment; this seemed to occur only in the last decade of the period under study. *CMAJ* 47 (1)(1942), 51; *CMAJ* 48 (3)(1943), 231-32.

126. *CMAJ* 14 (2)(1924), 139; Dudley, *The Principles of Gynecology*, 765; *CMAJ* 30 (4)(1934), 400; Davis, *Gynecology and Obstetrics*, vol. III, chap. 9, p. 11; *CMAJ* 37 (3)(1937), 234; Ryberg, *Health, Sex and Birth Control*, 181; *MMR* 29 (3)(1949), 125; Curtis and Huffman, *A Textbook of Gynecology*, 562. See also the discussion of sterility in males above. It should be noted that some of the physiological problems did have a volitional source; for example, blocked passages for the sperm were often a result of venereal infection.

127. *CL* 40 (1)(1906), 8; *CMAJ* 37 (3)(1937), 235; *CMAJ* 47 (1)(1942), 51; Curtis and Huffman, *A Textbook of Gynecology*, 567; *AMB* 14 (2)(1949), 28. See also Morton, *Genito-Urinary Diseases*, 477; Edgar, *The Practice of Obstetrics*, 28; Dudley, *The Principles and Practice of Gynecology*, 765; Graves, *Gynecology*, 658-69; Novak, *Textbook of Gynecology*, 590, 609; Scott and Van Wyck, *The Essentials of Obstetrics and Gynecology*, 338-40.

128. Davis, *Gynecology and Obstetrics*, vol. III, chap. 9, p. 1; Novak, *Textbook of Gynecology*, 590; *MMR* 29 (3)(1949), 125.

129. *CMAJ* 14 (2)(1924), 138; *CMAJ* 63 (4)(1950), 345.

130. *MMJ* 32 (2)(1903), 101; Morton, *Genito-Urinary Diseases*, 477; Edgar, *The Practice of Obstetrics*, 28; Dudley, *The Principles and Practice of Gynecology*, 765; Kerr et al., *Combined Textbook of Obstetrics*, 730.

131. Walker, *Surgical Diseases*, 799; *CMAJ* 14 (2)(1924), 139; *MMR* 29 (3)(1949), 125.

132. *CL* 33 (12)(1900), 679; *CL* 40 (1)(1906), 12; *CMAJ* 14 (2)(1924), 139; *CMAJ* 24 (5)(1931), 662; *CMAJ* 30 (4)(1934), 400; *CMAJ* 37 (3)(1937), 234; Ryberg, *Health, Sex and Birth Control*, 282; *MMC* 3 (6)(1948), 44; *MMR* 29 (3)(1949), 124; *AMB* 14 (2)(1949), 28; *CMAJ* 63 (4)(1950), 344-45.

133. Pierce, *The People's Common Sense Medical Adviser*, 749-50.

134. Garrigues, *A Text-Book of Diseases*, 125.

135. *English Herbal Dispensary* (1910), 13. The relationship between masturbation and ill health had long been posited. The medical literature of the nineteenth century focussed predominantly on male masturbation, although it recognized the existence of female masturbation. Doctors believed that masturbation led to weakness and to shunning of the opposite sex, both of which would lead to lack of procreation. A direct link with sterility, however, was quite rare, particularly with respect to women.

136. W. Goodell, *Lessons in Gynecology* (Philadelphia: F.A. Davis, 1890), 560-62; Garrigues, *A Text-Book of Diseases*, 125, 128-29; McGill University Archives, Records of the University Lying-in Hospital, patient admitted 19 May 1896 and discharged 24 May 1896.

137. Stockham, *Tokology*, 244.

138. *CMAJ* 24 (5)(1931), 660; *MMR* 29 (3)(1949), 122; *MMR* 30 (5)(1950), 290. The hallmark of the Victorian attitude toward female sexuality was control. Women should control their desires (which were natural) and only give in to them within marriage, and preferably for procreation. Early in the twentieth century, physicians

and lay people alike accepted that sex within marriage was healthy in and of itself; that is, sex and procreation had been separated. The emphasis on sex as an important ingredient for a happy marriage continued to be stressed in the following decades. What changed, however, was the degree to which sexual experimentation was countenanced before marriage. By the 1940s, sex manuals and popular periodical literature seemed accepting of "petting," but nothing beyond this.

139. For a discussion on the medical profession's attitudes toward birth control see Mitchinson, *The Nature of Their Bodies*, 125-51; Edgar, *The Practice of Obstetrics*, 38-39; *English Herbal Dispensary*, 13-14; E.E. Montgomery, *Practical Gynecology* (Philadelphia: Blakiston and Son, 1912), 23; Eden and Lockyer, *The New System of Gynaecology*, vol. II, 76-77.

140. *CMJ* 3 (1867), 226-67; *CHJ* 1 (5)(1870), 67-68; Napheys, *The Physical Life of Woman*, 98; Pierce, *The People's Common Sense Medical Adviser*, 734; *CMR* 17 (5)(1889), 98; Garrigues, *A Text-Book of Diseases*, 128-29; C.A.L. Reed, ed., *A Text-Book of Gynecology* (New York: D. Appleton, 1901), 10; Bourne, *Synopsis of Midwifery*, 414.

141. *PHJ* 7 (3)(1916), 139.

142. *CMAJ* 22 (6)(1930), 794.

143. *CMAJ* 53 (3)(1945), 298; Scott and Van Wyck, *The Essentials of Obstetrics and Gynecology*, 339.

144. *CPMR* 25 (1)(1900), 48; *CMAJ* 37 (3)(1937), 236-37; *Maclean's* 60 (1 April 1947), 62; Curtis and Huffman, *A Textbook of Gynecology*, 562.

145. *SJ* 1 (1874), 56; *CL* 6 (7)(1874), 233; *CMR* 7 (1879), 319; Lyman, *The Practical Home Physician*, 875-77; *CMR* 18 (2)(1889), 25-27; Goodell, *Lessons in Gynecology*, 549; *CP* 16 (6)(1891), 261; Garrigues, *A Text-Book of Diseases*, 125-29; *DMM* 3 (4)(1894), 112; *CPMR* 27 (11)(1902), 662; *CJMS* 11 (1)(1902), 2; C.B. Penrose, *A Text-Book of Diseases of Women*, 5th ed. rev. (Philadelphia: W.B. Saunders, 1905), 20. One aspect of higher education for women that many Canadian physicians disliked was the necessity of co-education, or competition with men. In the United States, doctors such as Mary Putnam Jacobi argued that education of women at schools such as Bryn Mawr was conducive to health. Such an argument would hold little weight in Canada because there were no women's universities. Also, statistics on college women revealed that they married later and had fewer children than their less educated sisters, neither of which was a positive endorsement for many Canadians.

146. *MMJ* 32 (2)(1903), 101.

147. *MMJ* 32 (2)(1903), 101-102.

148. *PHJ* 7 (7)(1916), 349; *PHJ* 7 (4)(1916), 189; Jewett, *The Practice of Obstetrics*, 342.

149. Davis, *Gynecology and Obstetrics*, vol. I, chap. 5, p. 7; *CMAJ* 37 (3)(1937), 235.

150. Eden and Lockyer, *The New System of Gynaecology*, vol. I, 297; C. Abeele, "Nations Are Built of Babies: Maternal and Child Welfare in Ontario, 1914-1940," Ph.D. dissertation, University of Guelph, 1987, 148.

151. *CMAJ* 35 (5)(1936), 572.

152. *Saturday Night* 58 (31 October 1942), 22; Adair, *Obstetrics and Gynecology*, 513.

153. See Mitchinson, *The Nature of Their Bodies*, 66-68.

154. *CPMR* 27 (11)(1902), 662; *CPMR* 30 (2)(1905), 92; Stockham, *Tokology*, 105.

155. *CLP* 74 (2)(1930), 41; see also *CMAJ* 55 (4)(1946), lxxv.

156. *CMAJ* 11 (9)(1921), 616; *CLP* 74 (2)(1930), 41-42; *CJMS* 75 (2)(1934), 41; *CMAJ* 39 (1)(1938), 76; *CMAJ* 47 (1)(1942), 18; *CMAJ* 46 (1)(1942), 5.

157. Eden and Lockyer, *The New System of Gynaecology*, vol. I, 412; Dudley, *The Principles and Practice of Gynecology*, 765; Bell, *The Principles of Gynecology*, 217.

158. *CL* 40 (1)(1906), 8; Dudley, *The Principles and Practice of Gynecology*, 765; Bell, *The Principles of Gynecology*, 217; *CMAJ* 5 (8)(1915), 667; *CMAJ* 14 (11)(1924), 1052; *PHJ* 18 (2)(1927), 95-96; Graves, *Gynecology*, 69; Adair, *Obstetrics and Gynecology*, vol. I, 508-12.

159. Crossen and Crossen, *Diseases of Women*, 878; A.C. Beck, *Obstetrical Practice* (Baltimore: Williams & Wilkins, 1947), 173.

160. *CPHJ* 30 (1)(1939), 9; *CMAJ* 40 (2)(1939), 134.

161. McGill University Archives, University Lying-in Hospital Records, patient admitted 19 May 1896 and discharged 24 May 1896; *CL* 40 (1)(1906), 8; *CMAJ* 12 (3)(1922), 163; *CMAJ* 17 (12)(1927), 1473; *CMAJ* 24 (5)(1931), 660; *CMAJ* 40 (2)(1939), 117; *MMC* 4 (10)(1949), 49.

162. Chavasse, *Advice to a Wife*, 22-23; *CPMR* 27 (8)(1902), 478.

163. *CL* 37 (10)(1904), 922; *CPMR* 30 (2)(1905), 92; Kelly et al., *Gynecology*, 158-59; *CMAJ* 24 (5)(1931), 660; *CMAJ* 40 (2)(1939), 117.

164. *CMAJ* 40 (2)(1939), 117.

165. *MMC* 4 (10)(1949), 49; Curtis and Huffman, *A Textbook of Gynecology*, 563.

166. *CMJ* 7 (1870-71), 185-86.

167. *MMR* 30 (5)(1950), 290. See also Bland-Sutton and Giles, *The Diseases of Women*, 423; Adair, *Obstetrics and Gynecology*, vol. I, 515.

168. Chavasse, *Advice to a Wife*, 89; *CL* 37 (10)(1904), 922; *Woman's Century* (October 1917), 9.

169. *CL* 37 (10)(1904), 922; Eden and Lockyer, *The New System of Gynaecology*, vol. I, 414; *CLNH* 63 (1)(1924), 2; Kerr et al., *Combined Textbook of Obstetrics*, 730; Ten Teachers, *Diseases of Women*, 125; *CMAJ* 40 (2)(1939), 116; *CMAJ* 42 (3)(1940), 243; Ryberg, *Health, Sex and Birth Control*, 174; *Canadian Home Journal* 40 (August 1943), 11; Scott and Van Wyck, *The Essentials of Obstetrics and Gynecology*, 339; *MMR* 29 (3)(1949), 125. One text pointed out that too great a difference in the ages of the spouses was also problematic. See Bell, *The Principles of Gynaecology*, 217.

170. Pierce, *The People's Common Sense Medical Adviser*, 762; *CL* 17 (1885), 320; *CL* 19 (1886), 72.

171. Garrigues, *A Text-Book of Diseases*, 129.

172. *CL* 34 (1)(1900), 20; *CMAJ* 14 (9)(1924), 797; Curtis and Huffman, *A Textbook of Gynecology*, 563.

173. See Mitchinson, *The Nature of Their Bodies*, 252-77.

174. *CMAJ* 14 (2)(1924), 139; Crossen and Crossen, *Diseases of Women*, 870-72; Curtis and Huffman, *A Textbook of Gynecology*, 564; Adair, *Obstetrics and Gynecology*, vol. I, 514.

175. Public Archives of Ontario, Canniff Papers, MU 490 Package 3; Canada Medical Association, 1882; reports from newspapers.

176. Lyman, *The Practical Home Physician*, 974; P. Mundé, *A Practical Treatise on the Diseases of Women* (Philadelphia: 1891), 42; *CMR* 26 (1898), 4. See also Mitchinson, *The Nature of Their Bodies*, 256-57.

177. *CMAJ* 1 (2)(1911), 131-32; *MMJ* 31 (4)(1904), 277; Penrose, *A Text-Book of Diseases*, 18-19.

178. *CMAJ* 10 (10)(1920), 901; *PHJ* 14 (6)(1923), 243; *CMAJ* 19 (2)(1928), 228; *CJMS* 66 (3)(1929), 71; Kerr et al., *Combined Textbook of Obstetrics*, 360; *Maclean's* 63 (15 July 1950), 49.

179. *CPHJ* 23 (12)(1932), 566; *CMAJ* 56 (2)(1947), 170.

180. Graves, *Gynecology*, 679.

181. *CMAJ* 25 (5)(1931), 584; *CMAJ* 48 (6)(1943), 546; Adair, *Obstetrics and Gynecology*, vol. I, 513.

182. Jewett, *The Practice of Obstetrics*, 342; Gilliam, *A Text-Book of Practical Gynecology*, 81; Dudley, *The Principles and Practice of Gynecology*, 765; Bell, *The Principles of Gynecology*, 217.

183. *CMJ* 7 (1870-71), 185-86; *CL* 34 (1)(1900), 23; *CL* 34 (8)(1901), 460-61; *CL* 37 (10)(1904), 922; *CL* 40 (1)(1906), 7; *English Herbal Dispensary*, 13.

184. *CL* 40 (1)(1906), 7.

185. *CMT* 1 (10)(1873), 78; Galabin, *The Student's Guide*, 340; *CMR* 17 (5)(1889), 98; *DMMOMJ* 8 (1897), 146; Garrett, *Textbook of Medical and Surgical Gynecology*, 11; *MMJ* 29 (3)(1900), 182; *MMJ* 29 (3)(1900), 178; *MMJ* 29 (4)(1900), 264; Reed, *A Text-Book of Gynecology*, 11; Hall, *Sexual Knowledge*, 140; Penrose, *A Text-Book of Diseases*, 18-19; *CL* 40 (4)(1906), 358; Morton, *Genito-Urinary Diseases*, 115; *CL* 40 (10)(1907), 932; Dudley, *The Principles and Practice of Gynecology*, 168; *CL* 43 (9)(1910), 657; Bell, *The Principles of Gynaecology*, 217; *CL* 45 (10)(1912), 781; *PHJ* 14 (6)(1923), 245; *CMAJ* 14 (9)(1924), 797; *CMAJ* 14 (2)(1924), 139; J.G. Fitzgerald, *An Introduction to the Practice of Preventive Medicine* (St. Louis: C.V. Mosby, 1926), 256; *CMAJ* 17 (12)(1927), 1473; Graves, *Gynecology*, 658; *CH* 37 (6)(1930), 257; Crossen and Crossen, *Diseases of Women*, 252; *MMR* 14 (7)(1934), 8; Davis, *Gynecology and Obstetrics*, vol. III, chap. 9, p. 32; Adair, *Obstetrics and Gynecology*, vol. I, 508-12; Ryberg, *Health, Sex and Birth Control*, 181; Scott and Van Wyck, *The Essentials of Obstetrics*, 340.

186. Dudley, *The Principles and Practice of Gynecology*, 168.

187. *CL* 40 (1)(1906), 8-9; *CL* 39 (12)(1906), 1078-79; Curtis and Huffman, *A Textbook of Gynecology*, 562.

188. *CL* 32 (6)(1900), 304; Jewett, *The Practice of Obstetrics*, 342; *MMJ* 32 (3)(1903), 101-102; *CL* 40 (1)(1906), 8; Gilliam, *A Text-Book of Practical Gynecology*, 81; *CMAJ* 11 (9)(1921), 616; *CMAJ* 12 (3)(1922), 163; *American Journal of Obstetrics and*

Gynecology (1922), 42; *CLNH* 60 (2)(1923), 73; *PHJ* 14 (6)(1923), 245; *PHJ* 15 (10)(1924), 452; *CMAJ* 17 (12)(1927), 1473; *CH* 37 (6)(1930), 257; *CMAJ* 24 (3)(1931), 391; *CMAJ* 42 (5)(1940), 477.

189. *CL* 32 (6)(1900), 304; *CPHJ* 14 (6)(1923), 245.

190. *CMAJ* 38 (5)(1938), 448; *CMAJ* 41 (4)(1939), 357.

191. *CL* 34 (1)(1900), 21.

192. *WCMJ* 1 (7)(1907), 302.

193. *CL* 40 (1)(1906), 7; *CPMR* 33 (12)(1908), 758-59; Dudley, *The Principles and Practice of Gynecology*, 768; Bell, *The Principles of Gynecology*, 217; *English Herbal Dispensary*, 13; *CL* 45 (10)(1912), 781; Hirst, *A Text-Book of Obstetrics*, 91; *CL* 48 (2)(1914), 79; Bourne, *Synopsis of Midwifery*, 415; *PHJ* 18 (2)(1927), 95-96; Kelly et al., *Gynecology*, 160; Graves, *Gynecology*, 677; Crossen and Crossen, *Diseases of Women*, 879; *CMAJ* 23 (1)(1930), 20; *CMAJ* 24 (5)(1931), 660; *CMAJ* 30 (4)(1934), 402; *CMAJ* 31 (5)(1934), 526; *CJMS* 79 (1)(1936), 17; *CMAJ* 37 (3)(1937), 234; *CMAJ* 40 (2)(1939), 118; Adair, *Obstetrics and Gynecology*, vol. I, 523-24; *CMAJ* 49 (3)(1943), 168; Novak, *Textbook of Gynecology*, 611; *MMR* 26 (1)(1946), 14; *MMC* 3 (6)(1948), 44; *MMR* 39 (3)(1949), 122; Curtis and Huffman, *Textbook of Gynecology*, 222; *CMAJ* 62 (1)(1950), 51.

194. Kerr et al., *Combined Textbook of Obstetrics*, 735.

195. Garrett, *Textbook of Medical and Surgical Gynaecology*, 128; Galabin, *The Student's Guide*, 412-13; *CL* 34 (1)(1900), 20; Bland-Sutton and Giles, *The Diseases of Women*, 69; *CL* 40 (1)(1906), 7; Dudley, *The Principles and Practice of Gynecology*, 766; *English Herbal Dispensary*, 13; Montgomery, *Practical Gynecology*, 23; *CMAJ* 5 (8)(1915), 668; *PHJ* 18 (2)(1927), 95-96; Kelly et al., *Gynecology*, 160; Graves, *Gynecology*, 655; *CMAJ* 30 (4)(1934), 400; *CMAJ* 44 (1)(1941), 69; Ryberg, *Health, Sex and Birth Control*, 181; *CMAJ* 49 (3)(1943), 167.

196. Reed, *A Text-Book of Gynecology*, 289; *DMM* 20 (2)(1903), 82; *MMJ* 32 (3)(1903), 101-102; Allbutt et al., *A System of Gynaecology*, 114; *CPMR* 33 (12)(1908), 758; *CL* 45 (10)(1912), 781; Hirst, *A Text-Book of Obstetrics*, 90; *CL* 48 (2)(1914), 79; Eden and Lockyer, *The New System of Gynaecology*, vol. II, 615; *DMM* 48 (3)(1917), 63; *CMAJ* 14 (9)(1924), 797; Kelly et al., *Gynecology*, 160; Crossen and Crossen, *Diseases of Women*, 870-72; *CMAJ* 23 (6)(1930), 763; *CMAJ* 25 (5)(1931), 584; *CMAJ* 30 (4)(1934), 400; *CMAJ* 37 (3)(1937), 236; *CMAJ* 41 (2)(1939), 117; Adair, *Obstetrics and Gynecology*, vol. I, 508-12; *CMAJ* 48 (6)(1943), 515-16; Novak, *Textbook of Gynecology*, 610; Scott and Van Wyck, *The Essentials of Obstetrics and Gynecology*, 339.

197. A reading of the twentieth-century literature could lead to the conclusion that any health problem had the potential to lead to sterility. Certainly from the late nineteenth century onward there was a recognition that abdominal growths, especially fibromyomata, interfered with conception and with the ability to carry a child to term. A strange note on this theme was sounded in 1950 in the *Manitoba Medical Review*. In an article on "Psychosomatic Considerations in Gynaecology" the author reported that "Kehrer, a German gynaecologist ... states that fibroma and sterility are co-ordinate sequelae of the same fundamental conditions; chronically disturbed psychosexuality, with resulting chronic disturbances in abdominal blood and lymph distribution. He finds that women leading satisfactory sexual lives

remain free from fibromata, whereas every patient with a fibroma has a history of chronic psychosexual disturbances." As was the case with lifestyle factors, the patient was held responsible for her infertility. *CP* 12 (10)(1887), 310; *CL* 34 (1)(1900), 20; *CJMS* 10 (3)(1901), 182; *MMJ* 32 (3)(1903), 101-102; *CPMR* 33 (12)(1908), 758-59; *CL* 50 (6)(1917), 265; Kelly et al., *Gynecology*, 160; Graves, *Gynecology*, 677; *CMAJ* 26 (6)(1932), 749; *CMAJ* 30 (4)(1934), 400; *CJMS* 75 (2)(1934), 41; Adair, *Obstetrics and Gynecology*, vol. I, 508-12; *CMAJ* 53 (4)(1945), 366; *MMR* 30 (5)(1950), 290.

198. *CPMR* 27 (11)(1902), 662.

199. Allbutt et al., *A System of Gynecology*, 94; *English Herbal Dispensary*, 13; Kelly et al., *Gynecology*, 160; Eden and Lockyer, *Gynecology for Students*, 129.

200. Galabin, *The Student's Guide*, 412-13; Garrett, *Textbook of Medical and Surgical Gynecology*, 128; *CL* 34 (1)(1900), 20; Eden and Lockyer, *The New System of Gynaecology*, vol. I, 405; Crossen and Crossen, *Diseases of Women*, 879; Davis, *Gynecology and Obstetrics*, vol. III, chap. 9, p. 27; *CMAJ* 40 (2)(1939), 118; *CMAJ* 40 (6)(1939), 542; Adair, *Obstetrics and Gynecology*, vol. I, 528; Novak, *Textbook of Gynecology*, 600.

201. Graves, *Gynecology*, 685; *CJMS* 78 (4)(1935), 106; *CMAJ* 40 (1)(1939), 36; *CMAJ* 56 (3)(1947), 345; *MMC* 2 (8)(1947), 31; *MMR* 30 (2)(1950), 74-75; Curtis and Huffman, *A Textbook of Gynecology*, 562.

202. *CMAJ* 56 (3)(1947), 345; *MMC* 2 (8)(1947), 31; Novak, *Textbook of Gynecology*, 610.

203. *CMAJ* 5 (8)(1915), 667; *CMAJ* 30 (4)(1934), 400; *CMAJ* 40 (2)(1939), 117.

204. *CMAJ* 14 (9)(1924), 797; Kelly et al., *Gynecology*, 158-59; Graves, *Gynecology*, 679; Crossen and Crossen, *Diseases of Women*, 894; *CMAJ* 24 (5)(1931), 660; *CMAJ* 40 (1)(1939), 41; Adair, *Obstetrics and Gynecology*, vol. I, 508-12; *CMAJ* 49 (3)(1943), 167; *CMAJ* 49 (3)(1943), 170; Novak, *Textbook of Gynecology*, 593; *AMB* 13 (1)(1948), 67; *MMR* 29 (3)(1949), 122.

205. Eden and Lockyer, *The New System of Gynaecology*, vol. I, 413.

206. *CMAJ* 40 (2)(1939), 116.

207. *CL* 37 (10)(1904), 922; Gilliam, *A Text-Book of Practical Gynecology*, 81; Dudley, *The Principles and Practice of Gynecology*, 764; Bell, *The Principles of Gynecology*, 217; Eden and Lockyer, *Gynaecology for Students*, 128; Crossen and Crossen, *Diseases of Women*, 870; Davis, *Gynecology and Obstetrics*, vol. III, chap. 9, p. 13; Adair, *Obstetrics and Gynecology*, vol. I, 523-24; *MMR* 29 (3)(1949), 122; Eden and Lockyer, *The New System of Gynaecology*, vol. I, 413; Kerr et al., *Combined Textbook of Obstetrics*, 729.

208. Bonnicksen, *In Vitro Fertilization*, 12; *CMAJ* 40 (2)(1939), 116; McLaren, *A History of Contraception*, 261.

209. Napheys, *The Physical Life of Woman*, 90.

210. *Jayne's Medical Almanac* (Philadelphia: 1863), 17; R.V. Pierce, *Dr. Pierce's Neighborhood Gossip and Dream Book* (Bridgeburg: [1920?]), 31; *CPMR* 29 (3)(1904), 141.

211. *CPMR* 29 (3)(1904), 141; Hirst, *A Text-Book of Obstetrics*, 92; *PHJ* 18 (2)(1927), 95-96; Crossen and Crossen, *Diseases of Women*, 878; *CMAJ* 34 (3)(1936), 353;

CMAJ 34 (2)(1936), 140; *CMAJ* 43 (1)(1940), 93; Adair, *Obstetrics and Gynecology*, vol. I, 517; *CMAJ* 47 (1)(1942), 18; *CMAJ* 48 (3)(1943), 231; *AMB* 14 (2)(1949), 28; *CMAJ* 63 (4)(1950), 345.

212. *CPMR* 29 (3)(1904), 141. The limited existing documentation on infertility means that information about the men and women coming to physicians for problems of infertility remains unknown. Most likely, they were middle class, because the cost of consulting a physician would have been prohibitive for many working-class Canadians in a pre-medicare period. There is little doubt that physicians were more concerned about the fertility of the white middle class than that of the working class and visible minorities. In the late nineteenth and early twentieth centuries, many doctors and other Canadians feared what they termed racial suicide if working-class Canadians and new immigrants continued to maintain a high birth rate and the "respectable" classes did not. In the inter-war years, this fear supported the rise of the eugenics movement in Canada. See McLaren, *Our Own Master Race*.

213. H.T. Byford, *Manual of Gynecology* (Philadelphia: P. Blakiston and Son, 1895), 130; *CL* 34 (1)(1900), 23; *DMM* 20 (2)(1903), 82; *CL* 45 (3)(1911), 211; *CMAJ* 11 (11)(1921), 831; *CMAJ* 14 (2)(1924), 139; Kelly et al., *Gynecology*, 103; Eden and Lockyer, *Gynaecology for Students*, 131; Davis, *Gynecology and Obstetrics*, vol. III, chap. 9, p. 28; Sir Comyns Berkeley and V. Bonney, *A Textbook of Gynecological Surgery* (London: Cassell, 1942), 76.

214. Curtis and Huffman, *A Textbook of Gynecology*, 563.

215. Byford, *Manual of Gynecology*, 130; Hirst, *A Text-Book of Obstetrics*, 90; Kelly et al., *Gynecology*, 103; Davis, *Gynecology and Obstetrics*, vol. III, chap. 9, p. 28.

216. *CMAJ* 24 (5)(1931), 660; *CMAJ* 37 (3)(1937), 234; *CMAJ* 40 (6)(1939), 542; Adair, *Obstetrics and Gynecology*, vol. II, 673; Novak, *Textbook of Gynecology*, 600.

217. *PHJ* 18 (2)(1927), 95-96; *CMAJ* 23 (1)(1930), 20; Kerr et al., *Combined Textbook of Obstetrics*, 738.

218. Bourne, *Synopsis of Midwifery*, 415; Crossen and Crossen, *Diseases of Women*, 879; Adair, *Obstetrics and Gynecology*, vol. I, 527; Scott and Van Wyck, *The Essentials of Obstetrics and Gynecology*, 340.

219. *MMC* 3 (6)(1948), 44.

220. *AMB* 13 (1)(1948), 64; *MMC* 4 (10)(1949), 49; Novak, *Textbook of Gynecology*, 604-608.

221. *CL* 33 (12)(1900), 687.

222. See Mitchinson, *The Nature of Their Bodies*, 252-77, for a description of the rise of gynaecological surgery.

223. A. McLaren, "'The Creation of a Haven for Human Thoroughbreds': The Sterilization of the Feeble-Minded and the Mentally Ill in British Columbia," *Canadian Historical Review* 67 (June 1986): 127-50. Both British Columbia and Alberta had sterilization legislation. No research has emerged yet on native women. In the 1970s, however, Dr. Clarence Ekstrand noted a "surgery rate five times *higher* [on native peoples] than the general population, particularly for women and particularly for tubal ligations." R.F. Morgan, ed., *The Iatrogenics Handbook: A*

Critical Look at Research and Practice in the Helping Professions (Toronto: IPI Publishing, 1983), v-vi.

224. *CL* 34 (1)(1900), 23; *CL* 34 (9)(1901), 460-61; *CL* 37 (10)(1904), 922; *WCMJ* 1 (7)(1907), 302; *CPMR* 33 (12)(1908), 759; *DMM* 35 (2)(1910), 48; *PHJ* 18 (2)(1927), 95-96; *CMAJ* 30 (4)(1934), 401; Curtis and Huffman, *A Textbook of Gynecology*, 222.

225. *DMM* 33 (3)(1909), 92.

226. *DMM* 35 (2)(1910), 48; *CMAJ* 14 (2)(1924), 139; Kelly et al., *Gynecology*, 169.

227. *CMAJ* 14 (9)(1924), 798.

228. Graves, *Gynecology*, 680.

229. Curtis and Huffman, *A Textbook of Gynecology*, 222.

230. *DMM* 20 (2)(1903), 82; *CL* 45 (10)(1912), 731; Hirst, *A Text-Book of Obstetrics*, 90; *DMM* 48 (3)(1917), 63; Graves, *Gynecology*, 678; *CMAJ* 23 (1)(1930), 20; Davis, *Gynecology and Obstetrics*, vol. III, chap. 9, p. 28; *CMAJ* (1937), 236; Novak, *Textbook of Gynecology*, 610.

231. *CL* 3 (2)(1870), 46-47.

232. Webster, *A Text-Book of Diseases*, 700; Dudley, *The Principles and Practice of Gynecology*, 770.

233. Eden and Lockyer, *Gynecology for Students*, 131; Graves, *Gynecology*, 683-84; Crossen and Crossen, *Diseases of Women*, 880; Ten Teachers, *Diseases of Women*, 127; Davis, *Gynecology and Obstetrics*, vol. III, chap. 9, p. 27.

234. Tyrer, *Sex, Marriage and Birth Control*, 238-39.

235. Curtis and Huffman, *A Textbook of Gynecology*, 573; Adair, *Obstetrics and Gynecology*, vol. I, 528; Novak, *Textbook of Gynecology*, 613.

236. Around 1930, instances of ovarian grafting are mentioned in the literature — that is, the "surgical disposition of active ovarian tissue from one woman to another." These reports referred as well to a theoretical future when complete ovarian transplants could occur, with all the legal complications this would entail. Little reference was made to these procedures after that date, however. *CMAJ* 23 (1)(1930), 20; Graves, *Gynecology*, 683. The earliest mention of experiments "upon the lower animals, as well as upon human beings" was made in 1912 (Hirst, *A Text-Book of Obstetrics*, 92).

237. *CMAJ* 5 (8)(1915), 668; *CMAJ* 11 (11)(1921), 831.

238. *CMAJ* 23 (1)(1930), 21; *CMAJ* 34 (3)(1936), 297; *CMAJ* 37 (3)(1937), 236; Novak, *Textbook of Gynecology*, 612; S.E. Bell, "Changing Ideas: The Medicalization of Menopause," *Social Science and Medicine* 24 (1987), 537; *CMAJ* 63 (4)(1950), 346.

239. Graves, *Gynecology*, 679; Crossen and Crossen, *Diseases of Women*, vii; *CMAJ* 41 (1)(1939), 99; *CMAJ* 40 (1)(1939), 91; *CMAJ* 40 (6)(1939), 542; *CMAJ* 42 (6)(1940), 583; *CMAJ* 47 (1)(1942), 13, 23; *CMAJ* 49 (3)(1943), 167; *CMAJ* 48 (3)(1943), 231; Novak, *Textbook of Gynecology*, 609; *CMAJ* 55 (5)(1946), lxxxiii; Scott and Van Wyck, *The Essentials of Obstetrics and Gynecology*, 339; *MMC* 2 (2)(1947), 6; *AMB* 13 (1)(1948), 67; *MMC* 4 (10)(1949), 50.

240. *MMR* 29 (3)(1949), 124.

241. *CMAJ* 42 (6)(1940), 583, 585; Novak, *Textbook of Gynecology*, 559; *AMB* 13 (1)(1948), 67; *AMB* 14 (2)(1949), 27.

242. *CMAJ* 57 (4)(1947), 354.

243. Kelly et al., *Gynecology*, 161; Ten Teachers, *Diseases of Women*, 125.

244. Davis, *Gynecology and Obstetrics*, vol. III, chap. 9, p. 28.

245. *MMR* 29 (3)(1949), 125.

246. Novak, *Textbook of Gynecology*, 589-90.

247. *CPMR* 27 (8)(1902), 477; *CMAJ* 23 (4)(1930), 505; Kelly et al., *Gynecology*, 161.

248. B. Ehrenreich and D. English, *Complaints and Disorders: The Sexual Politics of Sickness* (Old Westbury: Feminist Press, 1973), 5.

Bibliography

Primary Sources

Medical Journals
Alberta Medical Bulletin (1935-50)
British American Journal of Medical & Physical Science (1845-50)
Canada Health Journal (1870)
The Canada Lancet (1870-1921)
Canada Lancet and National Hygiene (1922-24)
The Canada Lancet and Practitioner (1925-34)
Canada Medical and Surgical Journal (1872-88)
The Canada Medical Journal and Monthly Record of Medical and Surgical Science (1864-72)
The Canada Medical Record (1872-1904)
Canadian Health (1930-33)
Canadian Journal of Medicine and Surgery (1897-1936)
Canadian Medical Association Journal (1911-50)
The Canadian Medical Times (1873)
Canadian Practitioner (1888-98; 1922-24)
Canadian Practitioner and Medical Review (1899-1921)
Canadian Public Health Journal (1929-42)
Dominion Medical Monthly (1893-95)
Dominion Medical Monthly and Ontario Medical Journal (1898-1921)
Manitoba Medical Review (1934-50)
Modern Medicine of Canada (1946-50)
The Montreal Medical Journal (1888-1910)
The Public Health Journal (1910-28)
The Sanitary Journal (1874-83)
The Western Canada Medical Journal (1907-15)

Non-Medical Journals
Canadian Child Welfare News (1922-26)
Canadian Home Journal (1938-46)

Canadian Magazine (1900-46)
Maclean's (1905-20; 1938-46)
Saturday Night (1900-50)
Woman's Century (1915-21)

Books

Adair, F.L., ed. *Obstetrics and Gynecology*. Philadelphia: Lea & Febiger, 1940.

Allbutt, T.C., W.S. Playfair, and T.W. Eden, eds. *A System of Gynaecology*. London: MacMillan, 1906.

Ayers, H. *Ayers' Everyman His Own Doctor: Family Medical Advisor*. Montreal: 1884.

Beck, A.C. *Obstetrical Practice*. Baltimore: Williams & Wilkins, 1947.

Becklard, E. *Physiological Mysteries and Revelations in Love, Courtship and Marriage*. New York: 1842.

Bell, B.W. *The Principles of Gynaecology*. London: Longmans, Green, 1910.

Berkeley, Sir Comyns, and V. Bonney. *A Textbook of Gynaecological Surgery*. London: Cassell, 1942.

Bland-Sutton, J., and A.E. Giles. *The Diseases of Women: A Handbook for Students and Practitioners*. London: Rebman, 1906.

Bourne, A.W. *Synopsis of Midwifery and Gynaecology*. 3d ed. rev. Toronto: Macmillan of Canada, 1925.

Buchanan, J. *The Eclectic Practice of Medicine*. Philadelphia: 1867.

Byford, H.T. *Manual of Gynecology*. Philadelphia: P. Blakiston and Son, 1895.

Carpenter, W.B. *Principles of Human Physiology*. 7th ed. London: John Churchill and Son, 1869.

Cazeaux, P.A. *Theoretical and Practical Treatise on Midwifery*. Philadelphia: Lindsay and Blakiston, 1837.

Chavasse, P.H. *Advice to a Wife on the Management of Her Own Health and on the Treatment of Some of the Complaints Incidental to Pregnancy, Labour, and Suckling*. Toronto: Willing and Williamson, 1882.

Crossen, H.S., and R.J. Crossen. *Diseases of Women*. St. Louis: C.V. Mosby, 1930.

Curtis, A.H., and J.W. Huffman. *A Textbook of Gynecology*. 6th ed. Philadelphia: W.B. Saunders, 1950.

Davis, C.H., ed. *Gynecology and Obstetrics*. Hagerstown: W.F. Prior, 1935.

Dudley, E.C. *The Principles and Practice of Gynecology for Students and Practitioners*. Philadelphia: Lea & Febiger, 1908.

Dunbar, H.F. *Emotions and Bodily Changes*. 3d ed. New York: Columbia University Press, 1947.

Eden, T.W., and C. Lockyer, eds. *Gynaecology for Students and Practitioners*. London: J. & A. Churchill, 1928.

—. *The New System of Gynaecology*. Toronto: Macmillan, 1917.

Edgar, J.C. *The Practice of Obstetrics: Designed for the Use of Students and Practitioners of Medicine*. Philadelphia: P. Blakiston's Son, 1907.

Edis, A. *Diseases of Women: A Manual for Students and Practitioners.* Philadelphia: Henry C. Lea's Son, 1882.

English Herbal Dispensary (1910).

Fitzgerald, J.G. *An Introduction to the Practice of Preventive Medicine.* St. Louis: C.V. Mosby, 1926.

Flint, A. *The Physiology of Man.* New York: 1874.

Galabin, A.L. *Diseases of Women.* London: J.A. Churchill, 1893.

—. *A Manual of Midwifery.* Philadelphia: P. Blakiston and Son, 1886.

—. *The Student's Guide to the Diseases of Women.* London: 1884.

Garrett, R.W. *Textbook of Medical and Surgical Gynaecology.* Toronto: J.A. Carveth, 1897.

Garrigues, H.J. *A Text-Book of the Diseases of Women.* Philadelphia: W.B. Saunders, 1894.

Gilliam, G.T. *A Text-Book of Practical Gynecology.* Philadelphia: F.A. Davis, 1907.

Goodell, W. *Lessons in Gynecology.* Philadelphia: F.A. Davis, 1890.

Graves, W.P. *Gynecology.* Philadelphia: W.B. Saunders, 1928.

Hall, W.S. *Sexual Knowledge.* Toronto: McClelland and Stewart, 1921.

Hirst, B.C. *A Text-Book of Obstetrics.* Philadelphia: W.B. Saunders, 1898.

Jayne's Medical Almanac. Philadelphia: 1863.

Jefferis, B.G. *Search Lights on Health: Light on Dark Corners.* Toronto: J.L. Nichols, 1894.

Jewett, C., ed. *The Practice of Obstetrics.* New York: Lea Brothers, 1901.

Kelly, H.A., et al. *Gynecology.* New York: D. Appleton, 1928.

Kerr, J.M., et al. *Combined Textbook of Obstetrics and Gynaecology for Students and Medical Practitioners.* Edinburgh: E. & S. Livingstone, 1933.

Lyman, H., et al. *The Practical Home Physician and Encyclopedia of Medicine.* Guelph: World, 1884.

Montgomery, E.E. *Practical Gynecology.* Philadelphia: P. Blakiston and Son, 1912.

Morton, H.H. *Genito-Urinary Diseases and Syphilis.* 2d ed. Philadelphia: F.A. Davis, 1908.

Mundé, P. *A Practical Treatise on the Diseases of Women.* Philadelphia: 1891.

Napheys, G.H. *The Physical Life of Woman: Advice to the Maiden, Wife, and Mother.* Toronto: Rose Publishing, 1890.

Novak, E. *Textbook of Gynecology.* Baltimore: Williams & Wilkins, 1944.

Penrose, C.B. *A Text-Book of Diseases of Women.* 5th ed. rev. Philadelphia: W.B. Saunders, 1905.

Pierce, R.V. *Dr. Pierce's Neighborhood Gossip and Dream Book.* Bridgeburg: [1920?].

—. *The People's Common Sense Medical Adviser in Plain English.* Buffalo: 1882.

Reed, C.A.L., ed. *A Text-Book of Gynecology.* New York: D. Appleton, 1901.

Ryberg, P.E. *Health, Sex and Birth Control*. Toronto: Anchor Press, 1943.

Scott, W.A., and H.B. Van Wyck. *The Essentials of Obstetrics and Gynecology*. Philadelphia: Lea & Febiger, 1946.

Smith, W.T. *Parturition and the Principles and Practice of Obstetrics*. Philadelphia: Lea and Blanchard, 1849.

Stockham, A. *Tokology: A Book for Every Woman*. Toronto: McClelland, Goodchild and Stewart, 1916.

Ten Teachers. *Diseases of Women*, ed. C. Berkeley et al. London: Edward Arnold, 1935.

Thomas, T.G. *A Practical Treatise on the Diseases of Women*. Philadelphia: Henry C. Lea, 1868.

Tyrer, A.H. *Sex, Marriage and Birth Control*. 10th ed. Toronto: Marriage Welfare Bureau, 1943.

Walker, J.W.T. *Surgical Diseases and Injuries of the Genito-Urinary Organs*. London: Cassell, 1914.

Webster, J.C. *A Text-Book of Diseases of Women*. Philadelphia: W.B. Saunders, 1907.

Secondary Sources

Abeele, C. Comacchio. "Nations Are Built of Babies: Maternal and Child Welfare in Ontario, 1914-1940." Ph.D. dissertation, University of Guelph, 1987.

Achilles, R. "Desperately Seeking Babies: New Technologies of Hope and Despair." In *Delivering Motherhood: Maternal Ideologies and Practices in the 19th and 20th Centuries*, ed. K. Arnup, A. Lévesque, and R.R. Pierson. London: Routledge, 1990.

Bart, P. "Social Structure and Vocabularies of Discomfort." In *Life as Theatre*, ed. D. Brissett and C. Edgley. Chicago: Aldine, 1975.

Bell, S.E. "Changing Ideas: The Medicalization of Menopause." *Social Science and Medicine* 24 (1987): 535-42.

Berger, C. *Science, God and Nature in Victorian Canada*. Toronto: University of Toronto Press, 1983.

Bernard, J. *The Future of Motherhood*. New York: Penguin, 1975.

Bonnicksen, A.L. *In Vitro Fertilization: Building Policy from Laboratories to Legislatures*. New York: Columbia University Press, 1989.

Cook, R. *The Regenerators: Social Criticism in Late Victorian English Canada*. Toronto: University of Toronto Press, 1985.

Dally, A. *Inventing Motherhood: The Consequences of an Ideal*. New York: Schocken Books, 1983.

Devitt, H. "The Statistical Case for Elimination of the Midwife: Fact Versus Prejudice, 1890-1935." [Part 1] *Women and Health* 4 (1)(1979): 81-96.

Ehrenreich, B., and D. English. *Complaints and Disorders: The Sexual Politics of Sickness*. Old Westbury: Feminist Press, 1973.

Francis, R.D., R. Jones, and D.B. Smith. *Destinies: Canadian History Since Confederation.* 2d ed. Toronto: Holt, Rinehart and Winston of Canada, 1992.

Frisch, R.E. "Nutrition, Fatness and Fertility: The Effect of Food Intake on Reproductive Ability." In *Nutrition and Human Reproduction,* ed. W.H. Mosley. New York: Plenum Press, 1978.

Gee, E. "The Life Course of Canadian Women: An Historical and Demographic Analysis." *Social Indicators Research* 18 (1986): 263-83.

Goldman, M. *Gold Diggers and Silver Miners.* Ann Arbor: University of Michigan Press, 1981.

Hamowy, R. *Canadian Medicine: A Study in Restricted Entry.* Vancouver: Fraser Institute, 1984.

Kenneally, R. "The Montreal Maternity, 1843-1926: Evolution of a Hospital." M.A. thesis, McGill University, 1983.

Laqueur, T. *Making Sex: Body and Gender from the Greeks to Freud.* Cambridge: Harvard University Press, 1990.

Leonardo, R.A. *History of Gynecology.* New York: Froben Press, 1944.

McKeown, T. *Medicine in Modern Society: Medical Planning Based on Evaluation of Medical Achievement.* New York: Hafner Publishing, 1966.

McLaren, A. "'The Creation of a Haven for Human Thoroughbreds': Sterilization of the Feeble-Minded and the Mentally Ill in British Columbia." *Canadian Historical Review* 67 (June 1986): 127-50.

—. *A History of Contraception: From Antiquity to the Present Day.* Oxford: Basil Blackwell, 1990.

—. *Our Own Master Race: Eugenics in Canada, 1885-1945.* Toronto: McClelland and Stewart, 1990.

McLaren, A., and A.T. McLaren. *The Bedroom and the State: The Changing Practices and Politics of Contraception and Abortion in Canada, 1880-1980.* Toronto: McClelland and Stewart, 1986.

Mitchinson, W. *The Nature of Their Bodies: Women and Their Doctors in Victorian Canada.* Toronto: University of Toronto Press, 1991.

Morgan, R.F., ed. *The Iatrogenics Handbook: A Critical Look at Research and Practice in the Helping Professions.* Toronto: IPI Publishing, 1983.

Naylor, C.D. *Private Practice, Public Payment: Canadian Medicine and the Politics of Health Insurance, 1911-1966.* Montreal: McGill-Queen's University Press, 1986.

Oakley, A. *Women Confined: Towards a Sociology of Childbirth.* New York: Schocken Books, 1980.

Oxorn, H. *Harold Benge Atlee M.D.: A Biography.* Hantsport: Lancelot Press, 1983.

Prentice, A., et al. *Canadian Women: A History.* Toronto: Harcourt, Brace, Jovanovich, 1988.

Sandelowski, M. "Failures of Volition: Female Agency and Infertility in Historical Perspective." *Signs* 15 (1990): 475-99.

—. *Women, Health, and Choice*. Englewood Cliffs: Prentice-Hall, 1981.

Stewart, P. "Infant Feeding in Canada, 1910-1940." M.A. thesis, Concordia University, 1982.

Susser, M. "Ethical Components in the Definition of Health." *International Journal of Health Services* 4 (1974): 539-48.

Tannahill, R. *Sex in History*. London: Abacus, 1981.

Tolnay, S.E., and A.M. Guest. "Childlessness in a Transitional Population: The United States at the Turn of the Century." *Journal of Family History* 7 (1982): 200-19.

Valverde, M. *The Age of Light, Soap and Water: Moral Reform in English Canada, 1885-1925*. Toronto: McClelland and Stewart, 1991.

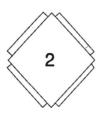

The Prevalence of Infertility in Canada, 1991-1992: Analysis of Three National Surveys

Corinne S. Dulberg and Thomas Stephens

Executive Summary

Three independent national telephone surveys were conducted in late 1991 and early 1992 on behalf of the Royal Commission on New Reproductive Technologies (RCNRT) by the Canada Health Monitor (CHM) and Decima. The primary objective was to obtain the data necessary to calculate one- and two-year infertility prevalences among Canadian women, aged 18-44, married or cohabiting for at least one year or two years.

A woman was defined as infertile if she and her husband/partner did not use any contraceptive method (non-surgical or surgical) but she was not pregnant during the specified time period of one or two years prior to the interview.

The prevalence estimates from the three surveys were highly consistent. The national estimates of the prevalence of infertility (with confidence intervals [CI] and sample sizes) among Canadian women aged 18-44, married or cohabiting for at least one year, were as follows:

This paper was completed for the Royal Commission on New Reproductive Technologies in July 1992.

CHM-6:   7.7% (95% CI: 4.4% - 11.0%) (n = 281)
CHM-7:   8.6% (95% CI: 5.8% - 11.4%) (n = 407)
Decima: 8.7% (95% CI: 6.6% - 10.8%) (n = 725)

The three national estimates of two-year prevalence of infertility were naturally somewhat lower than the one-year prevalence estimates, and were also consistent with each other:

CHM-6:   6.0% (95% CI: 3.0% - 9.0%) (n = 271)
CHM-7:   7.2% (95% CI: 4.5% - 9.9%) (n = 384)
Decima: 7.3% (95% CI: 5.4% - 9.2%) (n = 695)

The prevalence of one- and two-year infertility among women in Canada, 18-44 years of age, married or cohabiting for at least one or two years, from data combined across surveys, was as follows:

One-year infertility: 8.5% (95% CI: 7.0% - 9.9%) (n = 1 413)
Two-year infertility: 7.0% (95% CI: 5.6% - 8.4%) (n = 1 350)

When estimates of prevalence were recalculated to correspond exactly to the definition of infertility used in the U.S. National Survey of Family Growth (NSFG), the findings were very comparable. For one-year infertility, the prevalence estimates were as follows:

Canada
  1991-92: 8.0% (age 18-44, married/cohabiting, n = 1 488)
USA
  1988:   7.9% (age 15-44, married, n = 8 450)

The secondary objective of this project was to examine variation in prevalence of infertility as a function of demographic characteristics.

Both one- and two-year infertility prevalences were significantly associated with parity, dichotomized as no prior births versus any number of prior births. The odds of infertility among women who had never given birth were over five times the odds of infertility among those who had given birth previously. Specifically, the Mantel-Haenszel odds ratios (OR_{MH}) for infertility among nulliparous compared to multiparous women, adjusted for both age and survey, were as follows:

One-year infertility: OR_{MH} = 5.2 (95% CI: 3.5 < OR_{MH} < 8.4)
Two-year infertility: OR_{MH} = 6.3 (95% CI: 4.0 < OR_{MH} < 10.6)

While, overall, one- and two-year infertility prevalences were not significantly associated with age (18-29 versus 30-44), a significant age effect was observed when parity was statistically controlled. Adjusting for both parity and survey, the odds of infertility among women 30-44 years old were about twice the odds among women 18-29 years of age. The Mantel-Haenszel adjusted odds ratios were as follows:

One-year infertility: OR_{MH} = 1.8 (95% CI: 1.1 < OR_{MH} < 3.1)
Two-year infertility: OR_{MH} = 2.5 (95% CI: 1.4 < OR_{MH} < 5.1)

In the RCNRT surveys, one- and two-year infertility prevalences were not significantly associated with region of residence.

Introduction

Objectives

The primary objective of this project was to collect and analyze survey data to obtain national estimates of the prevalence of infertility in Canada.

The reference time periods for infertility were one year and two years, and the reference population was women between the ages of 18 and 44 years who had been married or cohabiting for at least one year (or two years) prior to the surveys, which took place in late 1991 and early 1992.

The secondary objective was to determine whether the prevalence of infertility varied as a function of age, previous childbearing, or geographic region of residence.

Background

The most comprehensive analysis of the national prevalence of infertility is the U.S. National Survey of Family Growth (NSFG), conducted in 1965, 1976, 1982 (Mosher and Pratt 1987), and 1988 (Mosher and Pratt 1990). Because of the thoroughness of the U.S. approach and the desirability of comparing Canadian and U.S. prevalence figures, the NSFG was adopted as a model for the current project. However, the U.S. approach was not completely appropriate, in its original form, for the current project. The adaptations that were necessary are described below.

In the NSFG, infertility was considered a "medical concept, used for diagnosis." Infertility was defined as the inability "to conceive after a year or more of unprotected intercourse" (Mosher and Pratt 1987, 13).

In order to define respondents as infertile for operational purposes, the first and second NSFG surveys focussed on married women and divided them into one of three categories of infertility status, as follows:

Infertile: "Couples who were not surgically sterile were classified as infertile if they (a) had been continuously married, (b) had not used contraception, and (c) had not become pregnant, for a year or more immediately preceding the interview" (Mosher and Pratt 1987, 45).

Fecund: This category consisted of "those not classified as sterile or infertile and is therefore a residual group" (Mosher and Pratt 1987, 45). This group included women who were pregnant during the year prior to the interview, couples using any form of birth control other than voluntary sterilization, women whose date of marriage was unknown, and any woman who could not be identified as falling into the other two categories of infertility status.

Surgically Sterile: This category included women who had had a tubal ligation or hysterectomy and whose husbands had had a vasectomy.

These categories were used by the NSFG to compute the prevalence of infertility as follows:

infertile/[infertile + fecund + surgically sterile]

This method is referred to in this report as "the NSFG approach." It provided the *conceptual* basis for the definition adopted in this project. Operationally, however, the current project defined the *fecund* group differently, as described below.

Since one of the objectives of the NSFG series was to compare changes in the prevalence of infertility over time, a modified approach was also used in the United States in 1982. Faced with the large increases from 1965 to 1982 in the proportion of women (or their partners) who had been surgically sterilized, infertility was also calculated excluding such cases. By thus adjusting for changing proportions in the surgically sterile, this method permitted comparisons to be made in prevalence estimates over time. Such an approach also allows for comparisons of infertility rates between national populations with very different rates of sterilization.

The prevalence of infertility using this approach (labelled here as "sterilization excluded") was computed as

infertile/[infertile + fecund]

It should be noted that while this report refers to infertile *women*, it might equally refer to infertile *couples* in which the woman is of childbearing age, since vasectomy, male contraceptive use, and male infertility were equally considered in the questions.

Methods

Questionnaire Development

Although the NSFG provided the conceptual basis for the current project, the RCNRT surveys were not precise replications of the NSFG. Because the primary focus of the NSFG was *fertility*, much of that questionnaire was not directly relevant to the key issue in the present project — assessing *infertility*. Therefore, RCNRT survey question design and data analysis were based on the subset of questions in the NSFG required to classify a couple's infertility status.

Since the results from the RCNRT surveys were also to be related to those from the Ontario Health Survey (OHS), the subset of NSFG questions relevant to infertility was edited and organized to follow closely the OHS questions. When questions from the NSFG and the OHS covered the same information, the wording of the OHS questions was used. In addition, the sequence of the OHS questions was followed as closely as possible. The RCNRT questions are provided in Appendix 1.

The current project departed from the original NSFG design in two other significant ways: the minimum age of 15 years in the NSFG was raised to 18, and coverage was extended to unmarried cohabiting women, whereas only married women were included in the estimates of infertility in the NSFG surveys. (Consideration was given to extending coverage to all adult women in long-term relationships, regardless of living arrangements, but no satisfactory means was found to identify such women.)

Design Considerations

Conducting a survey to calculate infertility raises the serious practical problem of the need to contact a very large number of individuals in order to obtain a reasonable number of female respondents who fulfil the entry criteria of age 18-44 and married or cohabiting.

As an example of the rapidly dwindling numbers from initial contact to final sample, consider the predicted number of women aged 18-44, married or cohabiting, among approximately 2 500 people contacted by Price Waterhouse for the fall 1991 Canada Health Monitor (CHM) Survey #6:

- 2 500 males and females are contacted and agree to participate;
- 55% of 2 500 are 18-44 years old — 1 375 males and females;
- 60% of 1 375 are married or cohabiting — 825 males and females;
- 50% of 825 are female — 413 females;
- 90% agree to be called back to answer all relevant questions — 371 females.

Thus, although the survey begins with a large number of telephone contacts, data from 371 or just 15% of the approximately 2 500 persons originally contacted (or 30% of females) would be anticipated as fulfilling the entry criteria and as providing data for the analysis of infertility. In addition, with a prevalence of infertility expected to be between 5% and 10% of this group (Mosher and Pratt 1987), the actual number of infertile women in the samples available for subgroup analysis could be very small indeed.

Such considerations would normally argue for a very large initial sample, which would also mean considerable expense. In the current project, an alternative strategy was adopted. The essence of this was to conduct three small independent surveys, by piggy-backing on activities that already were in progress for the RCNRT. The results from these surveys were assessed for consistency and combined for more detailed analysis, if statistically appropriate. The goal was not only to provide replications of the estimates of infertility, but also to enable the estimates to be combined (as weighted averages) to provide more precise prevalence estimates.

In addition to lower cost, the advantage of such an approach is that the data from three independent surveys may be of higher quality than those from a single survey of the same overall size. Consistent results from independent surveys, despite differences in interviewers, timing, details of sampling procedures, and so forth, are evidence of reliability. The risk of such an approach is that results from the three surveys would be inconsistent and thus inappropriate to combine. Nevertheless, this strategy was adopted, with the insurance of knowing that the very large OHS (n = 67 000) was being used in a separate project (Balakrishnan and Maxim 1993) to analyze infertility among subgroups of women.

Data Collection

In response to the practical problem of reaching large numbers of married or cohabiting women aged 18-44, the RCNRT used three mechanisms for collecting data.

CHM-6

Price Waterhouse, the data collection agency for the CHM, was contracted to call back the relevant subsample of the approximately 2 500 individuals in the sixth CHM (CHM-6) survey conducted in the fall of 1991. Demographic information obtained in that survey was used to identify all women fulfilling the entry criteria for age and marital status. Since all the original respondents had been advised of possible re-contact, this relevant subgroup of respondents could be readily re-interviewed. This approach was deemed to be both straightforward and cost-effective. Calls were made over the period 9-14 December 1991.

CHM-7

As the CHM is an ongoing, semi-annual telephone survey of the Canadian population, it was decided to include the infertility questions in their seventh survey (CHM-7) in order to reach a second, independent sample.

Price Waterhouse was contracted to ask the questions necessary to determine infertility status of all females aged 18-44, married or cohabiting, among the approximately 2 500 people contacted for CHM-7 from 12 December 1991 through 19 February 1992. Adding questions to an existing survey was viewed as a cost-effective procedure for identifying a subgroup of relevant respondents.

Decima

After these two surveys were initiated, the opportunity arose to collect relevant data from a third national sample, in concert with a survey on "Canadian Values and Attitudes" being undertaken by Decima on behalf of the RCNRT. Because of the considerable length of time necessary to develop the values questionnaire, Decima eventually recommended that the values survey be separated from their survey on infertility. Decima drew women from their pool of over 5 000 adults whose spouse/partner had participated in prior Decima surveys. Sufficient demographic data had been collected on individuals in this subject pool so that women fulfilling entry criteria could be selected for the infertility survey. Interviews were conducted during the period 1-14 March 1992.

All three surveys provide representative samples of the Canadian population living in households. While precise details of the sampling procedures varied (see Appendix 2), the samples can be regarded as equivalent. Data collection was by telephone in all cases, in English or French, and was computer-assisted in the case of the CHM. All surveys used the same entry criteria and the same questions to assess infertility. Response rates are reported below, under "Results."

Sample Selection and Weighting

Information provided by Price Waterhouse and Decima concerning survey methodology and sample selection procedures is provided in Appendix 2. Weights were used in the Canada Health Monitor surveys to adjust for differences in response rates according to province and community size. Respondents' weights from the original Canada Health Monitor surveys were provided for each woman in the RCNRT subsamples. On the recommendation of the RCNRT's consultant survey statistician, these weights were adjusted so that the sum of the weights for each RCNRT survey equalled the RCNRT sample sizes (see Appendix 3). These "normalized" weights were used for all descriptive and inferential statistical analyses.

For the Decima survey, selection was completed with quotas to achieve a sample proportional to the Canadian population with respect to region and city size. After reviewing the description of the sampling method for the Decima survey, the consultant statistician confirmed that no weights were necessary for analyses of Decima's data.

The consultant statistician also suggested the conservative use of an "adjustment factor" to take into account a possible design effect arising from the sampling procedures used in the CHM surveys (Appendix 3). This adjustment factor, incorporated into calculations of the confidence intervals around proportions, is equal to the sum of the squared normalized weights divided by the sample size and had values of 1.13 for CHM-6 and 1.09 for CHM-7. Use of this factor was not required for the Decima survey data.

To be included in any analysis, the respondent had to be a female 18-44 years of age, married or cohabiting. For the results reported in the body of this paper, women whose age was unknown or fell outside the given range and those not married or cohabiting were therefore excluded from all analyses. Furthermore, in order to be able to delineate clearly the population to whom the infertility estimates apply, women whose date of marriage or beginning date of cohabitation was unknown or whose date indicated a duration of marriage/cohabitation less than the required periods of at least one year or at least two years were excluded from calculations of infertility.

Primary Outcome Measures

Closely following the 1982 NSFG approach (Mosher and Pratt 1987, 1990; U.S. National Center for Health Statistics 1990), respondents to each survey were classified into one of three categories of infertility status, within the previous 12 (and 24) months, as follows:

Infertile: respondents reporting no contraceptive method use (surgical or non-surgical) and no pregnancy during the 12 (and 24) months prior to the interview. Absence of contraceptive use during the prior 12 (and 24) months was verified with information, where available, on month and year the woman reported last using any contraceptive method. When responses to the survey questions confirming absence of birth control use during the prior 12 (or 24) months conflicted with information provided on the month and year of last use of birth control, the date of last use took precedence over the yes/no response.

Fecund: respondents who were pregnant at the time of the survey, were pregnant within the past 12 (and 24) months, or used contraceptives during the past 12 (and 24) months. Also included in this residual category were respondents with missing responses to questions either on pregnancy or on contraceptive use, precluding classification into the category of infertile. Unlike the NSFG approach, respondents whose beginning date of cohabitation was unknown, or whose date indicated a duration of cohabitation less than the required periods of at least one year or at least two years, were excluded from calculations of infertility.

Surgically Sterile: respondents or partners who had had at least one surgical sterilization procedure, including tubal ligation, vasectomy, hysterectomy, and partial hysterectomy.

Using these operational definitions, the prevalence of one-year and two-year infertility for this report was calculated as

infertile/[infertile + fecund + surgically sterile]

The infertility rates provided in this report thus indicate the proportion of all women aged 18-44 who had been married or cohabiting for at least one year or two years, who had not used any contraceptive method, surgical or non-surgical, and whose husband/partner had not used any contraceptive method, surgical or non-surgical, during the year (or two years) prior to the interview, but who had not been pregnant during that time.

A second approach used was a direct replication of that used in the NSFG, differing from the definition above with regard to the handling of cases for which the woman's duration of cohabitation was either missing or less than the required time period. Rather than excluding such cases when calculating prevalence, the NSFG had included these cases in the residual "fecund" category of infertility status. NSFG calculations of prevalence of infertility thus eliminated these women from the numerator, but not from the denominator, of the proportion infertile.

In the NSFG approach, denominators of the proportions infertile contain the total numbers of women meeting the age and marital status entry criteria. On the basis of the NSFG approach, prevalence of infertility can be interpreted as follows: among all women 18-44 years of age, married or cohabiting for any duration of time, x% have been married or cohabiting for at least one year (or two years), have not used any form of contraception, and have not been pregnant during the prior year (or two years).

As a consequence of deleting cases from the numerator and adding cases to the denominator, using the NSFG approach produces proportions of one-year and two-year infertility that are slightly lower than those obtained using our principal method of calculation. While the NSFG method is conceptually less desirable than the principal approach, it is necessary in order to compare Canadian and U.S. prevalence rates. Canadian prevalence estimates replicating the NSFG definition are found in Appendix 4.

As indicated in the Introduction, the NSFG used yet another definition to calculate infertility among respondents (or partners) who had not reported surgical sterilization. Thus, these prevalence estimates indicate, among women aged 18-44 who had been married or cohabiting for at least one year or two years, who were not surgically sterilized and whose partners had not been surgically sterilized, the proportion who had not used any contraceptive method during the year (or two years) prior to the interview but who had not been pregnant during that time.

Restricting analysis of infertility to those who have not been surgically sterilized provides prevalence estimates that are not readily generalizable to the population and can thus be misinterpreted. For this reason, calculations using this approach are also placed in an appendix (Appendix 5).

Analyses

Price Waterhouse and Decima provided the RCNRT with SPSS/PC+ system files for each survey. Analyses were conducted using SPSS/PC+ Version 4.01 and BMDP PC-90 statistical software. Because these two programs handle weights differently, SPSS/PC+ was used to produce all weighted data in this report. Weighted frequencies produced with SPSS were analyzed using BMDP to calculate adjusted odds ratios and tests of homogeneity. Epi Info Version 5 was used to obtain confidence intervals around individual odds ratios.

Analysis Plan

The primary objectives of the analyses were:

1. to provide descriptive and inferential statistics on data from each of the three national telephone surveys; and

2. to provide descriptive and inferential statistics summarizing data across the three independent surveys.

Individual Surveys

Descriptive statistics are provided on the distributions of parity (i.e., number of prior births) and age, the two demographic factors suggested by NSFG results as being associated with prevalence of infertility (Mosher and Pratt 1987). Distributions of respondents are also provided by geographic region.

For each survey, estimates of the one-year and two-year prevalence of infertility were calculated. In addition, variations in prevalence as a function of parity and age were computed in the form of odds ratios. Odds ratios (which are conceptually similar to relative risk and, for phenomena of the magnitude of prevalence of infertility, numerically similar as well) summarize the risk or odds of an event in one group in relation to the odds of the event in a comparison group. Cramer's phi coefficients (ϕ), interpretable as correlation coefficients, were calculated to provide measures of strength of associations between prevalence and age in six groups and between prevalence and geographic region.

Lastly, 95% confidence intervals (95% CI) were calculated for each estimate of prevalence and odds ratio. The 95% CI indicates the range of possible population values of prevalence that would be expected in 95 out of 100 repeated surveys of equivalent sampling frame and sample size.

Examination of Data Across Surveys

Prior to combining data across surveys, several analyses were conducted to ensure that it was appropriate to do so. Because of their association with prevalence of infertility, potential confounding by parity and age on prevalence estimates from the three RCNRT surveys was examined using chi square tests and Cramer's phi coefficients. These statistics provide both statistical significance and strength of associations between parity and survey and between age and survey.

The a priori criterion for combining data across surveys was an association between parity and/or age and survey that was neither statistically significant (i.e., $p > 0.05$) nor meaningful (phi coefficient less than 0.20). The criterion of 0.20 for Cramer's phi is the value intermediate between the conventions for a "small" and a "medium" effect size (Cohen 1988).

Similarity or homogeneity of the independent estimates of one-year and two-year prevalence of infertility from the three surveys was verified using the approach recommended by Fleiss for the comparison of proportions from several independent samples (Fleiss 1981). Since Fleiss does not provide a formula for the standard deviation of the overall weighted proportion, calculation of the standard deviation needed to compute the 95% confidence interval was based upon Cochran's formula #5.57 (with f_h substituted for W_h) (Cochran 1977).

Summary statistics are also provided on associations between prevalence and parity, controlling for survey and age, and between prevalence and age, controlling for survey and parity, using the Mantel-Haenszel approach (Fleiss 1981). The Mantel-Haenszel adjusted odds ratio is a weighted average of stratum-specific odds ratios, where the strata are two-by-two tables of counts of infertile respondents (e.g., yes/no) by demographic factor (e.g., older/younger) obtained for each level of the second demographic factor (e.g., parity 0/1+) within each survey. These odds ratios, adjusted for survey and for parity or age, were calculated along with their 95% confidence intervals.

Results

Numbers of Respondents

Of the 418 households contacted for the CHM-6 callback, 113 women (27%) refused to participate or were unavailable at the time of the telephone callback. Among the remaining 305 women, 8 (3%) failed to meet the age and/or marital status entry criteria, leaving a total of 297 respondents for the analyses. Thirteen (3%) of the 454 respondents contained in the CHM-7 data file were excluded on the basis of failing to meet the age criterion, leaving a total of 441 women for the analyses of infertility. Because of Decima's quota-based sample selection, all 750 respondents contained in the Decima data file fulfilled the age and marital status entry criteria.

Cases Excluded from Calculation of Prevalence

Any respondent whose starting date of cohabitation was either missing or less than the required time period (i.e., at least 12 or 24 months) was eliminated from the calculations of proportion infertile.

To estimate one-year prevalence of infertility, 15 cases (5% of 297) were eliminated from CHM-6, 34 (8% of 441) were dropped from CHM-7, and 25 (3% of 750) were eliminated from Decima for these reasons. The numbers similarly eliminated from the calculation of two-year prevalence of infertility were 26 (9%), 56 (13%), and 55 (7%), from the CHM-6, CHM-7, and Decima surveys, respectively.

These numbers increased marginally when weighting was applied: in CHM-6, for one-year infertility, the number excluded increased to 16; in CHM-7, for two-year infertility, the number increased to 57.

Demographic Characteristics of the Samples

Table 1 provides the weighted frequency distributions (expressed as percentages) of parity, grouped age, and region of residence for respondents from each of the three surveys and across surveys. Parity was dichotomized into no prior births versus any number of prior births. Age was calculated as the difference between year of interview and year of birth. Based on the NSFG, age was divided into six groups as well as into the dichotomy of 18-29 versus 30-44 years. Results from age dichotomized into 18-34 versus 35-44 years, which divides the respondents into approximately equal-sized groups, are provided in Appendix 6. Because of the relatively limited sample sizes, provinces were grouped into four regions: Atlantic (Prince Edward Island, Newfoundland, Nova Scotia, and New Brunswick), Quebec, Ontario, and West (Manitoba, Saskatchewan, Alberta, and British Columbia).

While statistically significant ($\chi^2 = 6.197$, df = 2, p = 0.045), the association between parity and survey was small (Cramer's phi = 0.06). Distributions of age and region did not vary either meaningfully or statistically significantly across surveys. In other words, the samples can be regarded as equivalent on at least these three characteristics.

Only 20% of all respondents reported never having given birth, and 80% had given birth at least once. Approximately 25% were between the ages of 18 and 29 and 75% were between the ages of 30 and 44. Overall, 9% of the respondents came from the Atlantic provinces, 26% from Quebec, 35% from Ontario, and 30% from the western provinces.

Estimated Prevalence of Infertility

The three national estimates of the proportion of infertile among women aged 18-44, married or cohabiting for at least one year, were as follows:

CHM-6:	7.7%	(95% CI: 4.4% - 11.0%)	(n = 281)
CHM-7:	8.6%	(95% CI: 5.8% - 11.4%)	(n = 407)
Decima:	8.7%	(95% CI: 6.6% - 10.8%)	(n = 725)

Figures 1 and 2 present the weighted percentages of respondents from each survey who fall into the three categories of one-year and two-year infertility status: infertile, fecund, and surgically sterile. Results are very similar for the three surveys, especially for the prevalence of infertility.

Combining data across surveys results in a prevalence of one-year infertility among women in Canada, 18-44 years of age, married or cohabiting for at least one year, of

8.5%   (95% CI: 7.0% - 9.9%)   (n = 1 413)

Table 1. Percent Distribution of Respondents, Within Each Survey and Combined Across Surveys, as a Function of Grouped Demographic Factors*

Factor	Survey			All surveys (n = 1 488)	Chi squared (p-value) Cramer's phi
	CHM-6 (n = 297)	CHM-7 (n = 441)	Decima (n = 750)		
Parity					
0	16.6	23.6	19.1	19.9	6.197
1+	83.4	76.4	80.9	80.1	(p = 0.045)
Total	100.0	100.0	100.0	100.0	φ = 0.06
Age					
18-19	0.0	0.6	0.1	0.2	
20-24	5.9	6.4	5.2	5.7	
25-29	20.5	18.3	18.3	18.8	
30-34	29.8	23.8	26.6	26.4	
35-39	22.5	29.1	28.8	27.6	10.589
40-44	21.3	21.8	20.9	21.3	(p = 0.390)
Total	100.0	100.0	100.0	100.0	φ = 0.06
18-29	26.4	25.2	23.7	24.7	0.938
30-44	73.6	74.8	76.3	75.3	(p = 0.626)
Total	100.0	100.0	100.0	100.0	φ = 0.03
Region					
Atlantic	10.8	8.3	9.1	9.2	
Quebec	24.0	26.2	25.9	25.6	
Ontario	34.4	33.5	36.0	34.9	2.997
West	30.7	32.0	29.1	30.3	(p = 0.809)
Total	100.0	100.0	100.0	100.0	φ = 0.03

* Sample sizes are the total numbers of respondents; numbers available for parity and age are slightly lower (for parity, n = 437 for CHM-7; for age, n = 747 for Decima).

Note: Totals may not add to 100.0 due to rounding.

The three national estimates of two-year prevalence of infertility were naturally lower than the one-year prevalence estimates. The proportions of infertile among women aged 18-44, married or cohabiting for at least two years, were as follows:

CHM-6:	6.0%	(95% CI: 3.0% - 9.0%)	(n = 271)
CHM-7:	7.2%	(95% CI: 4.5% - 9.9%)	(n = 384)
Decima:	7.3%	(95% CI: 5.4% - 9.2%)	(n = 695)

Combining information across surveys for women in Canada, 18-44 years of age, married or cohabiting at least two years, results in a prevalence of two-year infertility of

7.0%	(95% CI: 5.6% - 8.4%)	(n = 1 350)

It is interesting to note that the proportion who were fecund remains essentially unchanged from calculations covering one year to those covering two years; proportions of infertile and surgically sterile change by about one to two percentage points (Figures 1 and 2).

Similarity of the estimates of one- and two-year prevalence of infertility can be readily seen in Figures 3 and 4, which present proportions infertile calculated from each survey and across surveys, along with 95% confidence intervals. The confidence intervals reported for the two CHM surveys have been calculated incorporating the previously described adjustment factors. Because these adjustment factors were so close to 1.00 — i.e., 1.13 for CHM-6 and 1.09 for CHM-7 — their impact was quite small. Including these adjustment factors extended the upper and lower limits of the confidence interval by at most one-tenth of a percent.

One-Year Infertility by Demographic Characteristics

Table 2 provides the distributions of one-year prevalence of infertility (expressed in percentages) across levels of each of the demographic factors considered: parity, dichotomized as no prior births versus any prior births; age, divided into six levels and dichotomized as 18-29 versus 30-44; and province, grouped into four regions.

Parity

For each survey, the one-year prevalence of infertility was considerably higher among the nulliparous compared to the multiparous women, and there was variation in the strength of this association across surveys. The odds ratio was the highest in CHM-6: OR = 12.9. In CHM-7 and Decima, the odds of one-year infertility among women who had never previously given birth were three to four times the odds among women who had previously given birth at least once. The association between one-year infertility and parity was statistically significant within each survey.

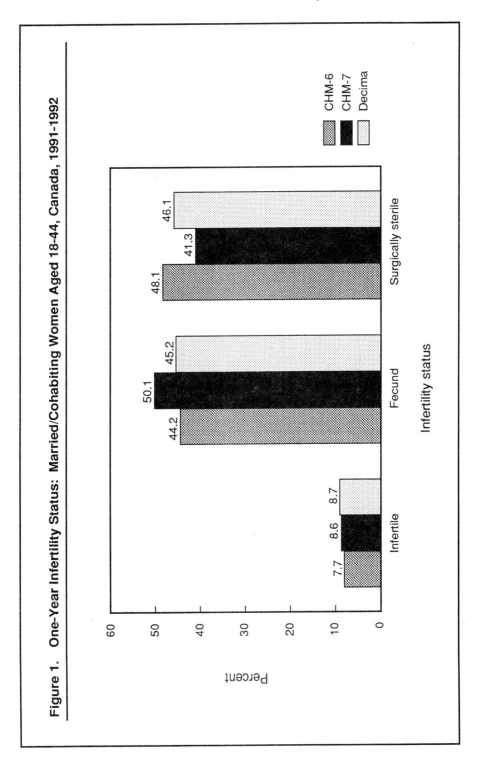

Figure 1. One-Year Infertility Status: Married/Cohabiting Women Aged 18-44, Canada, 1991-1992

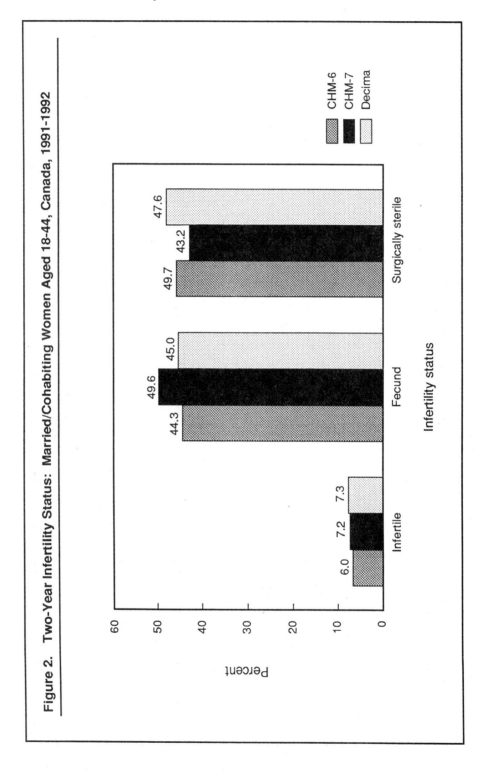

Figure 2. Two-Year Infertility Status: Married/Cohabiting Women Aged 18-44, Canada, 1991-1992

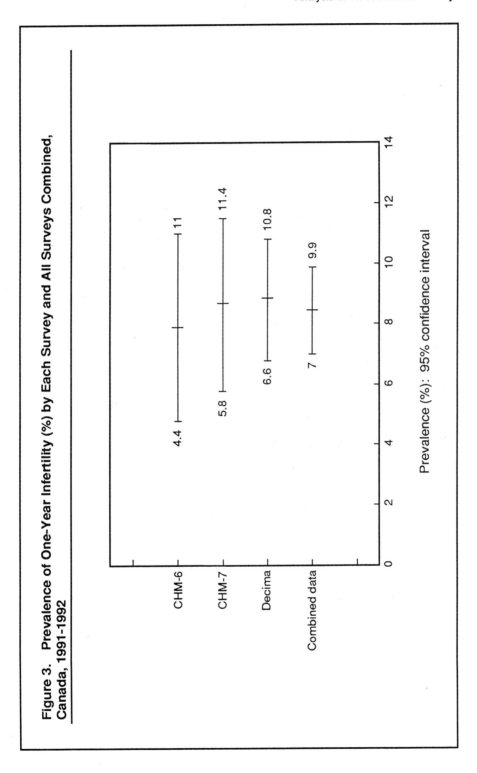

Figure 3. Prevalence of One-Year Infertility (%) by Each Survey and All Surveys Combined, Canada, 1991-1992

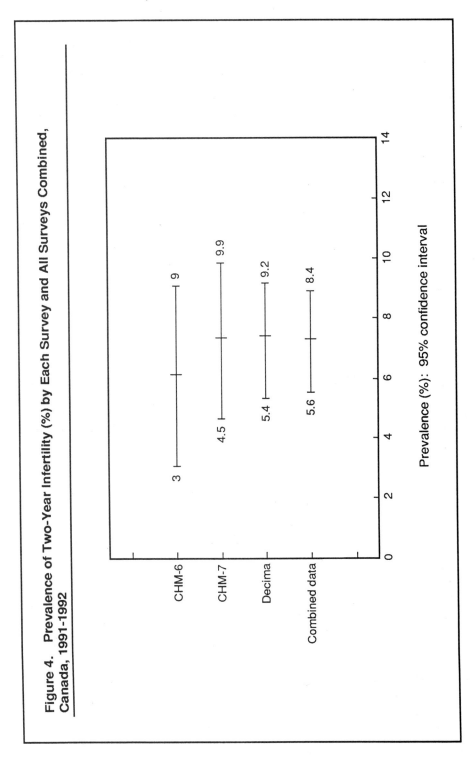

Figure 4. Prevalence of Two-Year Infertility (%) by Each Survey and All Surveys Combined, Canada, 1991-1992

The chi-square test for homogeneity of association between infertility and parity across surveys was of borderline significance (p = 0.05). This was a result primarily of the risk of infertility among nulliparous respondents to the CHM-6 survey, which was noticeably higher than the equivalent risks in the other two surveys. Data from the three surveys were therefore combined.

The Mantel-Haenszel odds ratio for infertility among nulliparous compared to multiparous women, adjusted for survey, was 4.4 (95% CI: $3.0 < OR_{MH} < 6.8$) and was statistically significant ($\chi^2_{MH} = 64.05$, p < 0.001). The magnitude of this association increased when the Mantel-Haenszel odds ratio was calculated adjusting simultaneously for both survey and age (dichotomized): $OR_{MH} = 5.2$; 95% CI: $3.5 < OR_{MH} < 8.4$ ($\chi^2_{MH} = 69.24$, p < 0.001).

Age

While prevalence of infertility varied across age groups, this variation was inconsistent across the three surveys. The association between one-year infertility and age divided into six levels was not statistically significant within any survey, and the low Cramer's phi coefficients indicated the associations were not meaningful.

Among respondents to the two CHM surveys, the proportion of one-year infertility among women 30-44 years of age was about twice that observed in those 18-29. Unexpectedly, the reverse was observed in the Decima survey. None of the three odds ratios was significant and the chi square test for homogeneity did not indicate significant variability in associations across surveys, indicating that the variability was essentially random. The data were therefore combined over surveys. The Mantel-Haenszel odds ratio for infertility among 30-44-year-olds compared to 18-29-year-olds, adjusted for survey, was 1.0 (95% CI: $0.6 < OR_{MH} < 1.7$) and was not statistically significant.

While, overall, one-year infertility was not associated with age, a different picture emerged when the age association was examined controlling for parity. Among the 258 nulliparous respondents, the percentage infertile increased from 15.3% in those aged 18-29 to 26.1% in those aged 30-44, whereas among the 1 151 multiparous women, the percentage infertile increased only slightly: from 4.1% in those aged 18-29 to 5.9% in those aged 30-44.

While the absolute difference in percentage infertile was clearly greater among nulliparous as compared to multiparous women, the relative age effects were similar in both parity groups. The Mantel-Haenszel odds ratio for infertility among those aged 30-44 compared to those aged 18-29, adjusted for survey, was 2.0 among nulliparous respondents and 1.5 among the multiparous.

With the data analyzed stratifying simultaneously by both survey and parity, the chi square test for homogeneity did not approach significance. Data were therefore combined to provide a single, adjusted measure of the effect of age. Adjusting for both survey and parity, the Mantel-Haenszel odds ratio for infertility among 30-44-year-olds compared to 18-29-year-olds was 1.8 (95% CI: $1.1 < OR_{MH} < 3.1$), which was statistically significant ($\chi^2_{MH} = 5.28$, $p = 0.022$). Parity was a confounding variable for the association between age and infertility, masking the association.

Region

As can be seen in Table 2, there was some variability, within each survey, in one-year prevalence of infertility across regions. In CHM-6, the percentages infertile ranged from 7.2% (western provinces) to 8.3% (Quebec); in CHM-7, from 6.4% (Quebec) to 11.6% (Atlantic); and in Decima, from 7.0% (Quebec) to 10.8% (Atlantic). These are essentially random variations that illustrate the value of multiple surveys. In no survey did the association between percentage of one-year infertility and region approach significance. Furthermore, the strength of associations between infertility and region, as measured by Cramer's phi, was very small: none exceeded 0.06.

Table 2. Prevalence of One-Year Infertility by Demographic Factors, for Each Survey and Across Surveys*

	Prevalence of one-year infertility (%)				Mantel-Haenszel chi squared (p-value)
	Survey				
Factor	CHM-6 (n = 281)	CHM-7 (n = 407)	Decima (n = 725)	All surveys (n = 1 413)	
Total	7.7	8.6	8.7	8.5	
Parity					
0	31.1	17.2	20.5		
1+**	3.4	6.2	6.2		69.24
odds ratio	12.9	3.1	3.9	5.2	(p < 0.001)
95% CI	4.6<OR<37	1.4<OR<7.0	2.2<OR<7.0	3.5<OR_{MH}<8.4	
Age					
20-24***	0.0	3.1	0.0		
25-29	5.3	7.4	13.5		
30-34	13.0	11.3	6.2		
35-39	7.6	10.4	9.4		
40-44	4.9	5.6	7.8		
Cramer's phi	0.14	0.09	0.11	0.7	

Table 2. (cont'd)

	Prevalence of one-year infertility (%)				Mantel-Haenszel chi squared (p-value)
	Survey				
Factor	CHM-6 (n = 281)	CHM-7 (n = 407)	Decima (n = 725)	All surveys (n = 1 413)	
18-29**	4.2	6.4	11.1		
30-44	9.0	9.3	7.9		5.28
odds ratio	2.3	1.5	0.7	1.8	(p = 0.022)
95% CI	0.6<OR<9.9	0.6<OR<4.2	0.4<OR<1.3	1.1<OR$_{MH}$<3.1	
Region					
Atlantic	7.7	11.6	10.8	10.3	
Quebec	8.3	6.4	7.0	7.0	
Ontario	7.7	9.8	9.5	9.2	
West	7.2	8.5	8.6	8.3	
Cramer's phi	0.02	0.06	0.04	0.04	

* Measures of strength of association are provided as odds ratios or Cramer's phi coefficients for each survey, and Mantel-Haenszel odds ratios adjusted for survey and for age or parity. Sample sizes are for total numbers of included respondents; number available for age, for Decima, is slightly lower (n = 722).
** Denotes baseline or comparison group for each OR.
*** Age group 18-19 deleted due to very small sample sizes.

Two-Year Infertility by Demographic Characteristics

Table 3 provides the distributions of two-year prevalence of infertility expressed in percentages across levels of each of the demographic factors: parity, age, and region. Patterns of two-year infertility as a function of demographic characteristics were similar to those observed for one-year infertility.

Parity

In each survey, the two-year prevalence of infertility was meaningfully and statistically significantly higher among the nulliparous compared to the multiparous women, with the greatest difference between parity groups observed in the CHM-6 survey. In this case, the chi square test indicated significant heterogeneity of associations between infertility and parity across surveys (p < 0.05).

Despite the significant heterogeneity, estimates from the three surveys were combined. The decision to do so was made on the following bases: the 95% confidence interval around the high proportion of infertile among nulliparous respondents to the CHM-6 overlapped the equivalent risks in the other two surveys; all odds ratios signified positive associations; and the 95% confidence intervals around the odds ratios from individual surveys overlapped one another.

The Mantel-Haenszel adjusted odds ratio for two-year infertility as a function of parity was 5.0 (95% CI: $3.2 < OR_{MH} < 8.1$), which was statistically significant ($\chi^2_{MH} = 61.11$, $p < 0.001$). Controlling simultaneously for both survey and age (dichotomized), the Mantel-Haenszel odds ratio increased: $OR_{MH} = 6.3$; 95% CI: $4.0 < OR_{MH} < 10.6$ ($\chi^2_{MH} = 74.56$, $p < 0.001$).

Age

As was the case for one-year infertility, the prevalence of infertility as a function of age was variable over the three surveys. Across surveys, the proportion of two-year infertility among women aged 30-44 was slightly higher than among women aged 18-29. The Mantel-Haenszel odds ratio for two-year infertility among the older compared to the younger respondents, adjusted for survey, was 1.4 (95% CI: $0.8 < OR_{MH} < 2.5$) and was not statistically significant.

Absence of an overall age effect on infertility was again found to be a result of confounding by parity. As age group increased from 18-29 to 30-44, two-year infertility increased from 12.9% to 25.3% among the 210 nulliparous women, and from 2.2% to 5.0% among the 1 136 multiparous women. In contrast to the differing absolute age effects between levels of parity, the relative effects were comparable. The Mantel-Haenszel odds ratio for infertility among 30-44-year-olds compared to 18-29-year-olds, adjusted for survey, was 2.5 and 2.6 for nulliparous and multiparous respondents, respectively.

Examination of the data stratified by both survey and parity did not indicate significant heterogeneity in the association between age and two-year infertility across strata. Adjusting for both parity and survey, the Mantel-Haenszel odds ratio for two-year infertility among the older compared to the younger respondents was 2.5 (95% CI: $1.4 < OR_{MH} < 5.1$), which was statistically significant ($\chi^2_{MH} = 8.61$, $p = 0.003$).

Region

Variability across region in two-year prevalence of infertility was observed in each survey. In CHM-6, the percentages infertile ranged from 3.9% (Atlantic) to 7.3% (Ontario); in CHM-7, from 4.5% (Atlantic) to 9.7% (Ontario); and in Decima, from 5.0% (Quebec) to 9.5% (Atlantic and Ontario). As was the case with one-year infertility, no association between percentage of two-year infertility and region approached significance, as reflected in the consistently small associations: Cramer's phi coefficients were all below 0.09.

Table 3. Prevalence of Two-Year Infertility by Demographic Factors, for Each Survey and Across Surveys*

| | Prevalence of two-year infertility (%) | | | | Mantel-Haenszel chi squared (p-value) |
| | Survey | | | | |
Factor	CHM-6 (n = 271)	CHM-7 (n = 384)	Decima (n = 695)	All surveys (n = 1 350)	
Total	6.0	7.2	7.3	7.0	
Parity					
0	28.9	14.7	20.2		
1+**	2.1	5.7	5.1		74.56
odds ratio	18.6	2.9	4.7	6.3	(p < 0.001)
95% CI	5.4<OR<67	1.2<OR<7.0	2.5<OR<9.0	4.0<OR_{MH} <10.6	
Age					
20-24***	0.0	0.0	0.0		
25-29	4.2	6.3	7.3		
30-34	11.8	7.7	4.7		
35-39	3.4	9.4	9.6		
40-44	3.8	5.7	7.9		
Cramer's phi	0.16	0.08	0.08	0.06	
18-29**	3.2	4.9	6.3		
30-44	6.7	7.6	7.5		8.61
odds ratio	2.2	1.6	1.2	2.5	(p = 0.003)
95% CI	0.5<OR<14	0.5<OR<5.6	0.5<OR<2.7	1.4<OR_{MH}<5.1	
Region					
Atlantic	3.9	4.5	9.5	7.0	
Quebec	6.2	5.4	5.0	5.4	
Ontario	7.3	9.7	9.5	9.1	
West	5.0	6.8	6.0	6.1	
Cramer's phi	0.05	0.07	0.08	0.06	

* Measures of strength of association are provided as odds ratios or Cramer's phi coefficients for each survey, and Mantel-Haenszel odds ratios adjusted for survey and for age or parity. Sample sizes are for total numbers of included respondents; number available for age, for Decima, is slightly lower (n = 692).

** Denotes baseline or comparison group for each OR.

*** Age group 18-19 deleted due to very small sample sizes.

Discussion

The principal conclusions of this project are that the current prevalence of infertility among married or cohabiting Canadian women aged 18-44 is 8.5% over the previous year, and 7.0% over the previous two years. Because these estimates are derived from three independent surveys of equivalent samples with identical questions, the reliability of these estimates is high.

These results exclude women who did not provide the starting date for living with a male partner. When such women are included, as in the "NSFG approach," the one-year and two-year prevalence rates are 8.0% and 6.4%. The one-year value is very similar to the one-year rate in 1988 in the United States, which was 7.9% (Mosher and Pratt 1990).

The one-year and two-year "sterilization excluded" rates for Canada are 15.4% and 13.2%, both of which are similar to the one-year rate of 13.9% reported by the 1982 NSFG for this definition (Mosher and Pratt 1987). Only this latter calculation provides support for the widely held view cited in much popular literature (e.g., University Hospital 1990) that one in six couples is infertile.

Not surprisingly, there was a significant difference in the prevalence of infertility according to previous childbearing. Women who have never given birth are far more likely to be infertile than those who have. This may be taken as evidence of the concurrent validity of the infertility estimates. The relative prevalence of one-year infertility in nulliparous compared to multiparous women is similar in magnitude to the U.S. figure (Mosher and Pratt 1987).

Although consistent increases in infertility with increasing age were reported in the 1965 and 1976 NSFG surveys (Mosher and Pratt 1987), an overall age effect was not observed in the RCNRT data. However, a significant association between infertility and increasing age was obtained when parity was controlled. There was no significant or meaningful difference in infertility among the four regions of Canada.

Despite the reliability of the estimated prevalence rates, they cannot be interpreted as applying to *all* women of childbearing years. Approximately 40% of women aged 18-44 are neither married nor cohabiting. While most of these women would be at the lower end of this age range, there is no reliable way to infer that their rates of infertility are similar to those reported here. Inclusion of such women will have to be addressed in a future study on this topic. Similarly, it should be acknowledged that the approach adopted here assumes that couples using contraception are fertile. While this is a reasonable assumption, it cannot be readily verified.

Finally, to provide some perspective on the prevalence of infertility, it should be remembered that only 15% of the total Canadian population fulfil the entry criteria for this project. Thus, the estimated prevalence of infertility calculated for this report refers to approximately 1% of the population as a whole.

Appendix 1. Infertility Survey Questions

1.   Since health practices are often related to age, we would like to know ... in what year were you born?

        _____

2.   Are you between the ages of 18 to 44?

        [ ] NO   → end of questionnaire.
        [ ] YES

3.   What is your marital status? Are you:

        [ ] living together as a couple?
        [ ] common-law marriage?
        [ ] married
        [ ] widowed   → end of questionnaire
        [ ] separated, or   → end of questionnaire
        [ ] divorced   → end of questionnaire
        [ ] single, never married. → end of questionnaire

4.   In what month and year did you and your husband/partner start living together?

        ‾‾ ‾‾
        MO YR

5.   Did you ever give birth to a child?

        [ ] Yes
        [ ] No

6. How many times have you been pregnant in your lifetime?

    _____ times   If 0 → Q11

7. Have you been pregnant since December 1986 (January 1987)?

    [ ] Yes
    [ ] No

    *If R volunteers that she is currently pregnant, repeat Q7 and add
    "... excluding your current pregnancy."*

8. Are you pregnant now?

    [ ] Yes   → end of interview
    [ ] No   → Q11 IF 5, 7 and 8 = NO.

9. What was the result of your last pregnancy?

    [ ] Birth of a child
    [ ] Stillbirth
    [ ] Miscarriage
    [ ] Abortion

10. What month and year did that happen?

    __ __
    MO YR

11. In the past year (that is, since Dec 1990/Jan 1991), what forms of
    birth control did you or your husband/partner use? Did you use ...

	Yes	No
a condom	[ ]	[ ]
a condom with foam	[ ]	[ ]
pills	[ ]	[ ]
a diaphragm	[ ]	[ ]
an IUD	[ ]	[ ]
a tubal ligation (tied tubes)	[ ]	[ ]
a vasectomy	[ ]	[ ]

other: (code but do not read)   [ ]   [ ]
[ ] foam, jelly, cream
[ ] douche
[ ] abstinence
[ ] withdrawal
[ ] rhythm method
[ ] breast-feeding
[ ] non-vaginal intercourse
[ ] other

IF TUBAL OR VASECTOMY → Q18
IF ANY OTHER METHOD (AND NOT TUBAL OR VASECTOMY) → Q22

12. So, just to confirm, you and your husband/partner did not use any form of birth control at all in the past 12 months. Is that correct?

    [ ] Yes
    [ ] No   → repeat Q11

13. Now, thinking back over the past two years, (that is, since Dec 1989/Jan 1990), did you or your husband/partner use any form of birth control, such as a condom, foam, the pill, a diaphragm, IUD, or anything else I have mentioned?

    [ ] Yes   → Q 15
    [ ] No

14. Have you ever used any form of birth control?

    [ ] No   → Q 16
    [ ] Yes

15. What month and year did you stop using all methods of birth control?

    __ __
    MO YR

16. Since you are not using a contraceptive method at present, which of the following best describes your situation?

    [ ] You want to become a parent   → end of questionnaire

[ ] You are unable to have children
[ ] Your husband/partner is unable to have children
[ ] Other (Specify:) _____ → end of questionnaire

17. What is the reason you or your husband/partner cannot have children?
Would it be ...

[ ] you've had a hysterectomy?   → end of questionnaire

IF AGE 40 OR MORE, ASK:

[ ] you're past child-bearing age (reached menopause) → end
[ ] some other physical condition affecting yourself?   → Q24
    (Specify: _____)
[ ] a physical condition affecting your partner?   → Q24
[ ] some other reason (Specify: _____)   → end

IF TUBAL LIGATION OR VASECTOMY REPORTED IN Q11, ASK ...

18. In what month and year did your tubal ligation take place?

    __ __
    MO YR

19. In what month and year did your vasectomy take place?

    __ __
    MO YR

20. Since your tubes were tied (your husband's/partner's vasectomy), have you ever felt any regret because you might have liked to have a(nother) child?

    [ ] No
    [ ] Yes   → Q 21

21. Do you think you would have tried to have a(nother) child if you/he were not sterilized?

    [ ] No   [ ] Yes

22. Have you ever discussed with a doctor the possibility of a procedure to help you become pregnant?

    [ ] No   [ ] Yes

23. As far as you know, has your husband/partner ever discussed with a doctor the possibility of a procedure to help you become pregnant?

    [ ] No   [ ] Yes

24. Do you think you would have tried to have a(nother) child if you were/your husband/partner was able to?

    [ ] No   [ ] Yes

25. Have you ever discussed with a doctor the possibility of a procedure to help you become pregnant?

    [ ] No   [ ] Yes

26. As far as you know, has your husband/partner ever discussed with a doctor the possibility of a procedure to help you become pregnant?

    [ ] No   [ ] Yes

Appendix 2. Descriptions of Survey Methodology

(Provided by Price Waterhouse and Decima)

Methodology: CHM-6

The Canada Health Monitor Survey #6 was carried out by Price Waterhouse of Ottawa.

Interviewing Dates, Sample Size, and Margin of Error

On behalf of the Canada Health Monitor, Price Waterhouse interviewed a representative sample of 2 723 Canadians, 15 years of age and older, between August and November 1991. Additional interviews were completed on 27 and 28 February 1992. For a sample of 2 723 the margin of error is plus or minus 1.88 percentage points in 19 samples out of 20. The margins of error are correspondingly higher for regional, demographic, and other subgroups.

Questionnaire Design

The questionnaire was designed by Dr. Earl Berger in consultation with Dr. Len Rutman, Dr. Tom Stephens, Dr. Neil Stuart, and Dr. Nancy Staisey. The Canada Health Monitor alone is responsible for the final version of the questionnaire. The instrument was pretested among 11 respondents approximately two weeks before the start of the fieldwork. The final questionnaire required, on average, 33 minutes to administer. Respondents were interviewed in either English or French, both versions residing simultaneously on Price Waterhouse's computer.

Telephone Interviewing

Experienced, professional telephone interviewers assisted in this survey. Prior to the fieldwork, each interviewer was briefed thoroughly about the nature of the study. The fieldwork was undertaken from Price Waterhouse's National Survey Centre in Ottawa, using computer-assisted telephone interviewing (CATI) technology.

Field supervisors were present at all times to ensure accurate and consistent interviewing and recording of responses. All responses were entered directly into Price Waterhouse's on-line Data General MV2000 minicomputer. This system of direct data entry automatically checks responses for appropriateness of range and logical consistency at the time of data entry.

At the conclusion of each night's interviewing, all interviews from that session were checked a second time for any possible errors. This procedure is equivalent to 100% keypunch verification when traditional paper and pencil methods are employed.

In addition, 10% of each interviewer's work was unobtrusively monitored in accordance with the verification standards of the Canadian Association of Marketing Research Organizations (CAMRO). A monitor listened to the interview over a one-way telephone while watching a terminal that simultaneously duplicated the interviewer's keystrokes.

Sample Selection

The sample for the Canada Health Monitor was generated using a stratified two-stage sampling technique. In the first stage, each province was allocated a quota proportional to its contribution to the population of Canada. In the second stage, each community in Canada was assigned to one of five community-size strata.

A quota then was established for each community-size stratum within each province. Montreal, Toronto, and Vancouver were treated separately in terms of the community-size strata.

A modified Waksberg-Mitofsky procedure was used to produce the actual sample frame. This method utilizes currently listed telephone numbers, and then randomly generates numbers around the initially selected numbers. This procedure ensures that the sample will include both unlisted numbers and numbers listed after directory publication. The original "seed" numbers are then discarded. A total of 20 164 telephone numbers were randomly generated using this technique to yield the final sample for the survey.

In households containing more than one eligible respondent, a single individual was selected using the Troldahl-Carter technique. This screening of respondents ensured that the sample accurately represented the population according to age and sex. Once a potential respondent was chosen by the Troldahl-Carter procedure, no other person in the household could be substituted.

The entire sampling procedure was designed to produce a probability sample to which all sample statistics are applicable.

Alberta Oversample

In addition to the proportional quota allocated to Alberta, a representative sample of 215 additional interviews were conducted. The Alberta oversample was drawn using the stratified two-stage sampling technique together with the Waksberg-Mitofsky procedure for randomly generating telephone numbers.

Weighting

At the conclusion of the survey and prior to the data analysis, the data for the Canada Health Monitor were weighted and verified against Statistics Canada information. Price Waterhouse used cell weights by province and community size in order to adjust for differences in response. The following table shows the sample distribution by province and community size with the weighting scheme used to correct the sample after interviewing.

Methodology: CHM-7

The Canada Health Monitor Survey #7 was carried out by Price Waterhouse of Ottawa.

Interviewing Dates, Sample Size, and Margin of Error

On behalf of the Canada Health Monitor, Price Waterhouse interviewed a representative sample of 2 725 Canadians, 15 years of age and older, between December 1991 and February 1992. For a sample of 2 725 the margin error is plus or minus 1.88 percentage points in 19 samples out of 20. The margins of error are correspondingly higher for regional, demographic, and other subgroups.

Questionnaire Design

The questionnaire was designed by Dr. Earl Berger in consultation with Dr. Len Rutman, Dr. Tom Stephens, Dr. Neil Stuart, and Dr. Nancy Staisey. The Canada Health Monitor alone is responsible for the final version of the questionnaire. The instrument was pretested among 11 respondents approximately two weeks before the start of the fieldwork.

The final questionnaire required, on average, 33 minutes to administer. Respondents were interviewed in either English or French, both versions residing simultaneously on Price Waterhouse's computer.

Telephone Interviewing

Experienced, professional telephone interviewers assisted in this survey. Prior to the fieldwork, each interviewer was briefed thoroughly about the nature of the study. The fieldwork was undertaken from Price Waterhouse's National Survey Centre in Ottawa using computer-assisted telephone interviewing (CATI) technology.

Field supervisors were present at all times to ensure accurate and consistent interviewing and recording of responses. All responses were entered directly into Price Waterhouse's on-line Data General MV2000 minicomputer. This system of direct data entry automatically checks responses for appropriateness of range and logical consistency at the time of data entry.

Table 2A. Canada Health Monitor, November 1991

	Population % of total	Sample unweighted n	Weight	Sample weighted n*
Newfoundland	2.25	48	1.2764	61
(n = 568 349)				
100 000+	0.64	12	1.4523	17
30 000 - 99 999	0.13	1	3.5399	4
10 000 - 29 999	0.24	8	0.8169	7
5 000 - 9 999	0.11	5	0.5991	3
<5 000	1.13	22	1.3986	31
Prince Edward Island	0.50	13	1.0473	14
(n = 126 246)				
100 000+	0.00	0	-	0
30 000 - 99 999	0.21	2	2.8592	6
10 000 - 29 999	0.06	3	0.5446	2
5 000 - 9 999	0.00	1	0.0000	0
<5 000	0.23	7	0.8947	6
Nova Scotia	3.46	77	1.2236	94
(n = 873 176)				
100 000+	1.65	17	2.6429	45
30 000 - 99 999	0.32	5	1.7427	9
10 000 - 29 999	0.43	18	0.6505	12
5 000 - 9 999	0.59	4	4.0164	16
<5 000	0.48	33	0.3961	13

Table 2A. (*cont'd*)

	Population % of total	Sample unweighted n	Weight	Sample weighted n*
New Brunswick	2.81	66	1.1593	77
(n = 709 442)				
100 000+	0.89	8	3.0293	24
30 000 - 99 999	0.40	23	0.4736	11
10 000 - 29 999	0.15	3	1.3615	4
5 000 - 9 999	0.32	6	1.4523	9
<5 000	1.06	26	1.1101	29
Quebec	25.89	520	1.3557	705
(n = 6 532 461)				
Montreal	11.58	232	1.3592	315
100 000+	4.84	97	1.3587	132
30 000 - 99 999	2.49	50	1.3561	68
10 000 - 29 999	1.03	20	1.4023	28
5 000 - 9 999	0.66	14	1.2837	18
<5 000	5.30	107	1.3488	144
Ontario	36.07	1 201	0.8178	982
(n = 9 101 694)				
Toronto	13.58	452	0.8181	370
100 000+	11.98	400	0.8155	326
30 000 - 99 999	3.53	117	0.8216	96
10 000 - 29 999	1.68	56	0.8169	46
5 000 - 9 999	1.58	52	0.8274	43
<5 000	3.72	124	0.8169	101
Manitoba	4.21	85	1.3487	115
(n = 1 063 016)				
100 000+	2.48	50	1.3506	68
30 000 - 99 999	0.15	3	1.3615	4
10 000 - 29 999	0.18	4	1.2254	5
5 000 - 9 999	0.28	6	1.2707	8
<5 000	1.12	22	1.3863	30
Saskatchewan	4.00	81	1.3447	109
(n = 1 009 613)				
100 000+	1.53	32	1.3019	42
30 000 - 99 999	0.31	6	1.4069	8
10 000 - 29 999	0.33	7	1.2837	9
5 000 - 9 999	0.07	1	1.9061	2
<5 000	1.77	35	1.3771	48

Table 2A. (cont'd)

	Population % of total	Sample unweighted n	Weight	Sample weighted n*
Alberta	9.38	402	0.6354	255
(n = 2 365 825)				
100 000+	5.77	248	0.6335	157
30 000 - 99 999	0.84	39	0.5865	23
10 000 - 29 999	0.43	19	0.6163	12
5 000 - 9 999	1.12	46	0.6630	30
<5 000	1.22	50	0.6644	33
British Columbia	11.43	230	1.3532	311
(n = 2 883 367)				
Vancouver	5.47	110	1.3541	149
100 000+	1.01	21	1.3096	28
30 000 - 99 999	2.26	45	1.3676	62
10 000 - 29 999	1.22	24	1.3842	33
5 000 - 9 999	0.63	13	1.3196	17
<5 000	0.83	17	1.3295	23
Canada	100.00	2 723		2 723
(n = 25 309 331)				

* Numbers may not add up to provincial totals due to rounding.

At the conclusion of each night's interviewing, all interviews from that session are checked a second time for any possible errors. This procedure is equivalent to 100% keypunch verification when traditional paper and pencil methods are employed.

In addition, 10% of each interviewer's work was unobtrusively monitored in accordance with the verification standards of the Canadian Association of Marketing Research Organizations (CAMRO). A monitor listened to the interview over a one-way telephone while watching a terminal that simultaneously duplicated the interviewer's keystrokes.

Sample Selection

The sample for the Canada Health Monitor was generated using a stratified two-stage sampling technique. In the first stage, each province was allocated a quota proportional to its contribution to the population of Canada. In the second stage, each community in Canada was assigned to one of five community-size strata.

A quota then was established for each community-size stratum within each province. Montreal, Toronto, and Vancouver were treated separately in terms of the community-size strata.

A modified Waksberg-Mitofsky procedure was used to produce the actual sample frame. This method utilizes currently listed telephone numbers, and then randomly generates numbers around the initially selected numbers. This procedure ensures that the sample will include both unlisted numbers and numbers listed after directory publication. The original "seed" numbers are then discarded. A total of 20 164 telephone numbers were randomly generated using this technique to yield the final sample for the survey.

In households containing more than one eligible respondent, a single individual was selected using the Troldahl-Carter technique. This screening of respondents ensured that the sample accurately represented the population according to age and sex. Once a potential respondent was chosen by the Troldahl-Carter procedure, no other person in the household could be substituted.

The entire sampling procedure was designed to produce a probability sample to which all sample statistics are applicable.

Alberta Oversample

In addition to the proportional quota allocated to Alberta, a representative sample of 200 additional interviews were conducted. The Alberta oversample was drawn using the stratified two-stage sampling technique together with the Waksberg-Mitofsky procedure for randomly generating telephone numbers.

Weighting

At the conclusion of the survey and prior to the data analysis, the data for the Canada Health Monitor were weighted and verified against Statistics Canada information. Price Waterhouse used cell weights by province and community size in order to adjust for differences in response. The following table shows the sample distribution by province and community size with the weighting scheme used to correct the sample after interviewing.

Sampling Methodology: Decima

Decima's samples are drawn using a modified random sampling technique based on geographic stratification and random digit dialling.

Using Statistics Canada data for the universe of interest (usually general population aged 18 and older) we calculate the proportionate number of interviews to be done in each province.

We further stratify each province into the smallest geographic level possible, which is the telephone switching area. A telephone switching area is a contiguous area served from a single central office consisting of one or more NXXs (the first three digits of the telephone number). Using information from the telephone companies and Statistics Canada enumeration area data we have matched census data to all 3 000 plus telephone switching areas in Canada. Using a fixed interval and random start we then calculate the correct number of interviews to complete in each switching area. This ensures a geographically balanced sample.

Within each switching area we have information about blocks of telephone numbers open for residential use. Using this information and generating the last digits of the telephone numbers allow us to reach telephone subscribers with unlisted numbers as well as recent movers with a chance proportionate to stable householders with listed numbers.

This sampling method allows us to consistently complete studies that are demographically balanced with the universe.

For all completed interviews, the telephone and demographics from the interview are stored in a data base. Because the majority of our samples are proportionate, either at the national or provincial level, our data base of completed interviews is close to proportionate to population nationally. The method used to draw samples from this demographic data base does produce a geographically correct sample by using switching area data to calculate the proportionate number of interviews for each of the 3 000 plus switching areas in Canada.

This two-tier method produces a true random sample. Because the initial tier includes unpublished numbers and recent movers, the second tier sample will also include those respondents; thus everyone in Canada with a telephone, regardless of mobility, listing of telephone number, or geography, has an equal chance of being selected for this survey.

In this data base, Decima has recorded age of respondent contacted. We will use this information to pull *all* possible respondents, and then a random sample will be taken from this subsample. Again, this method ensures that the sample is random, because of the large number of respondents in the data base.

Table 2B. Canada Health Monitor, February 1992

	Population % of total	Sample unweighted n	Weight	Sample weighted n*
Newfoundland (n = 568 349)	2.25	49	1.2513	61
100 000+	0.64	13	1.3415	17
30 000 - 99 999	0.13	3	1.1808	4
10 000 - 29 999	0.24	5	1.3080	7
5 000 - 9 999	0.11	4	0.7494	3
<5 000	1.13	24	1.2830	31

Table 2B. *(cont'd)*

	Population % of total	Sample unweighted n	Weight	Sample weighted n*
Prince Edward Island (n = 126 646)	0.50	10	1.3625	14
100 000+	0.00	-	-	-
30 000 - 99 999	0.21	4	1.4306	6
10 000 - 29 999	0.06	1	1.6350	2
5 000 - 9 999	0.00	-	-	-
<5 000	0.23	5	1.6350	8
Nova Scotia (n = 873 176)	3.46	77	1.2245	94
100 000+	1.65	36	1.2490	45
30 000 - 99 999	0.32	6	1.4533	9
10 000 - 29 999	0.43	9	1.3019	12
5 000 - 9 999	0.59	15	1.0718	16
<5 000	0.48	11	1.1891	13
New Brunswick (n = 709 442)	2.81	56	1.3674	77
100 000+	0.89	18	1.3474	24
30 000 - 99 999	0.40	8	1.3625	11
10 000 - 29 999	0.15	3	1.3625	4
5 000 - 9 999	0.32	6	1.4533	9
<5 000	1.06	21	1.3755	29
Quebec (n = 6 532 461)	25.89	530	1.3311	706
Montreal	11.58	234	1.3485	316
100 000+	4.84	103	1.2805	132
30 000 - 99 999	2.49	50	1.3571	68
10 000 - 29 999	1.03	22	1.2758	28
5 000 - 9 999	0.66	15	1.1990	18
<5 000	5.3	106	1.3625	144
Ontario (n = 9 101 694)	36.07	1 194	0.8232	983
Toronto	13.58	453	0.8169	370
100 000+	11.98	399	0.8182	326
30 000 - 99 999	3.53	117	0.8222	96
10 000 - 29 999	1.68	56	0.8175	46
5 000 - 9 999	1.58	48	0.8970	43
<5 000	3.72	121	0.8378	101

Table 2B. (cont'd)

	Population % of total	Sample unweighted n	Weight	Sample weighted n*
Manitoba	4.21	85	1.3497	115
(n = 1 063 016)				
100 000+	2.48	50	1.3516	68
30 000 - 99 999	0.15	3	1.3625	4
10 000 - 29 999	0.18	4	1.2263	5
5 000 - 9 999	0.28	6	1.2717	8
<5 000	1.12	22	1.3873	31
Saskatchewan	4.00	80	1.3625	109
(n = 1 009 613)				
100 000+	1.53	31	1.3449	42
30 000 - 99 999	0.31	6	1.4079	8
10 000 - 29 999	0.33	7	1.2846	9
5 000 - 9 999	0.07	1	1.9075	2
<5 000	1.77	35	1.3781	48
Alberta	9.38	411	0.6219	256
(n = 2 365 825)				
100 000+	5.77	252	0.6239	157
30 000 - 99 999	0.84	40	0.5723	23
10 000 - 29 999	0.43	19	0.6167	12
5 000 - 9 999	1.12	48	0.6358	31
<5 000	1.22	52	0.6393	33
British Columbia	11.43	233	1.3368	311
(n = 2 883 367)				
Vancouver	5.47	109	1.3675	149
100 000+	1.01	20	1.3761	28
30 000 - 99 999	2.26	45	1.3686	62
10 000 - 29 999	1.22	26	1.2787	33
5 000 - 9 999	0.63	15	1.1445	17
<5 000	0.83	18	1.2565	23
Canada	100.00	2 725		2 725
(n = 25 233 589)				

*   Numbers may not add up to provincial totals due to rounding.

Table 2C. The Canada Health Monitor — Survey 7, Final Report, March 1992

Number of interviews required	2 725
Interviews completed	2 725
Total telephone numbers dialled	21 424
Ineligible numbers	
Not valid/non-residential	1 513
Unusable call record	8
Not in service/wrong number	<u>5 752</u>
Total eligible telephone numbers	14 151
No answer/busy	4 502
Answering machine	1 183
Number of valid attempted interviews	8 466
Interview not completed	
Refused to participate (screening/introduction)	4 955
Refused to participate (incomplete interview)	176
Language barrier	339
Mental/physical disabilities	123
Does not meet study criterion	39
Respondent not available for duration of study	<u>109</u>
Completed interviews	2 725
Completion rate (2 725/8 466)	32.2%

Appendix 3. Recommendations from Consultant Survey Statistician

Weight Adjustments

The style of weights being used is such that the average expected weight is one, that is, the sum of the weights should be equal to the sample size. Said another way, they are not "expansion" weights for the estimation of population totals, but are altogether equivalent for the estimation of proportions, as in the present study. As such, there is no primary need to adjust them at all. However, the estimation of the design effect is perhaps seen more clearly if the weights are normalized first. I suggest that this be done only once for each sample, at the Canada level, and not separately by province *unless* estimates and design effects are desired by province, which seems inadvisable given the sample sizes involved.

The sum of the weights as given is slightly larger or smaller than the sample size: call this sum S. The desired total weight is the sample size, n. The "algorithm" given is simply to multiply all the present weights by n/S. More formally, if the individual weights as they now stand are w_i, then:

(1) $\quad \sum_{1}^{n} w_i = S$

Putting $w_i' = w_i * n/S$, we get

(2) $\quad \sum_{1}^{n} w_i = \sum_{1}^{n} (w_i * n/S)$

$\quad\quad = n/S * \sum_{1}^{n} w_i$

$\quad\quad = n/S * S$

$\quad\quad = n$, as desired.

Design Effect

In the absence of other information related to possible correlation between the weights and the variable of interest (and indeed under the assumption that this correlation is near zero, corresponding essentially to the absence of a regional effect on infertility), the contribution of weighting to the design effect may be estimated as a multiplicative factor that inflates the variance calculated under the supposition of simple random sampling. In the present simple case, where the average value of the weights is unity (i.e., the renormalized case), this factor is simply equal to the sum of the squared weights, divided by the sample size. Thus, we call this inflation factor D, and we have:

$$D = \frac{1}{n} * \sum_1^n w_i'^2$$

Following the development of the previous section and expressing the weights w_i', this is easily seen to be equivalent to:

$$D = \frac{1}{n} * \sum_1^n (n/S^2 * w_i^2)$$

$$= \frac{1}{n} * \frac{n^2}{S^2} * \sum_1^n w_i^2$$

$$= \frac{n}{S^2} * \sum_1^n w_i^2$$

so that this calculation could be done directly using the un-normalized weights.

I have worked out a few cases, at national and province levels, and it seems that D will range between 1.1 and 1.3, being smaller when national data are pooled and larger for a few provinces. In practice, this means an increase of 20% or so in the variance, or a relative broadening of about 10% for confidence intervals (since here it is the square root of D that inflates the standard error). This corresponds closely to the design effect of 1.2 quoted by Ms. Dulberg.

Clearly, when there are many records and few distinct weights, all the above algebra may be modified to sum over the distinct classes, using the corresponding frequencies. However, since I presume that these calculations will be done by a computer program that reads records one at a time, this may not be relevant. In any case, the formulation is obvious.

Appendix 4. Prevalence of Infertility Calculated Using the NSFG Approach

Method

The NSFG approach diverged from the approach used in the report by including cases in which the woman's duration of cohabitation was either missing or less than the required time period (i.e., at least one or two years). Prior to their exclusion in the set of calculations for the report, the following numbers of respondents were classified as infertile: one in CHM-6 for both one-year and two-year prevalences; three in CHM-7 for both one and two-year prevalences; and in Decima, three and five cases, for one- and two-year prevalences, respectively. Hence, the major difference between the two approaches to calculating proportion infertile is the numbers in the denominators.

Results

As would be expected, the NSFG prevalence estimates, based upon the smaller numerators and larger denominators, were slightly lower than the estimates obtained using the principal approach. Among all women 18-44 years of age, married or cohabiting for any duration of time, the percentage who have been married or cohabiting for at least one year, have not used any form of contraception, and have not been pregnant during the year prior to the interview was as follows:

CHM-6:	7.3%	(95% CI: 4.2% - 10.4%)	(n = 297)
CHM-7:	7.9%	(95% CI: 5.3% - 10.5%)	(n = 441)
Decima:	8.4%	(95% CI: 6.4% - 10.4%)	(n = 750)

Among all women 18-44 years of age, married or cohabiting for any duration of time, the percentage who have been married or cohabiting for at least two years, have not used any form of contraception, and have not been pregnant during the prior two years was as follows:

CHM-6:	5.4%	(95% CI: 2.7% - 8.1%)	(n = 297)
CHM-7:	6.3%	(95% CI: 3.9% - 8.7%)	(n = 441)
Decima:	6.8%	(95% CI: 5.0% - 8.6%)	(n = 750)

Combining data across surveys, the prevalence of one- and two-year infertility among women in Canada, 18-44 years of age, using the NSFG approach was as follows:

One-year infertility:	8.0%	(95% CI: 6.7% - 9.4%)	(n = 1 488)
Two-year infertility:	6.4%	(95% CI: 5.1% - 7.6%)	(n = 1 488)

Appendix 5. Prevalence of Infertility Calculated Excluding Surgically Sterile Women/Partners

Method

For the "sterilization excluded" approach, women falling into the surgically sterilized category of infertility status were excluded from calculations. In each survey, large percentages of respondents or their partners were reported as having undergone surgical sterilization: 48% (135 of 281) in CHM-6, 41% (168 of 407) in CHM-7 (weighted values), and 46% (334 of 725) in Decima.

Results

Eliminating these large numbers of cases from the calculation of the proportion infertile drastically reduces the denominator and leads to meaningfully higher percentages of infertile.

The three national estimates of the proportion of one-year infertility among women aged 18-44, married or cohabiting for at least one year, excluding those surgically sterilized or whose husbands/partners were surgically sterilized, were as follows:

CHM-6:	14.8%	(95% CI: 8.7% - 20.9%)	(n = 146)
CHM-7:	14.6%	(95% CI: 9.9% - 19.3%)	(n = 238)
Decima:	16.1%	(95% CI: 12.5% - 19.7%)	(n = 391)

The three national estimates of two-year prevalence of infertility among those not surgically sterilized were lower than the one-year prevalence estimates:

CHM-6:	11.9%	(95% CI: 6.1% - 17.7%)	(n = 136)
CHM-7:	12.7%	(95% CI: 8.1% - 17.3%)	(n = 218)
Decima:	14.0%	(95% CI: 10.4% - 17.6%)	(n = 364)

Combining data across surveys, the prevalence of one- and two-year infertility among women in Canada, 18-44 years of age, married or cohabiting for at least one or two years, not surgically sterilized, was as follows:

One-year infertility:	15.4%	(95% CI: 12.8% - 17.9%)	(n = 775)
Two-year infertility:	13.2%	(95% CI: 10.7% - 15.7%)	(n = 718)

Appendix 6. Results of Analyses: Age Grouped as 18-34/35-44

Table 6A. Percent Distribution of Respondents, Within Each Survey and Combined Across Surveys, as a Function of Grouped Age*

| | Percentage of respondents | | | | |
| | Survey | | | | Chi squared |
Factor	CHM-6 (n = 297)	CHM-7 (n = 441)	Decima (n = 750)	All surveys (n = 1 488)	(p-value) Cramer's phi
Age					
18-34	56.2	49.1	50.3	51.1	4.003
35-44	43.8	50.9	49.7	48.9	(p = 0.135)
Total	100.0	100.0	100.0	100.0	φ = 0.05

* Sample sizes are the total numbers of respondents; numbers available for age are slightly lower for Decima (n = 747).

Table 6B. Prevalence of One-Year Infertility by Age, Grouped as 18-34/35-44, for Each Survey and Across Surveys*

| | Prevalence of one-year infertility (%) | | | | |
| | Survey | | | | Mantel-Haenszel |
Factor	CHM-6 (n = 281)	CHM-7 (n = 407)	Decima (n = 725)	All surveys (n = 1 413)	chi squared (p-value)
Total	7.7	8.6	8.7	8.5	
Age					
18-34**	8.9	8.9	8.4		
35-44	6.2	8.3	8.7		0.07
odds ratio	0.7	1.0	1.0	0.9	(p = 0.79)
95% CI	0.2<OR<1.7	0.5<OR<2.0	0.6<OR<1.8	0.6<OR_{MH}<1.4	

* Odds ratios (OR) for each survey and Mantel-Haenszel odds ratios (OR_{MH}) adjusted for survey are provided. Sample sizes are for total numbers of respondents. Numbers available for age are slightly lower for Decima (n = 722).

** Denotes baseline or comparison group for each OR.

Table 6C. Prevalence of Two-Year Infertility by Age, Grouped as 18-34/35-44, for Each Survey and Across Surveys*

| | Prevalence of two-year infertility (%) | | | | Mantel-Haenszel chi squared (p-value) |
| | Survey | | | All surveys (n = 1 350) | |
Factor	CHM-6 (n = 271)	CHM-7 (n = 384)	Decima (n = 695)		
Total	6.0	7.2	7.3	7.0	
Age					
18-34**	8.5	6.4	5.4		
35-44	3.9	7.6	8.9		0.59
odds ratio	*0.4*	*1.2*	*1.7*	*1.2*	*(p = 0.44)*
95% CI	*0.1<OR<1.4*	*0.5<OR<2.9*	*0.9<OR<3.2*	*0.8<OR$_{MH}$<1.9*	

* Odds ratios (OR) for each survey and Mantel-Haenszel odds ratios (OR$_{MH}$) adjusted for survey are provided. Sample sizes are for total numbers of respondents. Numbers available for age are slightly lower for Decima (n = 692).
** Denotes baseline or comparison group for each OR.

Acknowledgments

We owe thanks to a number of individuals who were helpful, particularly during the conceptual stage of this project: Louise Barnard, Duy Ai Kien, Margaret de Groh, and Nancy Miller Chénier of the Royal Commission staff, and William Mosher and William Pratt of the U.S. National Center for Health Statistics. Nevertheless, the responsibility for the analyses and interpretation of results is ours.

References

Balakrishnan, T.R., and P. Maxim. 1993. "Infertility, Sterilization, and Contraceptive Use in Ontario." In *The Prevalence of Infertility in Canada*. Vol. 6 of the research studies of the Royal Commission on New Reproductive Technologies. Ottawa: Minister of Supply and Services Canada.

Cochran, W.G. 1977. *Sampling Techniques.* 3d ed. New York: Wiley.

Cohen, J. 1988. *Statistical Power Analysis for the Behavioral Sciences.* 2d ed. Hillsdale: L. Erlbaum Associates.

Fleiss, J.L. 1981. *Statistical Methods for Rates and Proportions.* 2d ed. New York: Wiley.

Mosher, W.D., and W.F. Pratt. 1987. *Fecundity, Infertility, and Reproductive Health in the United States, 1982.* Vital and Health Statistics: Data from the National Survey of Family Growth, Series 23, No. 14. Hyattsville: U.S. Department of Health and Human Services.

—. 1990. *Fecundity and Infertility in the United States, 1965-88.* Advance Data from Vital and Health Statistics of the National Center for Health Statistics, No. 192. Hyattsville: U.S. Department of Health and Human Services.

United States. National Center for Health Statistics. 1990. *Public Use Data Tape Documentation.* National Survey of Family Growth, Cycle IV, 1988. Hyattsville: U.S. Government Printing Office.

University Hospital. Department of Gynaecology, IVF Program. 1990. *In Vitro Fertilization.* London: University Hospital.

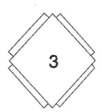

3

Infertility Among Canadians: An Analysis of Data from the Canadian Fertility Survey (1984) and General Social Survey (1990)

T.R. Balakrishnan and Rajulton Fernando

Executive Summary

Changes in reproductive behaviour, such as age at first marriage, late childbearing, family size, the option to be childless, and contraceptive use, in developed societies such as Canada's have led to low levels of fertility as well as to an increasing concern over infertility.

Only a limited number of surveys in Canada collect the relevant detailed information required on these important topics to estimate the prevalence of infertility. This study has made use of data gathered by the Canadian Fertility Survey in 1984 and the General Social Survey in 1990 to arrive at plausible estimates of infertility among Canadian women.

Obviously, the conclusions of any study on infertility cannot be quite definitive and will always be elusive,

1. especially in societies such as Canada's where contraception is practised almost universally;

This paper was completed for the Royal Commission on New Reproductive Technologies in May 1992.

2.   without examining trends in the prevalence of infertility as revealed in data collected through periodic surveys conducted at the national level;

3.   even if periodic surveys collect the necessary information, because of the very nature of the topic, which is not the common domain of perception and measurement; and

4.   without standardization of or agreement on the definition of "infertility" among the scientific community and the procedure adopted to measure it.

Given these limitations, this study has attempted to estimate the prevalence of infertility in Canada using the information available and has drawn some useful inferences for the purposes of national health planning.

Infertility

This study defines "infertility" as the inability to conceive over a period of 12, 24, or 36 months of exposure to becoming pregnant. This study also makes a major distinction between perceived infertility and inferred infertility, unlike other studies on infertility to date, which usually group them together. "Perceived infertility" refers to a self-report of an individual's (or woman's) perceptions of infertility and admission that he or she is infertile. "Inferred infertility" refers to the procedure of identifying individuals (or women) who are not using contraception at the time of the survey and following their union histories back 12, 24, or 36 months to determine whether, during this period, they were continuously exposed to the risk of pregnancy, did not use contraception, and did not become pregnant.

Both approaches have their strengths and weaknesses, and no study on infertility can rely on only one approach. Properly combined, these two approaches provide a plausible estimate of infertility, which is technically referred to in this study as "aggregate infertility."

•   Comparisons of infertility over three periods of exposure (12, 24, and 36 months) indicate that 24 months may be the optimum period to define infertility. Twelve months may be too short a period, giving a falsely high estimate. After 24 months, however, the proportions of infertility differ little. The following estimates, therefore, refer to a period of 24 months of exposure to the risk of pregnancy.

•   Close to 7% of married or cohabiting couples in Canada were infertile in 1984. This estimate is obtained from the 3 734 women in union out of the 5 315 women of reproductive age (age 18-49) interviewed by the Canadian Fertility Survey in 1984. This implies that out of about 4 800 000 couples nationwide in 1984 in which the female partner was 18-49 years of age, approximately 336 000 couples experienced infertility problems.

- Among childless couples, as many as 15% are estimated to be infertile. This proportion increased from 6% in the 18-29 age group to 17% in the 30-39 age group and to 44% among those over 40 years of age. At the national level, this would mean that about 95 000 childless couples experienced primary infertility.

- Among those with at least one child, 6% were infertile, increasing from 4% in the 18-29 age group to 5% in the 30-39 age group and to 7% among those over 40 years of age. This would mean that about 241 000 couples experienced secondary infertility on a national scale.

- Very high levels of contraceptive use at the younger ages and the fact that more than two-thirds of couples over the age of 35 years have been sterilized make it difficult to measure infertility accurately, especially at the higher ages. The result is to underestimate infertility. The above figures, therefore, are conservative lower bounds to the number of infertile couples in Canada.

- Infertility seems to be higher among those who are less educated.

Sterilization

- Sterilization has become the preferred method of birth control in Canada. Twenty-nine percent of women aged 18-49 years in union have undergone a tubal ligation. Not only are more women opting for tubal ligation, they are undergoing the operation at younger ages. More than one-third of the 35-39 age group have undergone this operation before age 35.

- When vasectomies are included, 41% of all couples have undergone a sterilization operation, a figure that reaches 60% in the 35-39 age group.

- The most important factor considered in the decision to undergo a sterilization operation is parity. Fifty-two percent of couples with two children have undergone sterilization operations, indicating a strong norm of two children in a family. Once they have had three children, 66% of couples are protected against pregnancy. Even in the youngest age group of 18-24 years, half of the couples with three children have had a tubal ligation or vasectomy.

- Even among those couples who have one child or none, more than one-third are sterilized when the woman is past the age of 35 years, indicating a strong reluctance to become pregnant later in life.

- Those who are least educated are most likely to be sterilized. Among couples in which the woman has had only some high school or less education, 59% have had a tubal ligation or vasectomy, whereas the corresponding proportions were 42% and 36% for those with 12-13 years of schooling and some university respectively. That the most educated are the least likely to resort to an extreme measure of birth control is an important finding of this study.

- Foreign-born women, especially those of non-European origin, are less likely to be sterilized than native-born women of European origin.

- Age and parity have a greater influence in the decision to become sterilized than education, ethnicity, and religion.

Contraceptive Use

- Contraceptive use in Canada is very high. Excluding those women who are pregnant or post-partum, seeking pregnancy, or non-contraceptively sterile, only 5% of currently married women do not use contraception. Among cohabiting single women, this proportion is even lower at 4.5%, and among cohabiting women who have been previously married, non-users account for only 1.2%. Women in union who do not desire additional births are not taking any chances.

- The levels of contraceptive use among single women who are not cohabiting (51%) suggest that at least half of the women in this group are sexually active.

- Women who have never married rely predominantly on the birth control pill (71% of users), whereas married women overwhelmingly rely on sterilization (59% of users, including 17% vasectomies of spouses).

- Surgical sterilization and the birth control pill, intrauterine device (IUD), diaphragm, and condom account for more than 95% of the contraceptive methods used.

- The birth control pill is now used in Canada, for the most part, only during the early years of a woman's reproductive life.

- Among single women not in cohabitation who use some contraceptive method, only 7.4% use the condom. This should have some negative implications for sexually transmitted diseases.

Introduction

Of the many changes that have taken place in Canadian society since the 1960s, none are more dramatic than the changes in the reproductive behaviour of Canadian women. Family size has rapidly decreased to the present level of less than two children on average per woman. Age at first marriage has increased and childbearing has been delayed. Childlessness, both voluntary and involuntary, has become more widespread. More and more couples are opting for sterilization operations to avoid unwanted pregnancies.

Even as fertility has been decreasing, there seems to be a growing concern over infertility. An increase in the number of visits to infertility clinics and a growing interest in various new technologies developed to help women who are experiencing infertility problems indicate this concern. There is clearly a need to examine the prevalence of infertility among Canadian men and women, especially because infertility is more likely to be experienced by women who postpone childbearing as part of the lifestyle pursued in many developed countries, such as in Canada.

Data to measure the prevalence of such phenomena as infertility, sterilization, and contraceptive use in Canada are extremely limited. Periodic surveys are not carried out at the national level, as they are in the United States, to gather information on these topics. The first and only large-scale national survey devoted exclusively to the reproductive behaviour of women in Canada was conducted in 1984. Since then, there have been a limited number of surveys, focussing on other topics, in which a few questions on reproductive behaviour have been included. One of these was the General Social Survey (Cycle 5) carried out in 1990.

The purpose of this study is to analyze data on infertility, sterilization, and contraceptive use collected during the 1984 Canadian Fertility Survey (CFS) and the 1990 General Social Survey (GSS).

This study has three main objectives:

- to measure the prevalence of infertility in Canada, as estimated from the Canadian Fertility Survey and General Social Survey, and to examine its demographic and socioeconomic correlates;

- to measure the prevalence of surgical sterilization among couples in Canada, based upon the Canadian Fertility Survey and General Social Survey, and to examine its demographic and socioeconomic correlates; and

- to analyze contraceptive use in Canada, using data from the Canadian Fertility Survey, to provide a demographic and socioeconomic profile of contraceptive users.

The Canadian Fertility Survey was conducted from April to June 1984. A national probability sample of 5 315 women of all marital statuses in the reproductive years of 18-49 were interviewed by telephone using a random dialling procedure. According to Statistics Canada, only about 2.1% of households did not have a telephone in 1984. All 10 provinces were covered in the survey. The Yukon and Northwest Territories, which contain only 0.2% of the nation's population, were not included in the survey. The response rate was 70%, including loss at the household contact (80% response) and eligible respondent (87% response) levels, a rate that is average or better than that obtained in similar telephone surveys and that is only slightly lower than that obtained in face-to-face interviews. The average interview lasted 36 minutes, during which time information was collected on most of the standard topics covered in fertility surveys, including contraceptive practice, birth histories and expectations, attitudes toward marriage, and socioeconomic status (Balakrishnan et al. 1985, 1993).

The General Social Survey (Cycle 5) was conducted from January to March 1990. The sample was selected by random digit dialling and included men and women aged 15 years and over throughout the 10 provinces. Interviewers dialled each computer-selected telephone number and completed a Selection Control Form for each one. When they contacted a private household, interviewers enumerated all members of the household on the form and then randomly selected and interviewed one member aged 15 or older. A total of 13 495 individuals answered the Family and Friends Questionnaire, yielding a response rate of approximately 80%. The survey collected the following types of information: aspects of the respondent's relationship with parents, grandparents, brothers, sisters, children, and friends; birth histories of the children; type of child care provided and contact with children living outside the household; fertility intentions; household help and support; marriage and common-law histories; satisfaction measures; and background socio-economic questions for classification purposes (Canada, Statistics Canada 1991).

Infertility

Measuring the prevalence of infertility in any population is complex because one needs not only to define what is meant by infertility, in other words to identify the infertile group, but also to specify the population base or what is often referred to as the "exposed-to-risk" population for which we are interested in estimating infertility. "Infertility" has been defined as the inability to conceive over some specified period of time, usually 12 or 24 months (Mosher 1985; Mosher and Pratt 1990b). "Impaired fecundity" has been defined as the inability to have a live-born child, which includes both difficulty in conceiving and difficulty in carrying the pregnancy to term (Mosher and Pratt 1990b). In this study, infertility is defined as the inability to conceive. An important question related to this definition is, how much time should elapse before a couple is considered to be infertile? One year, two years, or longer? In addition, a distinction has to be made between "primary" infertility and "secondary" infertility, referring to those who have never been pregnant and those who became infertile after having had at least one pregnancy respectively (for a good account of the various measures in use, see Larsen and Menken 1989).

Infertility can be measured using direct questions, or it can be measured indirectly using questions dealing with contraception, marriage, and pregnancy. In the former approach, women (or couples) are asked about their perception of infertility — that is, whether they can become pregnant and whether they have a problem in conceiving or delivering a baby. This is because in a society of contraceptive users, such as Canada's, absence of a child/live birth is not, in itself, an indication of infertility. A direct way of measuring infertility, therefore, requires a self-report on an individual's perceptions of infertility; a couple must have tested their "ability" and failed to conceive in spite of having regular intercourse for a few years without using any form of contraception. Estimating the proportions of infertility then becomes a simple matter of relating the answers (as numerators) to a relevant population base (as the denominator). This measure is referred to as "perceived infertility."

However, this measure based on direct responses may be biased for many reasons. The time frame before the couple think they have an infertility problem is subjective and need not be the 12 months that is commonly employed in the medical profession. On the one hand, those couples who are eager to have a child may see themselves as being infertile after a relatively short time even though they may actually be fertile. On the other hand, many couples who think they are fertile may, in fact, be infertile (Léridon 1991).

Indirect methods make use of the information obtained on pregnancy and birth histories in arriving at plausible estimates of infertility. Infertility can be inferred by observing the pregnancy history of a woman in relation to her exposure history. One can define as being infertile those women who, having had continuous exposure, did not become pregnant after a fixed period of time, such as 12, 24, or 36 months. The strategy then is to identify women who are not using contraception at the time of the survey and to backtrack one, two, or three years to determine whether, during this period, they were continuously exposed to risk, did not use contraception, and did not become pregnant. This measure is referred to as "inferred infertility."

Inferred infertility also has its own biases. Many who are inferred infertile may actually be fertile and may eventually become pregnant. In addition, excluding women who are using contraception as being "able to conceive" underestimates infertility, as some of these women may actually be infertile but they are unaware of it. It is also true that by this inference method, women will be defined as being infertile when it is actually their partner who is infertile, a bias that cannot be avoided given the constraints of the methodology used in the surveys.

Both approaches have been used in the United States in the National Survey of Family Growth (NSFG) (Mosher 1985; Mosher and Pratt 1990b). These authors emphasize the perceived measure, partly because they have an extensive set of direct questions on difficulties in conceiving and in carrying the pregnancy to term. The completeness of any perceived measure based on direct questions is, clearly, a function of how complete the questions on infertility are. No existing Canadian survey has such an extensive set of specific questions on infertility problems. The U.S. surveys also use an indirect measure of inferred infertility (for married couples only) defined as the inability to conceive after 12 months of marriage or cohabitation without contraception. Using this measure, about 8% of married couples in the United States were found to be infertile in 1982 and 1988.

In addition to the above two measures of perceived and inferred infertility, a third measure can be constructed by combining the information from the direct questions on infertility and the information from the birth and contraceptive histories. This measure is, in effect, a combination of perceived and inferred infertility, but it is not a simple addition of the two. Figure 1 presents the Venn diagram depicting the rationale of this third measure. In general, women can be classifed into three categories: fertile, perceived infertile, and inferred infertile (denoted by the circles F, P, and I, respectively, in Figure 1). It is possible that some women classified as "perceived infertile" can also be classified as "inferred infertile" by this procedure, which is depicted by the intersection of the two categories (denoted by the segment PI) in Figure 1. The overall proportion of infertile women can be derived as Prop (I) + Prop (P) − Prop (PI), which gives the best estimate of infertility. This measure is referred to as "aggregate infertility."

As the Venn diagram in Figure 1 illustrates, there can be combined segments of PF and IF as well (denoted as "error") — women classified as "perceived infertile" or "inferred infertile" who are actually fertile. These are biases that occur in the procedures adopted for this study based on the incomplete information obtained in the surveys. Although one should be aware of these biases, not much can be done to eliminate or estimate them.

Perceived Infertility

In the Canadian Fertility Survey, the following question was asked of all women who were not sterilized, not pregnant, and not using contraception at the time of the survey:

Q. Since you are not using any contraceptive method at the present time, which of the following statements best describes your situation? You are not using contraception because ...
... you do not have a husband/partner right now 1
... you want to become pregnant 2
... you think you are sterile 3
... you think your husband/partner is sterile 4
Other reason: _____

Those women who answered 3 or 4 are considered to be "perceived infertile" as defined earlier.

Figure 1.   Procedure for Infertility Analysis

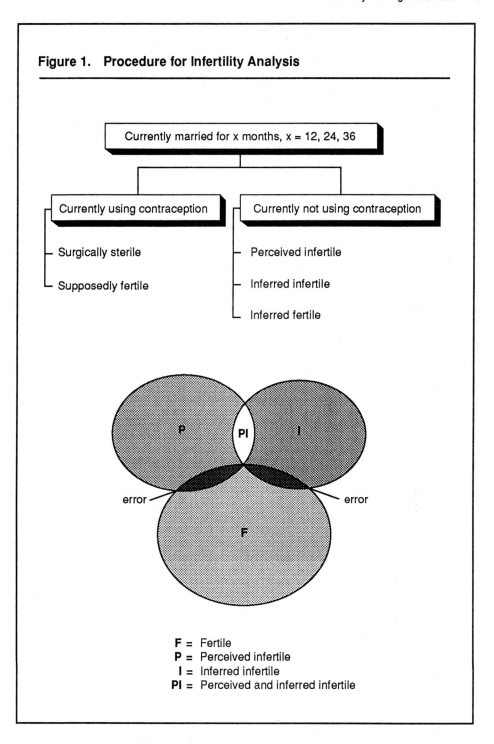

F = Fertile
P = Perceived infertile
I = Inferred infertile
PI = Perceived and inferred infertile

The fact that in the Canadian Fertility Survey not all women, but only those exposed to risk, were asked the question on possible infertility is a serious limitation. Of the 5 315 women of all marital statuses and 3 734 in union, only 1 219 women were asked this question. This selection process and the fact that there was only one question will underestimate the measure of infertility, something that should be kept in mind when comparisons are made, especially with the U.S. surveys, which asked a series of questions of all women. For example, in the U.S. surveys, even pregnant women are able to report, say, that it took them two years and thousands of dollars worth of medical care to become pregnant. The U.S. surveys also identify women who are using contraception or have been sterilized because it would be dangerous for them to become pregnant.

In the General Social Survey, the following question was asked of all respondents in the age group of 15-44 years who did not have an operation that made it impossible for them to conceive:

Q. Have you ever been told that you (or your partner) cannot have any (more) children?
    Yes_____ No_____

As in the case of the Canadian Fertility Survey, the General Social Survey will also underestimate infertility because not all women were asked the question on infertility. Moreover, the question implies that the couple must have visited a medical practitioner who has told them of their infertility problem. This means that those who have problems in becoming pregnant but who have not yet seen a physician will be excluded. The fact that the General Social Survey was not primarily concerned with fertility issues severely limits its usefulness for the present study.

Table 1 and Figure 2 present estimates of perceived infertility by parity and age, based on the Canadian Fertility Survey, for women legally married or in common-law union. Among these women in union who were not sterilized and whose husbands/partners were not sterilized, 6.1% aged 18-49 years for all parities reported that they thought that they or their husbands/partners were sterile (Table 1). Of the 6.1%, 5.0% reported that they might be infertile, with the remaining 1.1% attributing the infertility to their partners. Perceived infertility is higher among the childless (7.7%) than among those who have had at least one birth (5.3%). Infertility increases with age. Among the childless, only 2.0% of those aged 18-29 report perceived infertility. The percentage increases to 13.6% in the 30-39 age group. After age 40, there is a dramatic increase in perceived infertility, with 52.6% of childless women aged 40-44 and 75.0% of childless women in the oldest group, aged 45-49 years, reporting perceived infertility.

Perceived infertility also increases with age among those who have had a live birth, though the levels are much lower. Only 4.0% in the 30-39 age group, 11.1% in the 40-44 age group, and 26.9% in the 45-49 age group report perceived infertility.

Table 1. Percentage of Married or Cohabiting Women Who Report That They Think They or Their Partner Is Sterile Among Those Who Are Not Sterilized* (Canadian Fertility Survey 1984)

Parity and age of woman	Number of women		%
	Total	Think sterile	
Parity 0			
18-29	496	10	2.0
30-39	147	20	13.6
40-44	19	10	52.6
45-49	16	12	75.0
18-49	678	52	7.7
18-44	662	40	6.0
Parity 1+			
18-29	580	3	0.5
30-39	522	21	4.0
40-44	108	12	11.1
45-49	130	35	26.9
18-49	1 340	71	5.3
18-44	1 210	36	3.0
All parities			
18-49	2 018	123	6.1
18-44	1 872	76	4.1

* The couple has not had a tubal ligation, vasectomy, or any other sterilization operation.

The corresponding figures on perceived infertility based on the General Social Survey are presented in Table 2. One should be cautious in interpreting these figures. The upper age cut-off was 44 years, excluding the 45-49 age group in which infertility is likely to be high. Another more serious drawback of these figures is that it is not possible to identify who is infertile, the respondent or his/her partner. This creates a systematic underestimate in the infertility figures derived from the responses of male respondents. Because the husband or male partner is likely to be older than the wife or female partner by about two to three years, the effective age range for the female partner is more like 15-42, which means that in cases where the respondent is male, the infertility estimate will be lower.

Figure 2.   Perceived Infertility by Parity and Age* (Canadian Fertility Survey 1984)

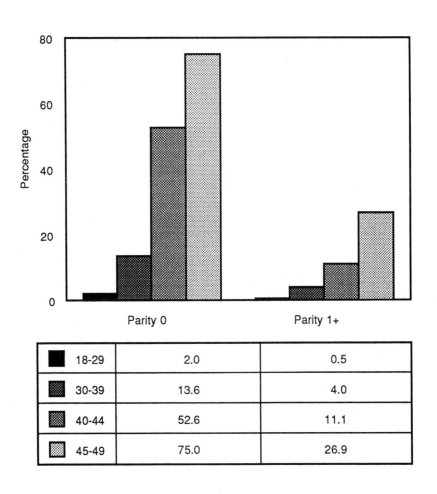

	Parity 0	Parity 1+
■ 18-29	2.0	0.5
▦ 30-39	13.6	4.0
▨ 40-44	52.6	11.1
▧ 45-49	75.0	26.9

* These are percentages of women in union who report that they think they or their partner is sterile.

Conversely, when the respondent is female, the male partner is likely to be older and the infertility estimates, therefore, will be higher. It is also possible that men may be more reluctant to admit to their own infertility problems and may also fail to report some operations performed on their partners that made them infertile. Moreover, selection by age and marital status reduces the sample size of the General Social Survey substantially. With these caveats in mind, the figures in Table 2 can be examined.

Perceived infertility estimates for couples based on female respondents amount to 3.3% for all parities. The figure is basically the same when the 18-44 age group is used, as there were only two respondents in the 15-17 age group who were in union. The comparable figure from the Canadian Fertility Survey for the 18-44 age group is 4.1%. One would expect the General Social Survey figure to be slightly lower due to the different ways in which the question was worded in the two surveys. In the General Social Survey, the question asked whether the respondents had been told that they could not have a/another child, whereas in the Canadian Fertility Survey, the question asked whether the respondents thought that they were infertile.

The patterns of infertility by parity and age based on the General Social Survey data are similar to those based on the Canadian Fertility Survey data, but in all categories the percentages are lower. For example, among all childless women aged 18-44 years, the estimate of perceived infertility based on the General Social Survey was 4.9% compared with 6.0% based on the Canadian Fertility Survey. Similarly, among those with at least one live birth, the General Social Survey estimate of perceived infertility was 2.3% compared with the Canadian Fertility Survey estimate of 3.0%.

The above estimates of the prevalence of perceived infertility were based on all women in union. These estimates will vary if the exposed-to-risk population (used as the denominator) is changed. For example, one may argue that those who are pregnant at the time of the survey or are in a post-partum period are not exposed to the risk of pregnancy. Similarly, those who are using contraception at the time of the survey are supposedly fecund and should not be considered as being exposed to risk. Because the Canadian Fertility Survey provides detailed data on contraceptive use, various refined populations exposed to risk can be used to estimate the prevalence of perceived infertility. This is not possible using the General Social Survey data.

Table 3 presents perceived infertility estimates for women in union using different exposed-to-risk populations. If all women in union are used as the base, the proportion who report perceived infertility amounts to 3.29%. If those who have been sterilized are excluded, the proportion increases to 6.10%. If those women who are currently pregnant or who have had a baby within the last two months are also excluded, the

Table 2. Percentage of Respondents Who Have Been Told That They (or Their Partner) Cannot Have Any (More) Children (i.e., Are Sterile) Among Those Who Are Not Surgically Sterilized* (General Social Survey 1990)

Parity and age of respondent	Men			Women		
	Total	Number sterile	%	Total	Number sterile	%
Parity 0						
18-29	274	1	0.4	364	6	1.6
30-39	170	7	4.1	135	15	11.1
40-44	24	2	8.3	30	5	16.7
18-44	468	10	2.1	529	26	4.9
Parity 1+						
18-29	201	1	0.5	273	2	0.7
30-39	442	7	1.6	413	11	2.7
40-44	139	4	2.9	114	5	4.4
18-44	782	12	1.5	800	18	2.3
All parities						
18-44	1 250	22	1.8	1 329	44	3.3

* The couple has not had a tubal ligation, vasectomy, or any other sterilization operation.

proportion increases further to 6.89%. Finally, if the exposed-to-risk population is defined very conservatively, namely those not sterilized, not pregnant, not in post-partum, and not using contraception, the estimated proportion reaches 22.82%. Of course, in this extreme case the exposed-to-risk population has already become selective in terms of higher infertility.

Inferred Infertility

As mentioned earlier, an estimate of infertility can be inferred indirectly by examining the exposure interval over which women have not become pregnant. Based upon Canadian Fertility Survey data, this measure has been estimated for three periods: 12, 24, and 36 months. Longer durations were also examined, but it was found that after 24 months there is no appreciable change in the estimates.

Table 3. Perceived Infertility Using Various Different Exposed-to-Risk Populations (Canadian Fertility Survey 1984)

Exposed-to-risk population	N	Perceived infertile (%)
All women in union	3 734	3.29
Women in union, not sterilized	2 018	6.10
Women in union, not sterilized, not pregnant, not in post-partum	1 785	6.89
Women in union, not sterilized, not pregnant, not in post-partum, not using contraception	539	22.82

The method consists of selecting women who are not pregnant and not using contraception at the time of the survey and backtracking one, two, or three years to determine whether, during this period, they were continuously exposed to risk, did not use contraception, and did not become pregnant. Some approximations had to be made. Although one can identify current contraceptive use from the Canadian Fertility Survey, there is no way of finding out the exact time periods when contraception was used during the previous one, two, or three years. Those who have been pregnant in the past and who have not used contraception since their last pregnancy are identified in the survey. Also, those who have never been pregnant and who have never used contraception are easily enumerated. However, data on those who have used contraception and have stopped are limited. It is possible to determine only whether and how long contraception was used during each pregnancy interval, not the exact dates when contraceptive use started or stopped. In these cases, the following rule was adopted. If the interval since the last pregnancy (or the date of marriage or commencing union, as the case may be, if there have been no pregnancies) is x months and the duration of contraceptive use is y months, then those women for whom the duration of non-use, i.e., x – y months, is greater than 12, 24, or 36 months are considered to be infertile (these durations have been used in the definition of infertility).

Table 4 and Figure 3 present estimates of inferred infertility for women who have been in union (legal marriage or common law) for at least 12, 24, or 36 months. As expected, the longer the duration of exposure, the lower the estimate of infertility. This is because the women have a longer period during which they can become pregnant. However, the difference between 24 and 36 months of exposure is much less than between 12 and 24 months. Therefore, there is a strong case to be made for waiting at least 24 months before being concerned about infertility. Taking all the

Table 4. Inferred Infertility Among Women Currently in Union Based on 12, 24, and 36 Months of Exposure, by Parity and Age (Canadian Fertility Survey 1984)

Parity and age of woman	Duration of exposure					
	12 months		24 months		36 months	
	N	%	N	%	N	%
Parity 0						
18-29	341	3.5	214	2.3	134	2.2*
30-39	162	9.9	145	8.3	132	8.3
40-44	36	16.7	36	16.7	36	16.7
45-49	21	47.6	21	42.9	21	42.9
18-49	560	7.9	416	7.7	323	9.0
18-44	539	6.3	395	5.8	302	6.6
Parity 1+						
18-29	700	5.6	642	3.6	569	3.3
30-39	1 247	5.5	1 226	4.6	1 196	3.8
40-44	502	3.8	491	3.9	489	3.7
45-49	457	3.9	449	3.8	443	3.8
18-49	2 906	5.0	2 808	4.1	2 697	3.7
18-44	2 449	5.1	2 359	4.2	2 254	3.7
All parities						
18-29	1 041	4.9	856	3.3	703	3.1
30-39	1 409	6.0	1 371	5.0	1 328	4.3
40-44	540	4.6	527	4.7	525	4.6
45-49	478	5.9	470	5.5	464	5.6
18-49	3 468	5.4	3 224	4.6	3 020	4.3
18-44	2 990	5.4	2 754	4.4	2 556	4.0

* Based on fewer than five cases.

Note: N denotes the number of women who have been in union for at least 12, 24, or 36 months at the time of the survey.

Figure 3. Inferred Infertility by Parity and Age* (Canadian Fertility Survey 1984)

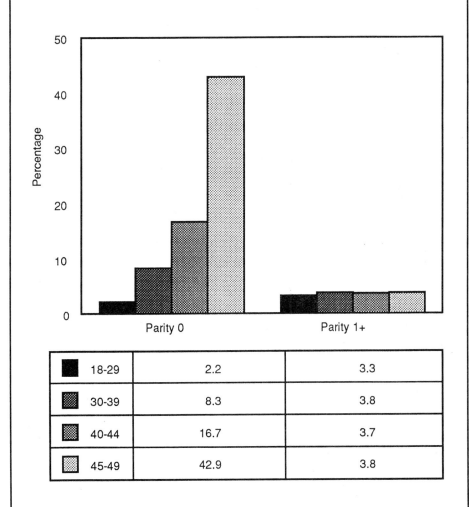

		Parity 0	Parity 1+
■	18-29	2.2	3.3
▨	30-39	8.3	3.8
▨	40-44	16.7	3.7
▨	45-49	42.9	3.8

* These are percentages of women currently in union and inferred to be infertile based on 36 months of exposure.

women aged 18-49 years in the sample and using a 12-month observation period gives an inferred infertility proportion of 5.4%. This proportion decreases to 4.6% for a 24-month period and further to 4.3% for a 36-month period. As was the case for perceived infertility, inferred infertility is higher among childless women than among those who have had at least one live birth. At the preferred duration of 24 months, infertility among childless women is 7.7% compared with 4.1% among those who have had at least one child. Inferred infertility increases significantly by age among childless women, but not among those who have had at least one birth. For example, based on 24 months of exposure, inferred infertility among childless women increases from 2.3% in the 18-29 age group to 8.3% in the 30-39 age group, 16.7% in the 40-44 age group, and 42.9% in the 45-49 age group. Among those women who have had at least one live birth, no age pattern was found, with the level of inferred infertility being almost constant. Here again, one should be aware of the effect of the changing nature of the denominator on the age-specific infertility estimates. For example, many women over the age of 30 are sterilized; hence, they are not exposed to the risk of pregnancy. They continue, however, to be included in the denominator when calculating the infertile proportion, thus making the estimate falsely low.

Aggregate Infertility

The expression "aggregate infertility" is used here to denote perceived and/or inferred infertility. Three types of women can be included: those who are perceived infertile only, those who are inferred infertile only, and those who are both perceived and inferred infertile. The sum of these groups should provide an upper limit of infertility. Tables 5 and 6 present these data based on the Canadian Fertility Survey sample of women and using 24 and 36 months of exposure respectively. These tables give the distribution of women by fertility status, that is, those who have been surgically sterilized, those who are infertile, and a residual group who can be considered to be fertile. Among the women who have been in union for at least two years, the proportion estimated to be infertile (aggregate infertility) is 6.8%, 14.9% among childless women and 5.6% among those who have had at least one live birth. As expected, the proportion increases with age. Among childless women, aggregate infertility increases from 6.0% in the 18-29 age group to 16.6% in the 30-39 age group, 30.6% in the 40-44 age group, and 66.7% in the 45-49 age group. Among those women with at least one child, the increase, though noticeable, is much less dramatic, increasing from 3.7 to 9.6% through the age groups.

The estimates are very similar when a 36-month period of exposure is used (Table 6; Figures 4 and 5). For these women, the proportion estimated to be infertile is 6.6%; 17.4% for childless women and 5.3% for those with at least one child. Age patterns are also very close to those observed for the 24-month period of exposure.

Table 5. Number of Women in Union for At Least 24 Months by Fertility Status of Couple and Parity and Age (Canadian Fertility Survey 1984)

Parity and age	N	Surgically sterile (%)	Perceived infertile (%)	Inferred infertile* (%)	Perceived and/or inferred infertile (%)	Fertile (%)
Parity 0						
18-29	214	3.7	3.7	2.3	6.0	90.3
30-39	145	22.8	11.7	8.3	16.6	60.6
40-44	36	47.2	27.8	16.7	30.6	22.2
45-49	21	23.8	57.1	42.9	66.7	9.5
18-49	416	15.1	11.3	7.7	14.9	70.0
18-44	395	14.7	8.9	5.8	12.2	73.1
Parity 1+						
18-29	642	21.8	0.3**	3.6	3.7	74.5
30-39	1 226	59.2	1.6	4.6	5.2	35.6
40-44	491	78.8	2.4	3.9	5.5	15.7
45-49	449	71.5	7.8	3.8	9.6	18.9
18-49	2 808	56.1	2.4	4.1	5.6	38.3
18-44	2 359	53.1	1.4	4.2	4.8	42.1
All parities						
18-29	856	17.3	1.2	3.3	4.3	78.4
30-39	1 371	55.4	2.7	5.0	6.4	38.2
40-44	527	76.7	4.2	4.7	7.2	16.1
45-49	470	69.4	10.0	5.5	12.1	18.5
18-49	3 224	50.8	3.6	4.6	6.8	42.4
18-44	2 754	47.6	2.5	4.4	5.8	46.6

* Inferred infertility is defined as those women who did not become pregnant during the last 24 months while being exposed to risk and not using contraception.
** Based on fewer than five cases.

Table 6. Number of Women in Union for At Least 36 Months, by Fertility Status of Couple and Parity and Age (Canadian Fertility Survey 1984)

Parity and age	N	Surgically sterile (%)	Perceived infertile (%)	Inferred infertile* (%)	Perceived and/or inferred infertile (%)	Fertile (%)
Parity 0						
18-29	134	3.7	5.2	2.2**	7.5	88.8
30-39	132	22.7	12.1	8.3	16.7	60.6
40-44	36	47.2	27.8	16.7	30.6	22.2
45-49	21	23.8	57.1	42.9	66.7	9.5
18-49	323	17.4	13.7	9.0	17.4	65.2
18-44	302	16.9	10.6	6.6	13.9	69.2
Parity 1+						
18-29	569	23.7	0.4**	3.3	3.5	72.8
30-39	1 196	59.5	1.6	3.8	4.5	36.0
40-44	489	78.5	2.5	3.7	5.3	16.2
45-49	443	71.3	7.9	3.8	9.7	19.0
18-49	2 697	57.4	2.5	3.7	5.3	37.3
18-44	2 254	54.6	1.5	3.7	4.4	41.0
All parities						
18-29	703	19.9	1.3	3.1	4.3	75.8
30-39	1 328	55.9	2.6	4.3	5.7	38.4
40-44	525	76.4	4.2	4.6	7.0	16.6
45-49	464	69.2	10.1	5.6	12.3	18.5
18-49	3 020	53.1	3.7	4.3	6.6	40.3
18-44	2 556	50.2	2.6	4.0	5.6	44.2

*   Inferred infertility is defined as those women who did not become pregnant during the last 36 months while being exposed to risk and not using contraception.

** Based on fewer than five cases.

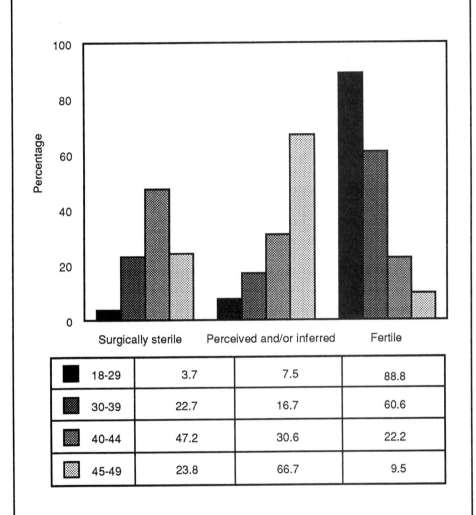

Figure 4.   Fertility Status of Childless Couples by Age* (Canadian Fertility Survey 1984)

		Surgically sterile	Perceived and/or inferred	Fertile
■	18-29	3.7	7.5	88.8
▦	30-39	22.7	16.7	60.6
▦	40-44	47.2	30.6	22.2
▦	45-49	23.8	66.7	9.5

* These are percentages of women grouped into surgically sterile, infertile (perceived and/or inferred, based on 36 months of exposure), and fertile.

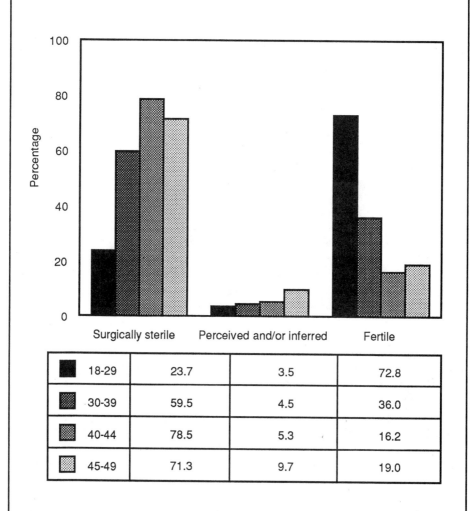

Figure 5. Fertility Status of Couples at Parity 1+ by Age* (Canadian Fertility Survey 1984)

		Surgically sterile	Perceived and/or inferred	Fertile
■	18-29	23.7	3.5	72.8
▨	30-39	59.5	4.5	36.0
▨	40-44	78.5	5.3	16.2
▨	45-49	71.3	9.7	19.0

* These are percentages of women grouped into surgically sterile, infertile (perceived and/or inferred, based on 36 months of exposure), and fertile.

Here again, one should be careful with the interpretation by age groups. Among older age groups, many women have already been surgically sterilized; hence, they should not be included in the denominator. One does not know how many women in the surgically sterile category would have been infertile or fertile when they reach a specified age had they not been sterilized. One might correctly argue that most sterilized women are likely to be fertile rather than infertile. This study clearly underscores the difficulties associated with accurately measuring infertility in societies, such as Canada's, where contraception is practised almost universally and there is uninhibited adoption of sterilization.

Some limited comparisons can be made between estimates of infertility in Canada based upon the Canadian Fertility Survey and estimates of infertility in the United States based upon the National Survey of Family Growth (Table 7). The data are not strictly comparable because of differences in the questions asked and estimation procedures used (Mosher and Pratt 1990b). There are at least three reasons why the estimates of infertility are lower for Canadian women than for women in the United States: (1) the Canadian survey asks only a subset of women the infertility question (i.e., those that are not sterilized, not pregnant, and not using contraception), whereas the U.S. survey asks a series of questions of all women; (2) the U.S. survey asks more questions, so more aspects related to fecundity and infertility problems are uncovered; and (3) the definition of aggregate infertility used in this study is narrower than the definition of "impaired fecundity" used by U.S. survey investigators (women are classified as having impaired fecundity if they experience difficulty in either becoming pregnant or carrying the baby to term, and as being infertile if they experience difficulty in conceiving only). The much lower infertility estimates for Canada are most likely due to those methodological differences between the surveys as there are no substantial differences between the two countries from socioeconomic or biological points of view.

Table 8 presents aggregate infertility by education, ethnicity, and religion. Small numbers in some of the cells make comparisons tenuous. However, infertility seems to be higher among the least-educated group. For example, among childless women with 11 years or less of schooling, infertility in the 18-34 age group is 15.0% compared with 6.3% and 5.5% among women with more education. There are even greater differences among the older age group, i.e., 35-49, with infertility ranging from 47.4% to 17.3%. Variations are lower among those who have had at least one child. There is no clear pattern by ethnicity of women when estimates of infertility are considered across parities and age groups. Differences in estimates of infertility by religious affiliation are also not significant.

Table 7. Percentage of Currently Married Women Who Are Infertile or Experience Impaired Fecundity in Canada and the United States, by Parity and Age

Parity and age of woman	Aggregate infertility, Canada (CFS)*	Impaired fecundity, United States (NSFG)**		
	1984	1988	1982	1976
Parity 0				
15-24		8.4	11.1***	10.6
18-24	—			
25-34	12.6	20.0	21.1	27.3
35-44	21.7	36.4	47.8	53.9
18-44	15.2			
15-44		20.5	21.7	21.4
Parity 1+				
15-24		7.1	7.2***	11.1
18-24	—			
25-34	4.4	8.3	7.3	13.2
35-44	4.8	8.8	10.0	16.8
18-44	4.5			
15-44		8.4	8.4	14.3

* Women married for at least three years. Aggregate infertility is defined as those women who think that they/their husband are infertile as well as those women/husbands who were not sterilized, not pregnant, and not using contraception and did not become pregnant during three years of exposure before the survey.

** Includes all married women. Women with "impaired fecundity" include (a) those who said that it was impossible for them to have a baby for some reason other than a sterilization operation, such as an accident, illness, or unexplained inability to conceive; (b) those who said that it was physically difficult for them to conceive or deliver a baby, or who had been told by a physician never to become pregnant again because the pregnancy would pose a danger to the woman, the baby, or both; and (c) those women or couples who were continuously married, did not use contraception, and did not become pregnant for 36 months or more (Mosher and Pratt 1990b).

*** Figure does not meet the standard of reliability or precision.

Note: —, too few cases.

Table 8. Aggregate Infertility Among Women Currently in Union for At Least 24 Months, by Parity and Age and Selected Socioeconomic Characteristics (Canadian Fertility Survey 1984)

	Age of woman							
	18-34				35-49			
	Parity 0		Parity 1+		Parity 0		Parity 1+	
Characteristic	N	%	N	%	N	%	N	%
Education								
≤11 years	40	15.0	385	5.7	38	47.4	676	7.2
12-13 years	126	6.3	528	3.8	33	30.3	468	7.1
≥14 years	127	5.5	346	4.6	52	17.3	404	3.5
Ethnicity								
French	68	13.2	305	3.9	35	28.6	354	4.5
British	100	11.0	464	4.7	44	36.4	589	5.8
Other	125	4.0	490	5.1	44	25.0	605	7.6
Religion								
Catholic	137	7.3	611	4.6	57	29.8	754	7.2
Protestant	96	7.3	441	4.3	43	37.2	594	5.2
Other	60	10.0	207	5.8	23	21.7	200	5.5
Total	293	7.8	1 259	4.7	123	30.9	1 548	6.2

Surgical Sterilization

In a report on infertility, it is necessary to discuss sterilization and contraception for a number of reasons. First, the most significant of all trends in the reproductive behaviour of Canadian couples is the rapid increase in the proportion who resort to a sterilization operation when a desired family size is reached, usually two children. Both tubal ligation and vasectomy, very rare even in the late 1960s, have become popular in a short span of about 20 years. This is all the more remarkable considering the fact that these two procedures are almost irreversible and couples have to be convinced of their decision not to have more children.   Second, because so many couples use sterilization and contraception, many have never tested their fertility. Therefore, they have no way of knowing whether they are fertile or infertile as they age. Third, apart from those who adopt sterilization as a contraceptive method, many women have other operations, such as a hysterectomy, that make them infertile. Most of these operations are not done by choice (but rather for medical reasons); however, though often done later in their reproductive years, such operations have a negative effect on childbearing if the woman has started bearing children later in life. Fourth, the extensive use of sterilization may create a demand for sterilization reversals, an extreme form of "infertility" treatment. There is also evidence, based upon the Canadian Fertility Survey, that 10% of the couples who have resorted to sterilization regret their decision. Ongoing medical research on reversible sterilization is worth noting in this regard.

Questions in the Canadian Fertility Survey and General Social Survey on Sterilization Operations

In the Canadian Fertility Survey, the following questions were asked:

Q. Have you or your husband/partner (if applicable) had an operation that would make it impossible for you to have children?
Yes___ No___

If the respondent answered yes to the first question, a second question was asked, as follows:

Q. Among the following operations, which one or ones did you, or your husband/partner (if applicable), have and when did they take place?

(a) tubal ligation?
Yes___ No___
If yes, month___ year___

(b) hysterectomy?
Yes___ No___

(c) another operation that made you sterile?
Yes___ No___
If yes, month___ year___

(d) (if applicable) has your husband/partner had a vasectomy?
Yes___ No___
If yes, month___ year___

Responses to these questions are used to identify sterilization operations performed for contraceptive and non-contraceptive reasons as well as the dates when they were performed.

In the General Social Survey, only one question was asked of respondents aged 44 years or younger:

Q. Have you (or your spouse/partner) had an operation that makes it impossible for you to have a/another child?
Yes_____ No_____

This question does not enable one to distinguish between operations performed for contraceptive reasons and those performed for non-contraceptive reasons. Nor can one identify tubal ligations or vasectomies. Because the respondent can be male or female, and the husband/partner is likely to be older than his wife/partner, the extent of sterilization will be underestimated when the respondent is male compared with the outcome when the respondent is female.

Sterilization by Age and Parity, Canadian Fertility Survey

Table 9 presents the percent distribution of women or their partners who had a sterilization operation for contraceptive or non-contraceptive reasons by age and marital status. Though from now on the focus will be only on women currently in union, it is worthwhile showing the distribution among ever-married women as well, given the largely irreversible nature of sterilization. It is clear that sterilization is strongly related to age. Looking at women currently in union, the proportion (self and/or partner) sterilized for all reasons increases from 4.9% in the 18-24 age group to 43.6% in the 30-34 age group and to 76.6% in the 40-44 age group. The proportion decreases slightly in the oldest age group (45-49 years) to 69.6%.

The drop in sterilization for contraceptive purposes in the oldest age group among married women is worth noting. In the 40-44 age group, 65.9% of married women were contraceptively sterile, whereas in the 45-49 age group, the proportion decreased to 55.4%. This is due to rapid increases in sterilization operations in the 1970s and 1980s. Women 45-49 years of age in 1984 were born between 1935 and 1939; thus, they were already 30-34 years old in 1965-1969, before the rapid increase in sterilization operations.

Most sterilization was performed for contraceptive reasons. For example, in the 30-34 age group, 42.2% of couples had operations for contraceptive reasons and only 1.5% for non-contraceptive reasons. In the 35-39 age group, 59.9% of operations were for contraceptive reasons and 5.5% were for non-contraceptive reasons. The proportion of operations for non-contraceptive reasons (such as hysterectomies) among women 40-44 and 45-49 years of age is not insignificant at 11.0% and 14.1%, respectively, and should be a cause for concern from a health point of view.

The Canadian Fertility Survey, unlike the General Social Survey, allows one to separate tubal ligations from vasectomies. Table 10 and Figure 6 give the percentages of tubal ligations and vasectomies performed among couples currently in union. Here, as throughout this report, the procedure of counting only the woman when both she and her husband/partner have undergone a sterilization operation has been

Table 9. Percentage of Women or Their Partners Who Underwent Surgical Sterilization for Contraceptive or Non-Contraceptive Reasons, by Age and Marital Status (Canadian Fertility Survey 1984)

Age of woman	Ever married			Currently married			Currently in union			
	N	CS	NCS	N	CS	NCS	N	CS	NCS	CS+ NCS*
18-24	362	6.1	0.8**	326	6.1	0.9**	494	4.3	0.6	4.9
25-29	736	20.4	0.8	645	19.5	0.8	753	18.1	0.9	19.0
30-34	805	43.4	1.6	679	42.6	1.6	754	42.2	1.5	43.6
35-39	795	58.7	5.9	663	60.1	5.7	705	59.9	5.5	65.4
40-44	617	65.3	10.2	513	65.9	10.3	547	65.6	11.0	76.6
45-49	569	54.6	15.3	457	55.4	13.6	481	55.5	14.1	69.6
18-49	3 884	43.7	5.6	3 283	43.4	5.2	3 734	40.9	5.0	45.9
18-44	3 315	41.9	3.9	2 826	41.4	3.9	3 253	38.7	3.7	42.4

*   Totals might not add due to rounding.
** Based on fewer than five cases.

Note: CS, contraceptively sterile (tubal ligation and vasectomy); NCS, non-contraceptively sterile (hysterectomy and other operations).

Table 10. Percentage of Women Currently in Union Who (or Whose Partners) Have Had a Sterilization Operation for Contraceptive Reasons, by Age of the Woman (Canadian Fertility Survey 1984)

Age of woman	N	Tubal ligation	Vasectomy	Either*
18-24	494	2.8	1.6	4.3
25-29	753	11.4	6.6	18.1
30-34	754	27.3	14.9	42.2
35-39	705	43.5	16.3	59.9
40-44	547	46.4	19.2	65.6
45-49	481	44.3	11.2	55.5

Table 10. (cont'd)

Age of woman	N	Tubal ligation	Vasectomy	Either*
18-49	3 734	29.0	11.9	40.9
18-44	3 253	26.7	12.0	38.7

*   Totals might not add due to rounding.

Note: In the few cases in which both the woman and the husband/partner are sterilized, only the woman's operation is counted.

Table 11. Percentage of Ever-Married Women Sterilized by Specific Ages and by Age at Interview

	Age at interview					
By end of age	18-24 n = 362	25-29 n = 736	30-34 n = 805	35-39 n = 795	40-44 n = 617	45-49 n = 569
24	3.3*	4.9	3.4	1.0	0.6	0.5
29	-	12.8*	17.9	12.8	6.2	2.1
34	-	-	28.2*	34.1	28.2	11.8
39	-	-	-	42.3*	42.0	31.6
44	-	-	-	-	45.5*	39.9
49	-	-	-	-	-	40.4*

*   These figures are an underestimate because some of the women in the cohort had not reached the end age at the time of the interview.

followed. This is necessary to avoid double counting. Of the 40.9% of couples who have had an operation for contraceptive reasons, 29.0% of the operations were tubal ligations and the remaining 11.9% were vasectomies. Though tubal ligations are performed more often than vasectomies, one can notice that the relative frequencies of vasectomies to tubal ligations have been increasing among the younger age groups. For example, in the oldest cohort, the ratio of tubal ligations to vasectomies was 4:1, whereas in the cohorts where the woman is less than 35 years of age, the ratio is more like 2:1.

Because the Canadian Fertility Survey collected information on the date a sterilization operation was performed on a woman, it is possible to examine for each cohort the cumulative proportion sterilized by various ages. Table 11 and Figure 7 present data on the proportion of ever-married women who have had a tubal ligation by selected ages. The data clearly show that not only are more women opting for tubal ligation but also that they are undergoing the operation at a younger age. For example, in the oldest cohort (45-49 years of age), only 11.8% were sterilized before the age of 35. This increased to 28.2% among the 40-44 cohort and 34.1% among the 35-39 cohort. It is surprising to see that among the 30-34 cohort, 17.9% are already sterilized before age 30, whereas in the oldest cohort this proportion is insignificant at 2.1%. If the trends continue, indications are that as many as half of the women in the younger cohorts may resort to tubal ligation before the end of their reproductive period. This analysis can only be done for tubal ligation. The extent of sterilization is greater when vasectomies are also included, which amount to approximately one-third the number of tubal ligations performed.

Apart from age, the factor most related to sterilization is parity. The relationship between parity and sterilization is examined in Table 12. More than half of the women are protected by sterilization through either a tubal ligation or a vasectomy on the part of their partner once they have had three children. This is true even in the youngest cohort of women 18-24 years of age (though the sample size is small, it fits into the pattern created by the other cohorts). Even after two children, more than half of the women are sterilized after age 30. The proportion reaches as high as 73.2% for the 40-44 cohort. What is more dramatic is the fact that, even among those who have had only one child or none at all, the proportion who are sterilized is more than one-third once the woman is past the age of 35. There seems to be a strong reluctance to become pregnant later in life even if the prevalent norm of two children has not been attained.

Figure 6.   Sterilization for Contraceptive Reasons* (Canadian
Fertility Survey 1984)

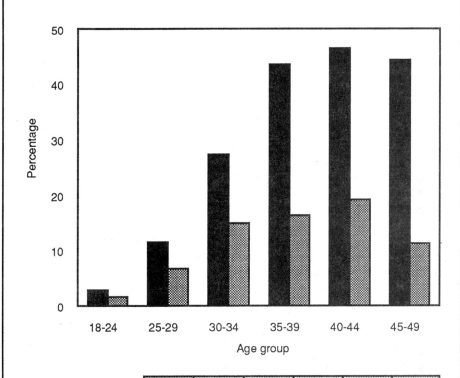

	18-24	25-29	30-34	35-39	40-44	45-49
■ Tubal ligation	2.8	11.4	27.3	43.5	46.4	44.3
▨ Vasectomy	1.6	6.6	14.9	16.3	19.2	11.2

* These are percentages of women currently in union who (or whose partners)
  have had a sterilization operation for contraceptive reasons.

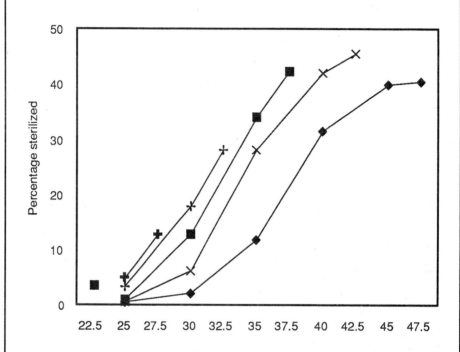

Figure 7.   Percentages of Women Sterilized Before Specific Ages (Canadian Fertility Survey 1984)

		22.5	25	27.5	30	32.5	35	37.5	40	42.5	45	47.5
■	18-24	3.3										
—+—	25-29		4.9	12.8								
—+—	30-34		3.4		17.9	28.2						
—■—	35-39		1.0		12.8		34.1	42.3				
—✕—	40-44		0.6		6.2		28.2		42.0	45.5		
—◆—	45-49		0.5		2.1		11.8		31.6		39.9	40.4

Sterilized before specific ages

Table 12. Percentage of Ever-Married Women Protected by Sterilization (Tubal Ligations Plus Vasectomies Without Double Counting), by Age at Interview and Number of Children

Number of children	Age at interview						
	18-24	25-29	30-34	35-39	40-44	45-49	18-49
0	0.6	1.1	13.7	23.6	33.3	8.0	8.8
1	0.8	6.3	18.8	47.6	45.2	44.9	20.9
2	20.1	32.3	49.7	64.7	73.2	50.4	52.2
3+	50.0	61.4	69.0	68.1	69.7	60.4	65.6
Total	6.1	20.5	43.3	58.7	65.2	54.5	43.8
	Base number of women						
0	166	188	102	89	42	25	612
1	119	206	160	103	73	49	710
2	63	254	372	334	194	134	1 351
3+	14	88	171	269	308	361	1 211
Total	362	736	805	795	616	570	3 884

Sterilization by Age and Parity, General Social Survey

Data on sterilization are limited from the General Social Survey. The only information known is whether an operation making it impossible to have a child was performed on the woman or the partner. It is not possible to distinguish those who had an operation for contraceptive reasons from those who had an operation for other reasons. It is also necessary to separate respondents by gender, so that one can examine patterns associated with age. Table 13 and Figure 8 present data on respondents currently in union by gender and age. Because there were only three respondents under the age of 17 years who were in union and none was sterilized, the results for the 15-44 age group are basically the same as those for the 18-44 age group, making comparisons with the Canadian Fertility Survey easier.

Table 13. Percentage of Male and Female Respondents Aged 15-44 Years Who Are Currently in Union and Report That They or Their Partners Have Had an Operation Making It Impossible for Them to Have A/Another Child, by Age (General Social Survey 1990)

Age of respondent	Male			Female		
	N	n	%	N	n	%
15-17	1	0	0.0	2	0	0.0
18-19	5	0	0.0	27	2	7.4
20-24	138	1	0.7	233	14	6.0
25-29	446	37	8.3	547	53	9.7
30-34	558	135	24.2	615	215	35.0
35-39	558	272	48.7	542	305	56.3
40-44	492	302	61.4	479	312	65.1
15-44	2 198	747	34.0	2 445	901	36.9
18-44	2 197	747	34.0	2 442	901	36.9

The sterilization figures for males are slightly lower than for females. Because respondents report both their operations and those of their partners, differences have to be attributed to possible under-reporting by men as well as the age difference referred to earlier between spouses as a source of systematic bias. Thirty-four percent of the males and 36.9% of the females report that they or their partners have had a sterilization operation. This compares with 42.4% (Table 9) for women in the 18-44 age group based on Canadian Fertility Survey information, a difference of 5.5 percentage points. Reporting of sterilization in the General Social Survey is probably incomplete because the question on sterilization is not explicit enough.

The direct relationship between sterilization and age is clear in the General Social Survey data as well. Below the age of 30, sterilization is relatively rare. After age 30, however, it increases dramatically. Among female respondents, the proportion sterilized (themselves or their partners) increases from 9.7% in the 25-29 age group to 35.0% in the 30-34 age group, 56.3% in the 35-39 age group, and 65.1% in the oldest age group (40-44 years). All of these figures are slightly lower than those obtained from the Canadian Fertility Survey sample. The norm of stopping at two children is also evident in the General Social Survey sample (Table 14). Among those with two or more children, 57.2% report that they or their partners have undergone a sterilization operation.

Figure 8. Voluntary Infertility* (Canadian Fertility Survey 1984 and General Social Survey 1990)

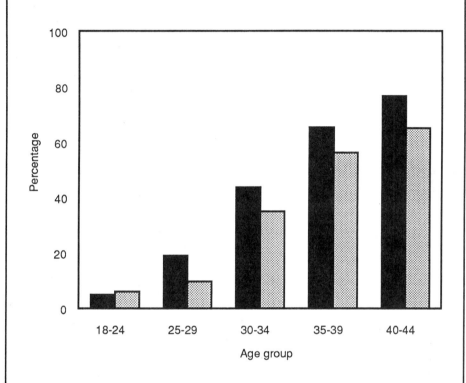

	18-24	25-29	30-34	35-39	40-44
■ CFS	4.9	19.0	43.6	65.4	76.6
▒ GSS	6.2	9.7	35.0	56.3	65.1

* These are percentages of women currently in union reporting that they or their partners have had an operation that makes it impossible for them to have a/another child.

Table 14. Percentage of Male and Female Respondents Aged 15-44 Years Who Are Currently in Union and Report That They or Their Partners Have Had an Operation Making It Impossible for Them to Have A/Another Child, by Parity (General Social Survey 1990)

Number of children	Male			Female		
	N	n	%	N	n	%
0	598	54	9.0	671	56	8.3
1	453	97	21.4	457	91	19.9
2+	1 147	597	52.0	1 317	753	57.2
Total	2 198	748	34.0	2 445	900	36.8

Socioeconomic Correlates of Surgical Sterilization

It is quite clear that sterilization has become the preferred method of birth control in Canada. Apart from the obvious demographic factors of age and number of children, it is useful to identify the characteristics of women who are more likely to undergo a sterilization operation compared to those who are not. Tables 15 and 16 present the extent of sterilization among various subgroups of the population of the Canadian Fertility Survey and General Social Survey respectively. Because the variables are correlated among themselves, one should be careful in making comparisons. Moreover, categories between the two surveys are not exactly the same. The differences by various regions of Canada are not significant. In the Canadian Fertility Survey, they are all within two or three percentage points of the national average of 45.9%. In the General Social Survey, the variation is slightly higher, but no clear pattern emerges.

Table 15. Percentage of Women Aged 18-49 Years Currently in Union Who or Whose Partners Have Been Sterilized, by Age and Selected Socioeconomic Characteristics (Canadian Fertility Survey 1984)

Characteristic	Age of woman									
	18-24		25-34		35-44		45-49		18-49	
	N	%	N	%	N	%	N	%	%	
Region of residence										
Atlantic provinces	46	13.0	141	37.6	111	76.7	41	53.7	48.7	
Quebec	149	2.0*	406	30.5	333	71.8	138	74.6	45.7	
Ontario	148	4.7	524	31.1	474	67.5	177	67.2	46.2	
Manitoba and Saskatchewan	43	7.0*	111	31.5	86	67.4	33	70.0	43.1	
Alberta	53	0.0	163	31.3	107	73.8	47	74.5	43.8	
British Columbia	55	12.7	164	29.3	142	71.1	45	77.8	47.0	
Religion										
Catholic	242	4.1	710	30.1	603	71.1	234	65.4	45.1	
Protestant	169	6.5	531	35.4	466	73.2	194	77.8	50.7	
Other or no religion	81	3.7*	263	26.2	182	61.0	52	61.5	36.8	
Church attendance										
Weekly	91	1.1*	359	35.1	416	67.3	187	61.5	49.8	
Sometimes	201	4.5	638	32.0	452	70.6	152	71.1	44.7	
Rarely or never	202	7.4	509	27.5	380	73.7	142	77.5	44.2	
Status										
Native born	456	5.3	1 314	32.6	1 015	73.4	385	71.4	46.4	
Foreign born	38	2.6*	193	11.9	237	57.4	96	62.5	42.6	

Table 15. (cont'd)

	Age of woman								
	18-24		25-34		35-44		45-49		18-49
Characteristic	N	%	N	%	N	%	N	%	%
Ethnicity									
British	162	6.8	562	35.4	486	73.5	181	70.7	50.0
French	126	3.2*	354	33.9	288	73.3	116	72.4	47.5
Other European	114	4.4	356	25.8	284	64.8	123	61.0	40.8
Non-European	29	3.4*	77	11.7	91	49.5	24	79.2	33.0
Education									
Some high school or less	140	11.4	366	47.3	471	76.4	269	70.6	59.1
12-13 years of school	243	3.7	605	34.0	405	69.6	110	72.7	42.2
Some university	111	0.9*	536	17.2	375	64.3	102	64.7	35.5
Total	494	4.9	1 507	31.3	1 252	70.3	481	69.6	45.9

* Based on fewer than five cases.

Note: Subgroup totals may not add to total due to item non-response.

Table 16. Percentage of Female Respondents Aged 15-44 Years Currently in Union Who or Whose Partners Have Had a Sterilization Operation, by Age and Selected Socioeconomic Characteristics (General Social Survey 1990)

	Age of female respondent						
	15-24		25-34		35-44		15-44
Characteristic	N	%	N	%	N	%	%
Region of residence							
Atlantic provinces	27	0.0	94	35.1	94	71.3	46.8
Quebec	86	5.8	321	26.2	251	67.3	39.0
Ontario	84	6.0	367	19.6	352	51.7	31.7
Manitoba and							
Saskatchewan	23	0.0	89	28.1	71	66.2	39.8
Alberta	28	14.3*	120	18.3	104	64.4	36.7
British Columbia	15	6.7*	130	19.2	126	60.3	38.2
Religion							
Catholic	132	6.8	546	24.2	483	61.3	37.5
Protestant	79	6.3	437	23.8	396	63.4	39.5
Other or no religion	47	2.1*	170	17.1	131	47.3	26.1
Church attendance							
At least once a week or							
at least once a month	70	5.7*	364	25.3	421	60.1	41.0
At least once a year or							
a few times a year	97	8.2	384	22.1	253	58.1	32.6
Not at all	58	6.9	271	22.1	244	64.8	38.8
Status							
Native born	234	6.0	983	25.0	794	66.2	39.1
Foreign born	28	7.1*	167	12.0	209	39.2	26.0
Ethnicity**							
British	117	6.0	556	22.5	460	66.3	39.2
French	112	6.3	367	30.8	322	69.6	42.9
Other European	68	4.4	329	18.2	309	52.8	32.1
Non-European	13	0.0	76	11.8	67	22.4	15.4

Table 16. *(cont'd)*

| Characteristic | Age of female respondent | | | | | | |
| | 15-24 | | 25-34 | | 35-44 | | 15-44 |
	N	%	N	%	N	%	%
Education							
Some high school or less	58	8.6	187	38.0	201	71.6	49.1
High school or diploma							
completed	102	8.8	459	25.1	385	63.6	39.0
Some university	102	1.0*	511	16.0	431	51.5	29.1
Total	263	6.1	1 162	23.1	1 021	60.4	36.8

*   Based on fewer than five cases.
** Subgroup total is greater than grand total due to multiple responses on ethnicity. Other subgroup totals may not add to grand total due to item non-response.

Protestants are more likely to be sterilized than other religious groups. In the Canadian Fertility Survey, the proportion of women who (or whose partners) had been sterilized was 50.7% among Protestants compared with 45.1% among Catholics. The proportion was much lower among other or non-religious groups at 36.8%. This pattern was noticeable in all age groups. It was also confirmed in the General Survey Social sample.

As far as religiosity (measured by church attendance) is concerned, the pattern is far from uniform within age groups. In the Canadian Fertility Survey, while in the 25-34 age group religiosity is positively associated with sterilization, in all the other age groups it is negatively associated. The reason for this reversal is not clear. The relationship between church attendance and sterilization is even weaker in the General Social Survey. One should be cautious with these interpretations as it is necessary to have proper controls before arriving at firm conclusions.

Native-born Canadians are more likely to be sterilized than immigrants. This is evident in both samples, but more so in the General Social Survey sample. In the Canadian Fertility Survey, 46.4% of native-born women reported that they or their partners had been sterilized compared with 42.6% of foreign-born women. The corresponding figures from the General Social Survey women were 39.1 and 26.0% respectively. The substantially higher incidence of sterilization among native-born women is also evident among the various age groups. Many immigrants come from cultures where the norms related to sterilization and vasectomy are different from those in Canada.

A breakdown by broad ethnic categories indicates that there is not much difference between the British and the French. In the Canadian Fertility Survey, the proportion sterilized among the British was 50.0% compared with 47.5% among the French. In the General Social Survey, the proportion sterilized among the French was slightly higher than among the British at 42.9 and 39.2% respectively. Other ethnic groups have much lower sterilization rates, especially non-European ethnic groups. Because the General Social Survey allowed multiple responses, comparisons between the two surveys are less than ideal.

Education has a strong negative relationship on sterilization. Those who are more educated are much less likely to resort to an irreversible operation, such as tubal ligation or vasectomy, to prevent unwanted pregnancies. In the Canadian Fertility Survey, among women who had at least some university education only 35.5% reported sterilization, whereas among those women with some high school or less education the proportion was 59.1%. The corresponding figures from the General Social Survey are 29.1 and 49.1% respectively. The higher incidence of sterilization among the least-educated group is clearly due to the fact that more of the older women are likely to be less educated than the younger women. Therefore, it is important to control this characteristic for age. Considerable differences can be noticed across age groups. Among those 35 years and older, the difference is present but not too great in the Canadian Fertility Survey sample. For example, among those aged 35-44 with less than 12 years of schooling, the proportion sterilized is 76.4% compared with 64.3% for those with some university education. In the General Social Survey data, however, this difference is significant, i.e., 71.6 and 51.5%. In the 25-34 age group the corresponding figures from the Canadian Fertility Survey are 47.3 and 17.2% respectively. Thus, it can be inferred that those with higher education resort to sterilization in fewer numbers and later in life than those with less education.

In summary, it can be concluded that the most important factors related to sterilization are age and number of children, and only to a much lesser degree such factors as education, ethnicity, and religion.

Canada-U.S. Comparisons in Surgical Sterilizations

Table 17 presents information on the proportion of currently married women respondents in the General Social Survey, Canadian Fertility Survey, and the U.S. National Survey of Family Growth who report that they or their husbands have had a sterilization operation. The data indicate that the incidence of sterilization in Canada is not very different from that in the United States. The U.S. data show that the greatest increase in sterilization for all age groups occurred during the period 1976-1982, with much smaller changes taking place during the 1982-1988 period (Mosher and Pratt 1990b). The overall rate of sterilization increased from 28.1% in 1976 to 38.9% in 1982 and 42.4% in 1988. Of course, rates have to slow down at the higher levels. The Canadian rate, as derived from the Canadian Fertility Survey, is slightly higher than that derived for the United States; the General Social Survey rate, on the other hand, is somewhat lower than the 1988 figure for the United States. Among currently married women aged 18-44 years in Canada, the Canadian Fertility Survey estimate of the proportion of sterilization was 45.6% compared with an estimate of 41.2% based upon the General Social Survey. The U.S. rate for 1988 fell in between these values at 42.4% for women between 15 and 44.

Table 17. Percentage of Currently Married Women (or Their Husbands) Who Are Surgically Sterile in Canada and the United States, by Age

	Canada		United States (NSFG)		
Age of woman	GSS 1990	CFS 1984	1988	1982	1976
15-24	8.9		6.0	7.2	3.9
18-24		7.0			
25-34	25.4	32.6	31.1	31.6	25.9
35-44	61.6	70.3	65.1	62.0	47.0
45-49		69.0			
18-49		48.7			
18-44	41.2	45.6			
15-44	41.0		42.4	38.9	28.1

Contraceptive Use*

An investigation of contraceptive use is an integral part of any study on infertility in a society such as Canada's for a number of reasons. First, contraception is widely used in Canada not only to limit family size but also to space children. Thus, contraception is widely used even before the birth of the first child and between first and second births. Some of the women using contraception may be infertile but may not know it. If all contraceptive users are treated as being fertile, one runs the risk of underestimating levels of infertility. The extent of contraceptive use and

---

* Much of this section has been published earlier in Balakrishnan et al. (1985).

the actual methods used, therefore, become relevant in any study on infertility.

One of the main purposes of the Canadian Fertility Survey was to ascertain the extent to which contraception is practised in Canada. Therefore, a great number of the survey's questions focussed on this topic. In contrast, no data were gathered on contraceptive use in the General Social Survey. As such, the discussion presented here will be based on Canadian Fertility Survey data and some comparisons with U.S. data.

Contraceptive status (including male and female sterilization) was measured at the time of the interview. If a woman was using more than one method of birth control, the most effective method was considered to be her current method. The hierarchy of effectiveness was based on the use of the following methods of contraception: female sterilization, male sterilization, birth control pill, intrauterine device (IUD), diaphragm, condom, foam, rhythm, and withdrawal. If both the woman and her husband or partner had been surgically sterilized, only the woman's procedure was counted in the contraceptive use estimates. This method was used in the U.S. surveys as well.

As shown in Table 18, among all Canadian women aged 18-49 years in 1984, 68% reported that they were practising birth control at the time of the interview. A further 9% were pregnant, post-partum, or seeking pregnancy, and 7% were non-contraceptively sterile. Fifteen percent were non-users. Table 18 reveals large differences in contraceptive prevalence by the woman's marital status. Currently married women show the highest overall level of use (73%), followed by previously married women (69%) and those who have never married (57%). Moreover, only 5% of currently married women are not using some method of birth control. The high level of contraceptive use among previously married women can be explained largely by the fact that these women are somewhat older than those who are married or who have never married and, therefore, are more likely to have been contraceptively sterilized while they were still married. Thirty-six percent of previously married women and 29% of currently married women were 40 years of age or older. Similarly, the higher average age of previously married women also helps account for the fact that these women reported a higher incidence of non-contraceptive sterility (mostly hysterectomy) than the other groups.

Levels of contraceptive use among single cohabiting women are high in Canada (83%), and even somewhat higher than the level reported among previously married women who are now living with a partner (79%). An interesting observation is that women in cohabiting unions have much higher levels of contraceptive use than women who are legally married. The levels of contraceptive use among single women who are not cohabiting (51%) suggest that at least half of the women in this group are sexually active. This finding indicates that there is no longer any justification for excluding single women from contraceptive prevalence surveys.

Table 18.   Percent Distribution of Women in Their Reproductive Years (18-49), by Current Contraceptive Status and Marital Status, Canada, 1984

	Total	Never married			Currently married	Separated, divorced, widowed		
		Total	In cohabitation	Not in cohabitation		Total	In cohabitation	Not in cohabitation
Number of women (sample)	5 315	1 431	289	1 142	3 283	601	162	439
Contraceptive users	68.4	57.4	83.1	50.8	73.1	68.8	78.9	65.2
Pregnant, post-partum, or seeking pregnancy	9.2	3.0	11.0	1.0	13.0	3.2	8.7	1.1*
Non-contraceptively sterile	7.0	1.5	1.4*	1.7	8.7	10.6	11.2	10.2
Non-users	15.4	38.1	4.5	46.6	5.2	17.4	1.2*	23.4
Total	100.0	100.0	100.0	100.0	100.0	100.0	100.0	100.0

* Denotes percentages with relative standard errors of 0.03 or more.

Note: Percentages may not add to 100.0 due to rounding.

Table 19 summarizes patterns of contraceptive use by method. The leading method in Canada — accounting for almost half of all use — is sterilization, both male and female. Birth control pills are the second most widely used method, accounting for 28% of all use, followed by the condom (9%) and the IUD (8%). The use of other methods is so low that they tend to be of no importance.

As Table 19 and Figure 9 illustrate, there are considerable differences between women who have never married and those women who are currently married in terms of the method of contraception used. Never-married women predominantly rely on the birth control pill (71%), whereas married women overwhelmingly rely on sterilization (59%, including vasectomies on spouses). The birth control pill, condom, and IUD are used considerably less among married women as ways of avoiding pregnancy (15%, 11%, and 8% respectively). Much of this pattern among currently married women, when compared with that among single women, is, of course, a function of the differing age structure of the two groups. The finding that a large proportion of married women resort to sterilization is consistent with the conclusions of an earlier study carried out in Quebec (Lapierre-Adamcyk and Marcil-Gratton 1981) and reflects the fact that many of these women have already had as many children as they want. The high level of female sterilization among previously married women reflects this same relationship. Reliance on male contraception methods (vasectomy and the condom) is, as one might expect, lower among separated, divorced, and widowed women than among those still living with their husbands.

Differentials in Contraceptive Use

Levels of contraceptive use according to method and selected background characteristics are presented in Table 20 for currently married women. Because cohabiting women behave very differently from married women with respect to contraceptive use, it was considered inadvisable to group them together. The data presented in Table 20 support the finding that a woman's age is by far the most important determinant in her choice of a contraceptive method. For example, among all currently married women, the proportion of contraceptive users who become contraceptively sterilized increases sharply after the age of 30; by age 30-34, 37% of users have undergone a tubal ligation, and by age 45-49, this proportion has climbed to 65%. If the incidence of vasectomy is also included, 85% of women in the 40-44 age group rely on sterilization to prevent pregnancy. Even among the 35-39 age group, combined male and female sterilization constitutes more than two-thirds of all contraceptive use. Correspondingly, reliance on the birth control pill among older women almost disappears, with only 2% of contraceptive users in 40-44 age group depending on this method. Even among women aged 30-34, use of the birth control pill

Table 19. Percent Distribution of Women in Their Reproductive Years (18-49) Practising Contraception, by Current Method and Marital Status, Canada, 1984

	Total	Never married			Currently married	Separated, divorced, widowed		
		Total	In cohabitation	Not in cohabitation		Total	In cohabitation	Not in cohabitation
Number of women	5 315	1 431	289	1 142	3 283	601	162	439
Number of users (sample)	3 635	821	241	580	2 400	414	128	286
			Distribution of users					
Female sterilization	35.3	4.3	4.1	4.3	41.8	59.7	53.5	62.4
Male sterilization	12.7	1.7	3.3*	1.0*	17.6	6.3	11.8	4.2
Birth control pill	28.0	71.2	66.0	73.4	15.0	17.4	16.5	17.8
IUD	8.3	7.9	9.5	7.2	8.0	10.6	11.0	10.5
Diaphragm	1.7	2.8	2.1*	3.1	1.4	1.2*	3.9*	0.0
Condom	9.1	7.9	9.1	7.4	10.8	2.2*	1.6*	2.1*
Foam	0.8	0.4*	0.4*	0.3*	0.7	2.2*	0.8*	2.8*
Rhythm	2.3	1.7	2.1*	1.4*	3.0	0.2*	0.0	0.3*
Withdrawal	1.2	1.3*	2.9*	0.7*	1.3	0.2*	0.8*	0.3*
Other	0.6	0.9*	0.4*	1.0*	0.6	0.0	0.0	0.0
Total	100.0	100.0	100.0	100.0	100.0	100.0	100.0	100.0

* Denotes percentage with relative standard errors of 0.03 or more.

Note: Percentages may not add to 100.0 due to rounding.

Figure 9. Types of Contraception Used Among Currently Married Couples (Canadian Fertility Survey 1984)

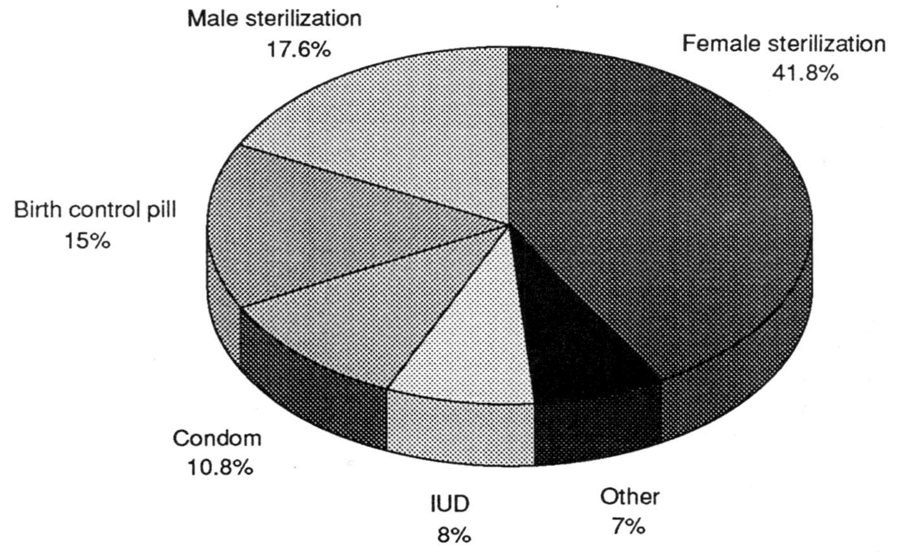

Female sterilization
41.8%

Male sterilization
17.6%

Birth control pill
15%

Condom
10.8%

IUD
8%

Other
7%

Note: Percentage totals may not add to 100.0 due to rounding.

amounts to only 13% of all contraceptive use. It is clear, then, that the birth control pill is now used in Canada only, for the most part, during the early years of a woman's reproductive life.

Table 20 indicates that 76% of all currently married women do not expect to have any more children (excluding the current pregnancy). Among these women, overall contraceptive use is very high (79%). Moreover, among users who do not expect to have any more children, 71% are protected against pregnancy by female or male sterilization.

The traditional differences observed between Catholics and Protestants have all but disappeared in Canada. Table 20 reveals that 72% of Catholics and 74% of Protestants were using some form of contraception at the time of the survey and that their choices of methods were remarkably similar. For example, 42% of female Catholic contraceptive users had been sterilized compared with 44% of female Protestant users.   No appreciable Catholic/Protestant differences could be seen in the use of vasectomies, the birth control pill, the IUD, or the condom. Moreover, the rhythm method, once widely relied upon by Catholics, accounts for only 3% of current use among Catholics compared with 1% among Protestants.   In fact, the differences found in the use of various methods between Catholics and Protestants are less than the differences observed between either of these two groups and other religious groups.

However, religiosity, as measured by church attendance, does appear to be associated with some differentials in contraceptive use. Married women who go to church at least once a week have lower overall levels of contraceptive use (69%) than women who attend church less often (74-75%). In addition, regular churchgoers report higher rates of sterilization and lower levels of birth control pill use than those who do not attend church regularly.

Wide differentials in the use of various contraception methods are found based upon educational level. Women with 8 years or less of schooling report the lowest overall level of contraceptive use (65%) and appear to depend heavily on tubal ligation (71% of all users in this educational level). The proportion sterilized among all users then decreases with rising levels of education, 50% among those with 9-11 years of schooling, 37% among women who attended school for 12-13 years, and 33% among those with 14 years or more of schooling. In contrast, use of the IUD and the condom rises with increased education and use of the birth control pill reaches its peak level among high school graduates. However, a strong relationship between educational level and method of contraception used cannot be inferred in the absence of controls for age. A long-term secular trend everywhere is for young women to be more educated than their older counterparts.   Therefore, the higher level of sterilization seen among less-educated women is due partly to the fact that older women are heavily represented in this group. A multivariate analysis is necessary to clarify these relationships.

Table 20. Contraceptive Use Among Currently Married Women, by Method and Selected Characteristics

Characteristic	Total number of women	Percentage using contraception	Total	Female sterilization	Male sterilization	Birth control pill	IUD	Condom	Other
							Percent distribution of users		
All women	3 283	73.1	100.0	41.8	17.6	15.0	8.0	10.8	7.0
Age group									
18-24	326	61.3	100.0	6.0	4.0	58.5	10.5	14.5	6.5
25-29	645	68.2	100.0	18.4	10.2	33.0	10.9	16.1	11.4
30-34	679	75.4	100.0	36.5	20.1	13.1	12.9	11.3	6.2
35-39	663	81.4	100.0	53.1	20.7	4.1	7.8	8.5	5.7
40-44	513	78.0	100.0	58.5	26.0	2.0	2.8	5.5	5.3
45-49	457	68.1	100.0	65.0	16.4	0.3	1.6	10.6	6.1
Children									
Expect more	761	53.2	100.0	0.0	0.0	49.0	12.5	23.0	15.5
Expect no more	2 509	79.4	100.0	50.2	21.2	8.1	7.1	8.1	5.3
Religious affiliation									
Catholic	1 544	72.2	100.0	42.2	17.4	16.2	7.8	8.8	7.6
Protestant	1 224	74.4	100.0	44.1	19.4	13.6	7.4	10.2	5.4
Other and no religion	511	73.6	100.0	34.4	13.8	14.8	10.1	18.0	9.0

Table 20. (cont'd)

Characteristic	Total number of women	Percentage using contraception	Total	Percent distribution of users					
				Female sterilization	Male sterilization	Birth control pill	IUD	Condom	Other
Church attendance									
Weekly	1 017	69.4	100.0	46.1	17.2	9.9	6.0	10.9	9.9
Sometimes	1 277	75.2	100.0	40.9	16.7	17.6	8.4	10.8	5.6
Rarely or never	985	74.3	100.0	38.6	19.2	16.6	9.4	10.5	5.6
Education									
8 years or less	296	64.9	100.0	71.0	11.9	7.3	2.6	4.7	2.5
9-11 years	810	73.1	100.0	50.3	22.1	11.5	5.2	5.9	5.0
12-13 years	1 174	73.8	100.0	37.0	19.0	19.0	8.1	10.1	6.8
14 years or more	1 003	74.8	100.0	32.6	13.8	15.2	11.5	16.8	10.1
Status									
Native born	2 751	73.3	100.0	42.0	18.3	16.3	8.2	9.2	6.0
Foreign born	532	72.4	100.0	40.5	14.0	8.6	7.0	18.7	11.2

Note: Subgroup totals may not add to total due to item non-response. Percentage totals may not add to 100.0 due to rounding.

A substantial portion of the Canadian population is made up of foreign-born residents. In the Canadian Fertility Survey sample, 16% of all currently married women were born outside Canada. During the last two decades, the countries of origin of immigrants to Canada have changed dramatically. A larger proportion are now coming from Asia and developing countries in other continents than from Western Europe, and this factor probably accounts for the somewhat different patterns of contraceptive use observed among foreign-born women and native-born women. Although overall levels of contraceptive use and the proportions relying on sterilization do not differ greatly, use of the birth control pill is much lower among foreign-born women than among native-born women (9% versus 16%) and condom use is much higher among foreign-born women (19% versus 9%).

Table 21 presents findings on contraceptive use among all unmarried women (never married and previously married) based upon age and religion. Because women who have never married tend to be concentrated among the younger age groups and previously married women among the older age groups, the age groups have been collapsed in this table into three categories: 18-24, 25-34, and 35-49. Two-thirds of single women fall into the 18-24 age group. Of these, 17% reported that they were living with a partner (cohabiting). Even if these cohabitants were removed from the denominator and the numerator, contraceptive prevalence among single women is as high as 49%. Eighty-four percent of single women aged 18-24 years and practising contraception use the birth control pill, whereas only 6% rely on the condom. Birth control pill use decreases with age, even among single women. However, because most single women are relatively young, the birth control pill is the dominant contraceptive used (71% of all use). The data presented in Table 21 reveal virtually no differences based upon religion in the contraceptive methods used by single women.

Except for patterns of use of male contraception methods and a somewhat higher recourse to female sterilization among previously married women, the use of birth control methods among previously married women is very similar to that observed among currently married women. As might be expected, very small proportions of previously married women rely on vasectomy or the condom. However, in the absence of any information on sexual activity, it is not possible to infer whether this pattern is a result of a preferred method of contraception or whether it stems from the fact that these women are not involved in a sexual relationship.

Canada-U.S. Comparisons in Contraceptive Status and Method Used

Current contraceptive status and percent distribution of methods used by currently married women based on the Canadian Fertility Survey and the U.S. National Survey of Family Growth are compared in Table 22 (Mosher and Pratt 1990a). The main observation is that Canadian women behave in a similar manner to their U.S. counterparts. Overall contraceptive use is almost identical. There is a slightly higher prevalence of surgical sterilization in Canada, which is compensated for by somewhat lower use of non-surgical methods. Once women who are not using contraception because they want to become pregnant are excluded, the proportion of non-users is only 4.6% in Canada, very close to the 1988 figure of 4.8% in the United States.

The proportion of non-surgically sterile women aged 18-44 years in the Canadian Fertility Survey is 2.4%. This crude measure of infertility is not significantly different from the 1.6% in the 1988 U.S. survey when one takes into account the nuances in the wording of the survey questions.

Regarding the use of particular contraception methods, certain differences are worth noting. The IUD is much more popular in Canada, the proportion of users being 6.6% compared with only 1.5% in the United States. On the other hand, the diaphragm is used much less in Canada than in the United States.

Conclusion

In societies such as Canada's, where there is almost universal use of contraceptives, it is very difficult to estimate the prevalence of infertility because most women cannot be observed for long enough periods of continuous exposure to the risk of pregnancy. One is often forced to depend upon the respondents' perception of their infertility. In this report, an attempt has been made to estimate infertility not only by this direct perception but also by indirectly inferring infertility by calculating the proportion of women who failed to become pregnant over a specified period, such as 24 or 36 months. This was possible using the Canadian Fertility Survey because sufficient information was available on contraceptive and pregnancy histories.

A crucial finding was that a one-to-one correspondence between perceived infertility and inferred infertility does not exist. Women fall into both categories, or only into one or the other. A combined measure of perceived and/or inferred infertility, therefore, is constructed as the upper limit of infertility. All measures increase with age, but perceived infertility is more strongly correlated with age, and there is a substantial difference by parity between perceived and inferred infertility.

Is infertility increasing in Canada and should it be a cause for concern? Without conducting identical studies over a period of time, something that has not been done in Canada, one cannot answer these

Table 21. Contraceptive Use Among Unmarried Women, by Method and Selected Characteristics

Characteristic	Total number of women	Percentage using contraception	Percent distribution of users						
			Total	Female sterilization	Male sterilization	Birth control pill	IUD	Condom	Other
Never married									
All women	1 431	57.4	100.0	4.3	1.7	71.2	7.9	7.9	7.0
Age group									
18-24	961	55.1	100.0	0.4*	0.8*	84.1	4.2	5.9	4.6
25-34	369	66.9	100.0	7.4	3.7	51.4	14.0	12.8	10.7
35-49	101	49.5	100.0	32.0	2.0*	24.0	18.0	6.0*	18.0
Religious affiliation									
Catholic	752	57.2	100.0	5.3	1.6	68.9	7.9	7.9	8.4
Protestant	428	60.5	100.0	2.7	2.3	74.5	8.1	8.1	4.3
Other and no religion	246	51.6	100.0	3.9	0.8*	74.0	7.8	7.1	6.4
Separated, widowed, divorced									
All women	601	68.8	100.0	59.7	6.3	17.4	10.6	2.2	3.8
Age group									
18-24	37	59.5	100.0	9.0	0.0*	59.1	27.3	4.5	0.0
25-34	217	75.1	100.0	43.6	7.4	27.0	14.1	3.7	4.2
35-49	347	66.3	100.0	76.1	6.1	6.5	6.5	0.4	4.4

Table 21. *(cont'd)*

Separated, widowed, divorced

Characteristic	Total number of women	Percentage using contraception	Total	Percent distribution of users					
				Female sterilization	Male sterilization	Birth control pill	IUD	Condom	Other
Religious affiliation									
Catholic	252	67.1	100.0	58.0	4.7	21.9	10.1	1.8	3.6
Protestant	219	73.5	100.0	64.0	7.5	14.3	8.7	0.6	5.0
Other and no religion	129	65.1	100.0	53.6	7.1	14.3	15.5	6.0	3.6

* Fewer than five women in the category.

Note: Percentages may not add to 100.0 due to rounding. Subgroup totals might not add to grand total due to item non-response.

Table 22. Percent Distribution of Currently Married Women in Their Reproductive Years, by Current Contraceptive Status and Method Used, Canada and the United States

Contraceptive status	Canada (CFS 1984) Age		United States (NSFG) Age		
	18-49	18-44	15-44 (1988)	15-44 (1982)	15-44 (1973)
Total	100.0	100.0	100.0	100.0	100.0
Sterile	52.1	47.7	44.0	40.9	23.9
Surgically sterile	49.2	45.9	42.4	38.9	22.9
Contraceptively sterile	43.4	41.4	36.2	29.5	16.4
Female	30.5	28.3	23.4	18.7	8.6
Male	12.9	13.1	12.9	10.8	7.8
Non-contraceptively sterile	5.2	3.9	6.1	9.3	6.5
Female	5.2	3.9	6.1	8.7	6.3
Male	0.0	0.0	0.0	0.6	0.2
Non-surgically sterile	3.5	2.4	1.6	2.0	0.9
Pregnant or post-partum	6.8	7.9	7.1	7.2	7.3
Seeking pregnancy	6.2	7.3	6.0	6.7	7.0
Non-user	5.1	4.6	4.8	5.0	8.7
Non-surgical contraception	29.7	32.5	38.1	40.1	53.2
Birth control pill	11.0	12.7	15.1	13.4	25.1
IUD	5.8	6.6	1.5	4.8	6.7
Diaphragm	1.0	1.2	4.6	4.5	2.4
Condom	7.9	8.0	10.6	9.8	9.4
Foam	0.5	0.5	1.0	2.0	3.5
Periodic abstinence	-	-	2.1	3.2	2.8
Rhythm	2.2	2.2	-	-	-
Withdrawal, douche, and other	-	-	3.2	2.3	3.4
Withdrawal	0.9	0.9	-	-	-
Other	0.4	0.4	-	-	-

Note: Percentages may not exactly add to totals due to rounding.

, questions. Though they are hardly comparable, the estimates of perceived infertility from the 1984 Canadian Fertility Survey and the 1990 General Social Survey do not show any upward trend. What is significant is that in both surveys, among women under 30 years of age, less than 2% report problems of infertility. In the Canadian Fertility Survey, even including inferred infertility, the estimate of aggregate infertility among these young women is less than 5%. The prevalence of infertility increases with age from 6.4% among women aged 30-39 to 9.5% among women over 40 years of age. Because the survey questions on infertility were not asked of all women and because the questions were not exhaustive, actual infertility rates may be somewhat higher than the estimates presented here. In Canada, over the last two decades, many women have delayed marriage and childbearing, which invariably results in an increasing incidence of infertility.

Bibliography

Balakrishnan, T.R., K.J. Krótki, and E. Lapierre-Adamcyk. 1985. "Contraceptive Use in Canada, 1984." *Family Planning Perspectives* 17: 209-15.

Balakrishnan, T.R., E. Lapierre-Adamcyk, and K.J. Krótki. 1993. *Family and Childbearing in Canada: A Demographic Analysis*. Toronto: University of Toronto Press.

Canada. Statistics Canada. 1991. *General Social Survey, Cycle 5: Family and Friends*. [Microdata file.] Ottawa: Statistics Canada.

Lapierre-Adamcyk, E., and N. Marcil-Gratton. 1981. *La stérilisation au Québec 1971-1979: Rapport de recherche, 1979-1981: Première phase*. Montreal: Université de Montréal, Département de démographie.

Larsen, U., and J. Menken. 1989. "Measuring Sterility from Incomplete Birth Histories." *Demography* 26: 185-201.

Léridon, H. 1991. "Stérilité et hypofertilité: du silence à l'impatience?" *Population* 46: 225-47.

Mosher, W.D. 1985. "Reproductive Impairments in the United States, 1965-1982." *Demography* 22: 415-30.

Mosher, W.D., and W.F. Pratt. 1990a. *Contraceptive Use in the United States, 1973-88*. Advance Data from Vital and Health Statistics of the National Center for Health Statistics, No. 182. Hyattsville: U.S. Department of Health and Human Services.

—. 1990b. *Fecundity and Infertility in the United States, 1965-88*. Advance Data from Vital and Health Statistics of the National Center for Health Statistics, No. 192. Hyattsville: U.S. Department of Health and Human Services.

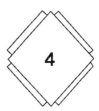

4

Infertility, Sterilization, and Contraceptive Use in Ontario

T.R. Balakrishnan and Paul Maxim

Executive Summary

This study analyzed data from a survey of general health in Ontario conducted in 1990, in order to quantify the extent of infertility and contraceptive use in the province. A sample of women aged 16-49 who were married and/or living with a partner at the time of the survey was selected for in-depth analysis. Based on their answers to a self-completed questionnaire, attempts were made to classify the women in the sample as infertile, surgically sterile, or fertile. The data are broken down by age and parity, and where possible by education and birthplace of the respondent.

To assess infertility, a distinction was made between women who perceive themselves as infertile (perceived infertility), women who are inferred to be infertile based on exposure to unprotected coitus with no resultant pregnancy (inferred infertility), and women who are classified as inferred infertile and/or perceived infertile (aggregate infertility). It is suggested that the latter is an upper limit of the estimate of infertility.

Among those aged 18-44, for all parities, sample results indicated a perceived infertility rate of 2.9%, an inferred fertility rate of 5.7%, and an aggregate infertility rate of 6.7%. Results also indicated that the rate of sterilization is very high in Canada and increases with age. Further, sterilization and the woman's education were found to be negatively

This paper was completed for the Royal Commission on New Reproductive Technologies in May 1992.

related, and the rate was lower among women born in Europe (outside the United Kingdom) and Asia. In general, contraceptive use is very high in Ontario — only 6.5% of married/cohabiting women aged 18-44 reported not using any birth control. After sterilization, the pill is the most widely used method, followed by condoms. Age and birthplace are important factors in determining which kind of contraceptive is used: the pill is the favourite method among younger women born in Canada, the United States, and the United Kingdom, but condoms are more widely used among younger women born in Asia.

Introduction

The objectives of this study were to measure the prevalence of infertility in Ontario and examine some of its sociodemographic correlates, to measure the prevalence of surgical sterilization among couples in Ontario and examine some of its sociodemographic correlates, and to analyze contraceptive use among couples in Ontario.

We analyzed data from the 1990 Ontario Health Survey (OHS) on infertility, sterilization, and contraceptive use among couples who were legally married or cohabiting at the time of the survey, and where the female partner was of reproductive age. Because the main focus of the survey was health and not fertility or family planning per se, it includes only a limited number of questions on these topics. The extent of our analysis, therefore, is dictated by this restriction.

Survey Method[1]

The 1990 OHS is a multi-purpose survey designed to collect baseline data on the health status, health determinants, and health-related attitudes of people in Ontario.[2] The content of the survey draws heavily from existing surveys, including the Canada Health Survey (CHS), the General Social Survey (GSS), and the Quebec Survey. Ancillary questions were composed by consultants and advisors from the provincial government and the private sector.

The data were collected through two procedures — a personal interview with a "knowledgeable household member," which provided demographic data, and a self-completed form that was left with household members aged 12 and over. Section J, on women's sexual health, was to be completed only by women aged 16 and over. The primary data for the present study were the self-completed questionnaires.

Sample Design

The target population for the OHS consisted of people who lived in private dwellings and who had resided in Ontario during the survey period of January through December, 1990.[3] For the self-completed questionnaire, the target population was restricted to those aged 12 years and over. The subsections dealing with sexual health were further restricted to individuals aged 16 years and older, with questions relating to women's health restricted to women.

The sample design employed was a multi-stage, stratified cluster sample. The province was initially stratified geographically according to the boundaries of 42 public health units (PHUs). Each PHU was stratified on a rural/urban basis, with the urban stratum defined as enumeration areas encompassed in a census metropolitan area (CMA) or census agglomeration and the rural stratum defined as any residual or non-urban enumeration areas. Enumeration areas and dwelling units within them were selected at random based on the 1986 census. Ultimately, 35 650 dwelling units were selected.

Because of the design of the survey and the extent of non-response, the survey is not self-weighting. Thus, all analyses of the data for this study are based on weighted observations. Base weights for the survey are related to the inverse of the probability of selecting a particular dwelling unit within an enumeration area for the rural and urban strata and the PHU. Adjustments were later made for non-response and to correct for PHU-age-sex groupings based on the 1986 census.

The overall response rate for the interviewer portion of the survey was 88%; for the self-completed portion it was reported to be 76%. Since not all the survey participants responded to all the questions (on questions relating to contraceptive use, for example, the response rate was approximately 84%), there was considerable variability in the level of coverage of particular items.

Since our focus is on women of childbearing age, we initially subdivided the data to include only women between the ages of 16 and 49. This resulted in a sample of 16 219 women. We then further narrowed the sample to include only women "at risk" — that is, women who were married and/or living with a partner.[4] This produced a sample of 7 765 women.

Infertility

Infertility can be measured using direct questions, or it can be measured indirectly using questions on contraception, marriage, and pregnancy. In the former approach, women (or couples) are asked about their perception of their infertility: whether they can get pregnant and whether they have a problem in conceiving or delivering a baby (Mosher 1985; Joffe 1989; Léridon 1991). Estimating the proportion of infertile couples is then a simple matter of relating the answers (the numerator) to a relevant population base (the denominator). We will refer to this measure as *perceived infertility*.

Indirect methods use the information obtained on pregnancy and birth histories in relation to exposure history to arrive at a plausible estimate of infertility. One can define as infertile those women who, after continuous exposure, did not get pregnant after a fixed period of time — 12 months, for example. The strategy, then, is to identify women who are not using contraception at the time of the survey and follow them back one year to determine whether they were continuously exposed to risk, did not use contraception, and did not get pregnant during this period. We will refer to this measure as *inferred infertility*.

It is possible that some women who perceive themselves to be infertile may not be inferred infertile and vice versa. Therefore, we constructed a third measure — *aggregate infertility* — to denote those who are perceived infertile and/or those who are inferred infertile. The highest estimate of infertility will therefore be this aggregate measure.

Perceived Infertility

Perceived infertility is measured solely on the basis of whether or not the respondent believes that she or her partner is incapable of having children. This knowledge could be based on a number of factors, such as a formal medical diagnosis, long-term experience with unprotected coitus, or simply a hunch. The indicator of perceived infertility in the OHS was question F5Q95:

Q. Since you are not using a contraceptive method at present, which of the following best describes your situation?
1. You or your partner are past childbearing age
2. You want to become a parent
3. You or your partner are unable to have children
4. Other _____(specify)

Respondents who chose option three were considered to perceive themselves as infertile.

This question is less than ideal, of course, since it self-selects those who do not use contraceptives. Optimally, it should have been asked of all women, both those who use and those who do not use contraceptives. The selective phrasing of the question undoubtedly meant that perceived infertility and actual infertility (to the extent that perceived infertility proxies actual infertility) were underestimated. This fact should be kept in mind when these data are compared with results from surveys — particularly U.S. surveys — that ask questions about perceived infertility of all women.[5]

In total, 248 women perceived themselves as unable to have children. Since there is some ambiguity as to what the appropriate denominator for this count ought to be, we estimated rates of perceived infertility using different base populations (Table 1). If all women at risk in our subsample are considered, the proportion of perceived infertility is 3.19%. Excluding women who have been sterilized, the proportion is higher, at 5.55%. It is 8.10% when pregnant and post-partum mothers are excluded, and reaches a level of 51.35% when contraceptive users are excluded.

Perceived infertility is broken down by parity and age in Table 2 and Figure 1. The base is all women at risk (i.e., those aged 16-49, married and/or living with a partner).

Table 1. Perceived Infertility in Various Populations at Risk, Ontario, 1990

Population at risk	N	Perceived infertile %
All women in union	7 765	3.19
Women in union, not sterilized	4 467	5.55
Women in union, not sterilized, not pregnant, not post-partum mothers	3 061	8.10
Women in union, not sterilized, not pregnant, not post-partum mothers, and not using contraception in year before survey	483	51.35

Source: Ontario Health Survey, 1990.

There are age and parity gradients; perceived infertility is substantially higher among women with no children than among those with one child or more. Among the childless, perceived infertility is only 1.12% in the 16-29 age group, 8.14% in the 30-39 age group, and 15.00% in the 40-44 age group. The corresponding figures among women who had at least one child were 1.08%, 2.15%, and 5.23%, respectively.

Inferred Infertility

Inferred infertility is estimated by examining the exposure interval during which a woman has not become pregnant. Unlike the analyses of the Canadian Fertility Survey (CFS) and the GSS, the period of exposure examined in the OHS was limited to approximately 12 months. Women who reported that neither they nor their partner were sterilized, that they had not used any form of contraception in the year prior to the survey, and that they were not currently pregnant or post-partum mothers were inferred infertile.

Table 2. Perceived Infertility by Parity and Age, Ontario, 1990

	n	Base	Perceived infertile %
Parity 0			
16-29	10	893	1.12
30-39	32	393	8.14
40-44	15	100	15.00
45-49	19	69	27.54
16-44	58	1 387	4.18
16-49	76	1 456	5.22
18-44	58	1 384	4.19
18-49	76	1 453	5.23
Parity 1+			
16-29	12	1 114	1.08
30-39	62	2 882	2.15
40-44	66	1 262	5.23
45-49	31	892	3.48
16-44	140	5 257	2.66
16-49	172	6 149	2.79
18-44	140	5 254	2.66
18-49	172	6 146	2.80
All parities*			
16-29	22	2 053	1.07
30-39	95	3 358	2.83
40-44	82	1 381	5.94
45-49	50	974	5.13
16-44	198	6 804	2.91
16-49	248	7 765	3.19
18-44	198	6 798	2.91
18-49	248	7 759	3.20

* Differences between totals for all parities and sum of 0 and 1+ parities are due to non-response.

Source: Ontario Health Survey, 1990.

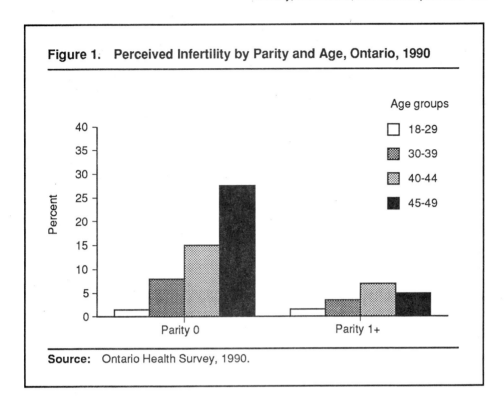

Figure 1. Perceived Infertility by Parity and Age, Ontario, 1990

Source: Ontario Health Survey, 1990.

Our attempt to classify women into three groups — infertile, surgically sterile, and fertile — relies on the responses to the following questions:

Q.93 In the past year what form of birth control did you or your partner(s) use?

	Yes	No
Condom		
Condom and foam		
Pills		
Diaphragm		
IUD		
Vasectomy and tubal ligation (tubes tied)		
Other_____		

Q.94 In the past year, how often did you or your partner(s) use some form of birth control?

Never
A few times
Often
Always

Unfortunately, these indicators of contraceptive use turned out to be less than ideal for a number of reasons. First, unlike the CFS, the OHS has no questions identifying the date that contraceptive use began. Second, with the exception of the global question (Q.94), respondents were not asked about the consistency with which they used the various types of birth control identified. The responses to Q.94 were often not consistent with the responses to the questions on forms of birth control used.

Third, it was not possible to determine which partner actually used which form of birth control. While self-evident for most methods, this was a particular problem for separating male and female surgical sterilization. Finally, the non-response rate for the birth control questions was extremely high — approximately 16% of all women considered to be at risk. Since the non-response rate was approximately two to three times some estimates of overall infertility rates, there is clearly considerable room for bias in some estimates.

For the sample of all women at risk (those aged 16-49), the uncorrected inferred infertility rate was 6.66%. Breakdowns for different age groups and parities are presented in Table 3 and Figure 2. There are, however, some factors that might influence the accuracy of the estimates. Beyond normal sampling error, the primary limitation of this aspect of the OHS is the high non-response rate of approximately 16% of the target sample. Initial analysis indicated that the two factors most likely related to differentials in infertility are age and parity; these variables were also strongly related to non-response rates. Consequently, we "corrected" the initial estimates of inferred infertility by standardizing the estimates on the age-parity distribution of the non-respondents. There are therefore two sets of estimates in Table 3 — "uncorrected" estimates, which ignore the issue of non-response, and "corrected" estimates, which correct for the differences between the age-parity distributions of the non-respondents and the respondents.

Correcting for the characteristics of the non-respondents slightly increases the absolute rates of inferred infertility. For women between the ages of 16 and 49 at all parities, the uncorrected proportion of infertile women was 6.22%; corrected, it was 6.66%. For the age groups 18-44 and 18-49, the uncorrected proportions of inferred infertility were 5.46% and 6.23%; corrected, they were 5.74% and 6.66%, respectively.

Regardless of the estimate used, however, inferred infertility increases with age, particularly for childless women. Overall, inferred infertility rates were twice as high among childless women as among women with at least one child. The corrected rates for the age category 18-44 show inferred infertility among childless women as 9.75%, compared with 4.35% among those with one or more children. Infertility steadily increases with age at all parities. However, the absolute increase is most dramatic among

Table 3. Inferred Infertility by Age and Parity, Ontario, 1990

	Uncorrected			Corrected		
	n	Base	%	n	Base	%
Parity 0						
16-29	49	893	5.49	53	974	5.44
30-39	56	393	14.25	70	492	14.23
40-44	23	100	23.00	36	158	22.78
45-49	22	69	31.88	36	113	31.86
16-44	128	1 387	9.23	159	1 624	9.79
16-49	150	1 456	10.30	195	1 737	11.23
18-44	127	1 384	9.18	158	1 620	9.75
18-49	149	1 453	10.25	194	1 733	11.19
Parity 1+						
16-29	32	1 114	2.87	34	1 195	2.85
30-39	113	2 882	3.92	129	3 311	3.90
40-44	82	1 262	6.49	101	1 558	6.48
45-49	89	892	9.98	124	1 241	9.99
16-44	228	5 257	4.34	264	6 064	4.35
16-49	315	6 149	5.12	388	7 305	5.31
18-44	228	5 254	4.34	264	6 064	4.35
18-49	315	6 146	5.12	388	7 301	5.31
All parities*						
16-29	86	2 053	4.19	95	2 241	4.24
30-39	178	3 358	5.30	216	3 893	5.55
40-44	107	1 381	7.75	142	1 763	8.05
45-49	112	974	11.45	164	1 370	11.98
16-44	371	6 804	5.45	453	7 897	5.74
16-49	483	7 765	6.22	617	9 267	6.66
18-44	371	6 798	5.46	453	7 891	5.74
18-49	483	7 759	6.23	617	9 261	6.66

* Differences between totals for all parities and sum of 0 and 1+ parities are due to non-response.

Source: Ontario Health Survey, 1990.

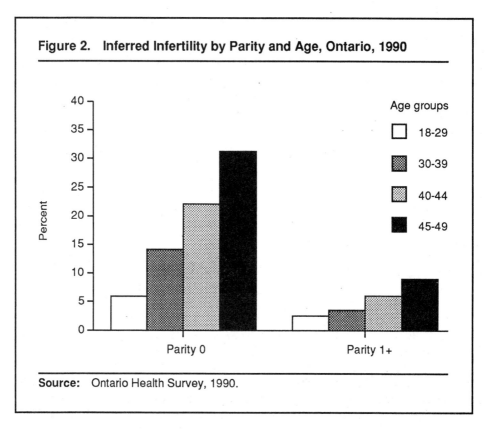

Figure 2. Inferred Infertility by Parity and Age, Ontario, 1990

Source: Ontario Health Survey, 1990.

childless women, where the rate is 5.44% in the 16-29 age group, 14.23% in the 30-39 age group, 22.78% in the 40-44 age group, and 31.86% in the 45-49 age group. The corresponding figures for women with at least one child are 2.85%, 3.90%, 6.48%, and 9.99%, respectively.

Aggregate Infertility

Aggregate infertility is defined as the combination of those who perceive themselves to be infertile and those who are inferred infertile. From the sample of women at risk, we estimate that 248 women perceive themselves to be infertile, whereas 483 women are inferred infertile. Of those two groups, only 130 women are classified as both inferred and perceived infertile. The groups can be broken down as follows:

Inferred infertile only	353
Both inferred and perceived infertile	130
Perceived infertile only	118

Thus, a total of 601 women can be classified in the aggregate infertility category. Aggregate infertility can be considered the upper limit of the estimate of infertility within the sample, since it is the broadest definition of the concept.

A detailed breakdown of aggregate infertility by parity and age is presented in Table 4. For the whole sample, those aged 16-49, the proportion of aggregate infertility is estimated at 7.74%. For women aged 18-44 and 18-49, the proportions are 6.72% and 7.75%. As is to be expected, all of these figures are higher than the corresponding ones for either perceived or inferred infertility alone.

When the trends are examined, it is evident that aggregate infertility follows the pattern of its constituent components: it increases with age and parity. Overall, the aggregate infertility rate of women in the 45-49 age group is 13.66%, almost three times that of the 16-29 age group (4.58%). Women with at least one child have an aggregate infertility rate of about half that of those with no children. The steepest gradient, though, is among those at parity 0. Aggregate infertility increases from 5.59% in the 16-29 age group, to 17.30% in the 30-39 age group, to 27.00% in the 40-44 age group, and 36.23% in the 45-49 age group. The corresponding figures among women with at least one child are 3.41%, 5.34%, 9.11%, and 11.88%, respectively.

Table 5 presents the infertility estimates derived from the OHS data and those from the CFS of 1984 and the GSS of 1990. It is important to note that the questions in the surveys were very different, and this invariably affects the estimates. For example, in the case of perceived infertility, in the OHS the respondents were asked whether they or their partner were unable to have children, in the GSS they were asked whether they had been told that they could not have more children, and in the CFS they were asked whether they thought they or their partner were sterile. Estimates of inferred infertility are also plagued by the problem of how to accurately measure the duration of exposure in the previous year.

The overall infertility figures reported in the three surveys are not too different from one another. Among the 18-44 age group, perceived infertility among all women in union at the time of the survey was 2.2% in the CFS, 2.9% in the OHS, and 3.3% in the GSS. All of these figures probably underestimate the true level of infertility, since only women who were not using any contraception, not sterilized, and not pregnant were asked these questions.

Since the GSS did not contain information on contraceptive use in the year leading up to the survey, inferred infertility could be estimated only from the CFS and the OHS. Overall estimates of inferred infertility among women aged 18-44 were quite close: 5.4% in the CFS and 5.7% in the OHS. Aggregate infertility, the upper limit in our estimation procedures, was 6.8% in both the CFS and the OHS among women aged 18-49 in union. In the 18-44 age group, aggregate infertility amounted to 6.1% in the CFS and 6.7% in the OHS.

Table 4. Aggregate Infertility by Parity and Age, Ontario, 1990

	n	Base	%
Parity 0			
16-29	50	893	5.59
30-39	68	393	17.30
40-44	27	100	27.00
45-49	25	69	36.23
16-44	145	1 387	10.45
16-49	170	1 456	11.68
18-44	144	1 384	10.40
18-49	170	1 453	11.70
Parity 1+			
16-29	38	1 114	3.41
30-39	154	2 882	5.34
40-44	115	1 262	9.11
45-49	106	892	11.88
16-44	307	5 257	5.84
16-49	413	6 149	6.72
18-44	307	5 254	5.84
18-49	413	6 146	6.72
All parities*			
16-29	94	2 053	4.58
30-39	231	3 358	6.88
40-44	144	1 381	10.43
45-49	133	974	13.66
16-44	467	6 804	6.86
16-49	601	7 765	7.74
18-44	457	6 798	6.72
18-49	601	7 759	7.75

* Differences between totals for all parities and sum of 0 and 1+ parities are due to non-response.

Source: Ontario Health Survey, 1990.

Surgical Sterilization

Estimates of surgical sterilization were determined from a positive response to Q.93. As mentioned previously, however, it is impossible to disaggregate surgical sterility by sex within the OHS. A positive response indicates that either the male or the female partner or both have been sterilized. Furthermore, one cannot be sure how many couples in the sample are surgically sterile through operations other than tubal ligation

Table 5. Infertility Status by Parity and Age, as Reported in the OHS (1990), CFS (1984), and GSS (1990)

	OHS %	CFS %	GSS %
Perceived infertility			
Parity 0			
18-44	4.2	4.9	4.9
18-49	5.2	6.3	-
Parity 1+			
18-44	2.7	1.4	2.3
18-49	2.8	2.3	-
All parities			
18-44	2.9	2.2	3.3
18-49	3.2	3.1	-
Inferred infertility			
(12 months' duration)			
Parity 0			
18-44	9.8	6.3	-
18-49	11.2	7.9	-
Parity 1+			
18-44	4.4	5.1	-
18-49	5.3	5.0	-
All parities			
18-44	5.7	5.4	-
18-49	6.7	5.4	-
Aggregate infertility			
(perceived and/or inferred,			
12 months' duration)			
Parity 0			
18-44	10.4	8.0	-
18-49	11.7	9.7	-
Parity 1+			
18-44	5.8	5.5	-
18-49	6.7	6.1	-
All parities			
18-44	6.7	6.1	-
18-49	6.8	6.8	-

Source: Ontario Health Survey, 1990; Canadian Fertility Survey, 1984; and General Social Survey, 1990.

or vasectomy (e.g., through hysterectomy). Thus, our inference from Q.93 may underestimate the true figure.

We know that rates of sterilization among women are very high, increasing with age and parity. This trend is borne out in the present analysis. Table 6 and Figure 3 present surgical sterility broken down by parity and age. Over 42% of women at risk in the 16-49 age group report that they or their partner are sterilized. The figure for those aged 16-44 is almost 39%. Since no women in the 16-17 age group of our sample were sterilized, the proportions for those aged 18 and over differ only negligibly. The lowest overall rates of sterilization are among women at parity 0 in the 16-29 age group, of whom 1.79% report that either they or their partner have been sterilized. For childless women, the rates increase to 13.49% in the 30-39 age group, 37.00% in the 40-44 age group, and 39.13% in the 45-49 age group. Naturally, the rates are much higher among those with at least one child. Most women in Canada do not want more than two children; the rates in Table 6 clearly support this. Almost half the women in the 30-39 age group and close to 70% of women aged 40-49 report sterilization of either themselves or their partner.

Table 7 reports sterilization by education and place of birth. Data from the OHS reveal, as do those of other surveys, that a woman's education is negatively related to sterilization. Among younger women aged 18-29, those with only primary or some secondary education are more likely to resort to sterilization. About one-fifth of these women (or their partners) in the lower educational categories are sterilized, whereas only about 5% among those with some or completed post-secondary education are sterilized. Among older women aged 30-49, though, the pattern is much weaker. Sixty-four percent of these women (or their partners) with some secondary education are sterilized, compared to about 50% of those with some or completed post-secondary education.

It can also be seen that sterilization is less popular among those born outside Canada, especially those born in Asia. Among the younger women born in Ontario, the proportion who are sterilized is about 12%. It is about the same for younger women born in the United Kingdom, but only about 6% among those born in Europe. Among younger women born in Asia, none reported sterilization. Among older couples (women aged 30-49) there is also a clear pattern of sterilization. Among those born in Ontario, the proportion of older couples who rely on sterilization is very high, at 58.7%. The proportion who are sterilized among the older couples born in Europe is lower at 48.5%, and among the Asian couples it is only 21.7%. It is quite possible that values acquired in the country of birth play a role in the reproductive behaviour of immigrants.

Table 6. Surgical Sterility by Parity and Age, Ontario, 1990

	n	Base	%
Parity 0			
16-29	16	893	1.79
30-39	53	393	13.49
40-44	37	100	37.00
45-49	27	69	39.13
16-44	106	1 387	7.64
16-49	133	1 456	9.13
18-44	106	1 384	7.66
18-49	133	1 453	9.15
Parity 1+			
16-29	182	1 114	16.34
30-39	1 429	2 882	49.58
40-44	876	1 262	69.41
45-49	622	892	69.73
16-44	2 487	5 257	47.31
16-49	3 109	6 149	50.56
18-44	2 487	5 254	47.34
18-49	3 109	6 146	50.59
All parities*			
16-29	200	2 053	9.74
30-39	1 519	3 358	45.24
40-44	928	1 381	67.20
45-49	658	974	67.56
16-44	2 640	6 804	38.80
16-49	3 298	7 765	42.47
18-44	2 640	6 798	38.84
18-49	3 298	7 759	42.51

* Differences between totals for all parities and sum of 0 and 1+ parities are due to non-response.

Source: Ontario Health Survey, 1990.

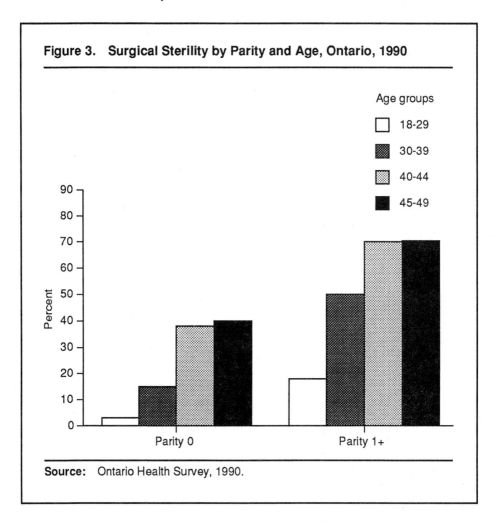

Figure 3. Surgical Sterility by Parity and Age, Ontario, 1990

Age groups
☐ 18-29
▨ 30-39
▨ 40-44
■ 45-49

Percent

Source: Ontario Health Survey, 1990.

Table 7. Surgical Sterility (Vasectomy or Tubal Ligation) by Education and Birthplace of the Female Partner, Ontario, 1990

	Age 18-29		Age 30-49	
	N	%	N	%
Education				
Primary	33	18.2	212	48.6
Some secondary	336	22.3	975	64.4
Completed secondary	649	13.9	1 859	57.8
Some post-secondary	294	4.8	752	52.9
Completed post-secondary	716	5.3	1 967	46.1
No response	12	8.3	46	47.8
Total	2 040	11.0	5 811	53.9
Birthplace				
Ontario	1 442	12.3	3 446	58.7
Canada (outside Ontario)	227	7.9	802	58.6
United Kingdom	62	11.3	303	53.5
United States	25	16.0	110	49.1
Europe	105	5.7	445	48.5
Asia	72	0.0	230	21.7
Caribbean	41	17.1	83	48.2
Other	69	4.3	286	39.9
No response	3	0.0	5	80.0
Total	2 046	10.9	5 710	54.9

Source: Ontario Health Survey, 1990.

Fertility Status

The findings on infertility and sterilization are summarized in Table 8 and Figure 4, which show the distribution of women by fertility status. The proportion who are fertile (the last column of Table 8) is a residual category derived by subtracting those who are either aggregate infertile or surgically sterile from 100. The data by age cohort should be interpreted with care, however. Among the older cohorts, many women are already surgically sterilized. We do not know, therefore, how many women in the surgically sterile category might have been infertile or fertile when they reached a specified age if they had not been sterilized. It might be reasonably argued that sterilized women are more likely to be fertile than infertile. Our attempts clearly underscore the difficulty of accurately measuring infertility in societies like Canada, where contraception is almost universal and the adoption of sterilization uninhibited.

Table 8. Fertility Status by Parity and Age, Ontario, 1990

	Infertility status			Surgically	
	Perceived (%)	Inferred (uncorrected) (%)	Aggregate (%)	sterile (%)	Fertile (%)
Parity 0					
16-29	1.12	5.49	5.59	1.79	92.62
30-39	8.14	14.25	17.30	13.49	69.21
40-44	15.00	23.00	27.00	37.00	36.00
45-49	27.54	31.88	36.23	39.13	24.64
16-44	4.18	9.23	10.45	7.64	81.91
16-49	5.22	10.30	11.68	9.13	79.19
18-44	4.19	9.18	10.40	7.66	81.94
18-49	5.23	10.25	11.70	9.15	79.15
Parity 1+					
16-29	1.08	2.87	3.41	16.34	80.25
30-39	2.15	3.92	5.34	49.58	45.08
40-44	5.23	6.49	9.11	69.41	21.48
45-49	3.48	9.98	11.88	69.73	18.39
16-44	2.66	4.34	5.84	47.31	46.85
16-49	2.79	5.12	6.72	50.56	42.72
18-44	2.66	4.34	5.84	47.34	46.82
18-49	2.80	5.12	6.72	50.59	42.69
All parities					
16-29	1.07	4.19	4.58	9.74	85.68
30-39	2.83	5.30	6.88	45.24	47.88
40-44	5.94	7.75	10.43	67.20	22.37
45-49	5.13	11.45	13.66	67.56	18.78
16-44	2.91	5.45	6.86	38.80	54.34
16-49	3.19	6.22	7.74	42.47	49.79
18-44	2.91	5.46	6.72	38.84	54.44
18-49	3.20	6.23	7.75	42.51	49.74

Source: Ontario Health Survey, 1990.

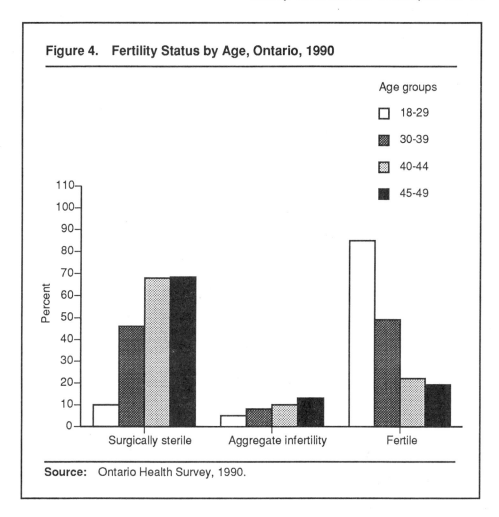

Figure 4. Fertility Status by Age, Ontario, 1990

Age groups

☐ 18-29

▨ 30-39

▨ 40-44

■ 45-49

Source: Ontario Health Survey, 1990.

Contraceptive Use

Just as with surgical sterilization, an investigation of contraceptive use should be an integral part of any study on infertility in an industrialized country like Canada. Many Canadians use contraception very early in life, even before their first birth, or between subsequent pregnancies for spacing purposes (Balakrishnan et al. 1985). Therefore, many women who use contraception may be infertile but unaware of it. Because of this, we may be underestimating overall infertility.

Regrettably, the measurement of contraceptive use is inadequate in the OHS. The only questions asked are Q.93, "In the past year what form of birth control did you or your partner(s) use?" and Q.94, "In the past year, how often did you or your partner(s) use some form of birth control?"

There is no way to estimate whether the couple used contraception for the whole year or only for a part of the year, or even started using it and then stopped in order to become pregnant. In other words, duration of exposure — which is vital in estimating infertility — cannot be calculated exactly. Also, where there is a multiple response, there is no way of knowing whether the methods were used simultaneously or sequentially.

Tables 9 and 10 and Figure 5 report contraceptive use among couples, by age. Table 9 allows multiple responses and indicates the distribution of the methods used. Because of multiple use, the totals exceed the number of women involved in the survey. In Table 10 and Figure 5, the methods are arranged in a hierarchical order of efficiency, and only the higher-order method has been counted where there is a multiple response. These data record use over the year preceding the survey and do not necessarily mean that the couples were using the method at the time of the survey. As mentioned, the percentages in Figure 5 are based only on those who report contraceptive use.

Table 9. Contraceptive Methods Used in the Year Prior to the Survey, Allowing Multiple Response, Ontario, 1990

Method	Age 18-44		Age 18-49	
	n	%	n	%
Sterilization (vasectomy or tubal ligation)	2 698	33.3	3 557	37.4
Pill	1 673	20.6	1 680	17.7
IUD	358	4.4	376	4.0
Diaphragm	175	2.2	177	1.9
Condom and foam	229	2.8	240	2.5
Condom	1 886	23.3	1 966	20.7
Other	415	5.1	511	5.4
Non-users	530	6.5	648	6.8
Not applicable	144	1.8	206	2.2
Non-response	1 181	14.6	1 550	16.3
Total (N)	8 111	114.2	9 515	112.6

Source: Ontario Health Survey, 1990.

It is clear that tubal ligation and vasectomy are the preferred methods of contraception among couples in the survey. A third of all the couples where the woman was aged 18-44 relied on these extreme methods of birth control. Next to sterilization, the condom and the pill are the most popular methods of birth control, with about 20% reporting their use in the year

Table 10. Contraceptive Methods Used in the Year Prior to the Survey, Counting Only the Most Efficient Method Indicated, Ontario, 1990

Method	Age 18-44		Age 18-49	
	n	%	n	%
Sterilization (vasectomy or tubal ligation)	2 698	33.3	3 357	35.3
Pill	1 605	19.8	1 611	16.9
IUD	304	3.7	321	3.4
Diaphragm	110	1.4	113	1.2
Condom and foam	146	1.8	156	1.6
Condom	1 116	13.8	1 192	12.5
Other	277	3.4	361	3.8
Non-users	530	6.5	648	6.8
Not applicable	144	1.8	206	2.2
Non-response	1 181	14.6	1 550	16.3
Total (N)	8 111	100.1	9 515	100.0

Note: Totals may not add up to 100 because of rounding.

Source: Ontario Health Survey, 1990.

preceding the survey. Although the IUD is a very effective method, it is not the preferred method in Ontario, with only 4.4% of women reporting its use. Only 6.5% of married or cohabiting women aged 18-44 reported not using any method, indicating that, overall, the use of birth control is high in Ontario among couples. It is unfortunate that non-response to the question of contraceptive use was high, at over 15% of the women sampled.

The distribution of couples who reported using several contraceptive methods, counting only the most effective method, is outlined in Table 10, in order of efficiency. The patterns are essentially the same as those illustrated in Table 9. Note, however, that here the pill is clearly more important than the condom. It is also evident that some couples are using condoms in addition to a more effective method.

Because data on various socioeconomic characteristics in the OHS are severely limited, we can examine the relationship only between contra-ceptive use and women's education and place of birth (Tables 11 and 12). Since age strongly influences the method of use, the results are reported for the 18-29 age cohort and the 30-49 age cohort. The main difference between the age groups is that within the younger group sterilization is low but pill use is high, a pattern that is reversed in the 30-49 age cohort. It

Table 11. Contraceptive Methods Used in the Year Prior to the Survey, Counting Only the Most Efficient Method Indicated, by Age and Education of the Female Partner, Ontario, 1990

Age and education	N	Sterilization	Pill	IUD	Diaphragm	Condom and foam	Condom only	Other	Non-user
						Method (%)			
Age 18-29									
Primary	33	18.2	42.4	15.2	0.0	0.0	12.1	0.0	12.1
Some secondary	336	22.3	42.9	2.1	1.5	1.8	17.0	3.6	8.9
Completed secondary	649	13.9	53.5	4.0	0.6	1.4	17.3	3.4	6.0
Some post-secondary	294	4.8	57.1	4.4	2.0	1.7	21.0	2.7	6.1
Completed post-secondary	716	5.3	59.8	2.1	0.4	2.0	22.2	2.4	5.9
Not specified	12	8.3	16.7	0.0	0.0	0.0	75.0	0.0	0.0
Total	2 040	11.0	54.1	3.2	0.9	1.7	19.8	2.9	6.5
Age 30-49									
Primary	212	48.6	2.8	2.4	13.6	0.5	11.3	3.3	17.5
Some secondary	975	64.4	4.6	3.5	5.0	0.5	6.8	5.9	9.2
Completed secondary	1 859	57.8	8.6	4.5	2.7	1.2	11.1	5.5	8.6

Infertility, Sterilization, and Contraceptive Use 185

Some post-secondary	752	52.9	10.2	4.1	1.1	2.0	16.6	5.1	8.0
Completed post-secondary	1 967	46.1	11.1	4.8	2.5	3.9	18.3	4.8	8.4
Not specified	46	47.8	6.5	15.2	0.0	8.7	13.0	4.3	4.3
Total	5 811	53.9	8.8	4.4	3.2	2.1	13.5	5.2	8.8

Note: Totals may not add up to 100 because of rounding.

Source: Ontario Health Survey, 1990.

Table 12. Contraceptive Methods Used in the Year Prior to the Survey, Counting Only the Most Efficient Method Indicated, by Age and Birthplace of the Female Partner, Ontario, 1990

Age and birthplace	N	Sterilization	Pill	IUD	Diaphragm	Condom and foam	Condom only	Other	Non-user
Age 18-29									
Ontario	1 442	12.3	55.2	2.8	1.0	1.7	17.5	3.4	6.0
Canada (outside Ontario)	227	7.9	60.4	4.8	0.9	2.2	12.8	2.2	8.8
United Kingdom	62	11.3	59.7	0.0	3.2	0.0	17.7	6.5	1.6
United States	25	16.0	60.0	0.0	0.0	4.0	16.0	0.0	4.0
Europe	105	5.7	35.2	4.8	4.8	1.0	36.2	0.0	12.4
Asia	72	0.0	23.6	1.4	0.0	0.0	62.5	1.4	11.1
Caribbean	41	17.1	48.8	9.8	0.0	0.0	19.5	0.0	4.9
Other	69	4.3	58.0	7.2	0.0	4.3	21.7	0.0	4.3
Not specified	3								
Total	2 046	10.9	53.9	3.2	1.2	1.7	19.7	2.9	6.6
Age 30-49									
Ontario	3 446	58.7	10.4	4.3	1.1	1.9	9.7	6.3	7.7
Canada (outside Ontario)	802	58.6	7.1	4.5	2.5	2.7	13.6	3.6	7.4
United Kingdom	303	53.5	4.6	5.0	1.0	3.3	15.8	3.3	13.5
United States	110	49.1	10.9	5.5	0.9	2.7	17.3	9.1	5.5

Method (%)

Europe	445	48.5	7.4	4.9	3.8	2.2	17.1	3.6	12.4
Asia	230	21.7	4.8	2.2	1.3	0.9	49.1	3.0	17.0
Caribbean	83	48.2	4.8	10.7	0.0	4.8	10.8	0.0	21.7
Other	286	39.9	7.3	4.9	2.8	2.1	27.6	4.2	11.2
Not specified	5								
Total	5 710	54.9	8.9	4.5	1.6	2.1	13.8	5.3	9.0

Note: Totals may not add up to 100 because of rounding.

Source: Ontario Health Survey, 1990.

is also apparent that education plays an important role in the method used. While sterilization is more popular among those with only secondary education than among those more highly educated, pill use increases with education. Among the younger cohort, the level of pill use is 42.9% among women with some secondary and 59.8% among those who have completed post-secondary education. Even though pill use is very low among women over the age of 30, the association with education is evident. Condom use, on the other hand, is less associated with education for this group.

We have already seen that place of birth is related to surgical sterilization. There is also an association between place of birth and other contraceptive methods (Table 12). For example, among younger women born in Canada, the United Kingdom, or the United States, the level of pill use is approximately 60%, whereas pill use is reported by 35% among those of other European origins, and by only 23.6% among women born in Asia. In contrast, use of the condom only is approximately 17% in young women born in Ontario, the United Kingdom, and the United States, whereas it is about 62% among Asian women. This same pattern of high condom use among people of Asian origin holds in the 30-49 age cohort as well. Here again, we see the influence of cultural factors and socialization on contraceptive choice.

Conclusions

The OHS was designed as a broad health monitoring survey and contains limited information on issues relating to fertility and birth control use. There was a high non-response rate in some areas, and many of the questions are either poorly worded or inadequately elaborated for our purposes. Despite these limitations, the overall results relating to the prevalence of infertility are generally consistent with other Canadian surveys.

For the age group 18-44, perceived infertility among all women in union at the time of the survey was 2.2% in the CFS (1984), 2.9% in the OHS (1990), and 3.3% in the GSS (1990). All these figures probably underestimate the true levels of infertility, since only women who were not using any contraception, not sterilized, and not pregnant were asked these questions.

Since the GSS does not contain information on contraceptive use during the year previous to the survey, we could estimate inferred infertility only from the other two surveys. The estimates of inferred infertility among women aged 18-44 were quite close — 5.4% in the CFS and 5.7% in the OHS. Aggregate infertility, the upper limit in our estimation procedures, was 6.8% in the CFS and the OHS among all women aged 18-49 and in union. Among the 18-44 age group, aggregate infertility amounted to 6.1% in the CFS and 6.7% in the OHS.

Canada has very high rates of sterilization, which was borne out by the OHS results. For married or cohabiting women between the ages of 18 and 49, the crude sterilization rate was 42.5%. There is considerable variability in the rate of sterilization by age and parity, however, with over 67% of women aged 40-49 reporting that either they or their partner had been sterilized. Childless women also reported significant rates of sterilization. The overall rate for women aged 18-49 was 9.15%, and 37-39% of women over the age of 40 reported that either they or their partner had been sterilized.

Many women reported multiple contraceptive use; however, the design of the questionnaire did not distinguish between simultaneous and sequential use within the reference period. We chose to analyze contraceptive use hierarchically based on presumed effectiveness. After sterilization, the pill is still the most popular choice among contraceptive users. Approximately 23% of contracepting women aged 18-49 reported using the pill (Figure 5). Overall, the pill is the most popular contraceptive method among younger women, and sterilization is preferred among older women.

Figure 5. Contraceptive Use (Determined Using Hierarchical Method) Among Married and Cohabiting Contraceptive Users Only, Aged 18-49, Ontario, 1990

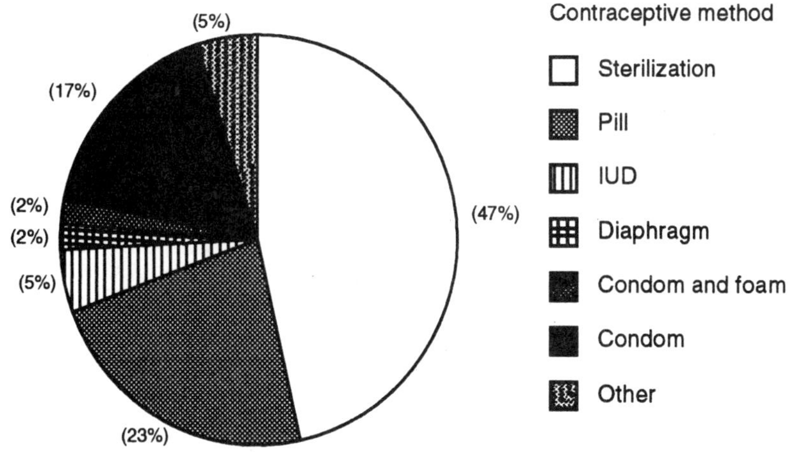

Contraceptive method

- ☐ Sterilization
- Pill
- IUD
- Diaphragm
- Condom and foam
- Condom
- Other

Note: Totals may not add up to 100 because of rounding.

Source: Ontario Health Survey, 1990.

The use of condoms and combined condoms and foam was reported by 17% and 2% of contraceptive users, respectively. Perhaps somewhat surprisingly, the use of the IUD is quite low in Ontario, with only about 5% of contracepting women reporting its use.

Notes

1. This discussion is drawn primarily from the "1990 Ontario Health Survey Documentation Report."

2. According to the "Ontario Health Survey Documentation Report," the survey was designed to be a comprehensive means of capturing data on such areas as health-related behaviours, risk factors, disability or reduced functioning, chronic health problems, and health-related attitudes, together with related socioeconomic indicators such as education, income, and housing.

3. Residents of Indian reserves, inmates of institutions, foreign service personnel, and residents of remote areas were excluded from the survey.

4. Specifically, the selection was based on a coding of 1 on questions Q14MS and F5Q58A.

5. The approach adopted in U.S. surveys, which ask a series of questions, is also not comparable to the "single" question method adopted in this survey.

Bibliography

Balakrishnan, T.R., K.J. Krótki, and E. Lapierre-Adamcyk. 1985. "Contraceptive Use in Canada, 1984." *Family Planning Perspectives* 17: 209-15.

Joffe, M. 1989. "Feasibility of Studying Subfertility Using Retrospective Self Reports." *Journal of Epidemiology and Community Health* 43: 268-74.

Johnson, G.D.R., et al. 1987. "Infertile or Childless by Choice? A Multipractice Survey of Women Aged 35 and 50." *British Medical Journal* 294: 804-806.

Léridon, H. 1991. "Stérilité et hypofertilité : du silence à l'impatience?" *Population* 46: 225-47.

Mosher, W.D. 1985. "Reproductive Impairments in the United States, 1965-1982." *Demography* 22: 415-30.

Mosher, W.D., and W.F. Pratt. 1990. *Fecundity and Infertility in the United States, 1965-88*. Advance Data from Vital and Health Statistics of the National Center for Health Statistics, No. 192. Hyattsville: U.S. Department of Health and Human Services.

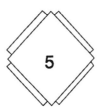

5

Adoption as an Alternative for Infertile Couples: Prospects and Trends

Kerry J. Daly and Michael P. Sobol

Executive Summary

Adoption has long been the traditional alternative for couples who are unable to conceive but who wish to become parents. This paper comments on adoption throughout history, then narrows the focus to Canadian adoption laws, policies, and practices from the turn of the twentieth century to today.

The authors examine the social and psychological issues for infertile couples who adopt, including views on infertility, societal expectations for parenthood, family identity, "blood ties" versus adoptive ties, and the long-term consequences of being an adoptive family. The formal and informal tasks in becoming adoptive parents are compared to the tasks in becoming biological parents, including parent-child relationships and a look at what the child should know of the adoption and the birth parents. Adoption alternatives are considered in light of new reproductive technologies available today.

Using data gathered through the National Adoption Study (funded by National Welfare Grants, Health and Welfare Canada, in 1990), the authors examine the demographics of adoptees and adoptive parents. For both public agencies and private adoption services, the authors describe the numbers of couples seeking to adopt, the availability of

This paper was completed for the Royal Commission on New Reproductive Technologies in November 1992.

adoptable children, the comparative availability of children under one year and older or special needs children, and domestic (including Native) adoptions compared to international adoptions.   Public and private adoptions are compared for accessibility.

Among the findings of this report are the following:

- In a majority of provinces, implementation policies, not adoption legislation, reinforce a parental model of a married, heterosexual couple.
- Infertile couples encounter strong cultural pressures to have children, but culture continues to emphasize the importance of blood ties for defining families.
- The adoption procedure is typically perceived as intrusive; it reinforces a sense of loss of control.
- The social parents and offspring of new reproductive technologies face many of the same identity challenges that adoptive parents and children encounter.
- Open adoptions are perceived by many service providers to be more successful.
- More than half of all infant adoptions are facilitated through private agencies or practitioners.
- The typical child placed through a public agency has special needs or is older than one year; the typical child placed privately is a healthy infant.
- Adopting a child privately happens faster (two years compared to six) but costs $3 000 to $4 000 (compared to almost nothing for public adoptions).
- For every infant who is placed for adoption in the public domain, there are eight waiting applicants, while in the private domain there are three applicants.

Introduction

Although the new reproductive technologies (NRTs) provide a range of options for infertile couples who wish to become parents, they are by no means viable or successful options for all couples. Due to various medical, ethical, financial, and social-psychological concerns, the NRTs may not provide appropriate avenues for some to follow. For other infertile couples, reproductive technologies are tried but unsuccessful options. Adoption has been the traditional alternative for those who are unable to conceive but wish to become parents. Yet, in recent years, the declining number of adoptable infants has restricted this option.

This report provides an overview of the state of adoption in Canada. Through an analysis of history, demographics, social-psychological and identity issues, and adoption alternatives, it provides some insight into the viability of adoption as an option for infertile couples in Canada. Specifically, this report addresses five objectives:

- It puts current adoption practice into historical perspective to highlight current trends in policy and service.

- It demonstrates, through an examination of the literature, the unique challenges facing adoptive parents in Canada, especially those experiencing fertility problems. The focus of this analysis is on the cultural context of adoption, the transitional tasks experienced by infertile couples going through an adoption process, and the nature of adjustment in adoptive families.

- It explores the parallel identity issues between adoption and the NRTs when at least one of the parents has no genetic link to the child.

- It provides a statistical overview of the state of adoption in Canada for the past 10 years based on the compilation of provincial data.[1] Specifically, this includes the number of domestic adoptions (excluding step and relative adoptions); the age and health characteristics of domestic adoptions; the number of public and private adoptions; the number of international adoptions; and the number of adoptive parent applicants.

- It reviews the options available to infertile couples who wish to adopt. These options include public adoptions through child welfare agencies, through which couples adopt either an infant or a special needs child; international adoptions, through either a child welfare agency or a private intermediary; and private adoptions arranged through an independent agency or private practitioner. The focus of this review is on the implications of these options for prospective adoptive parents.

Sources of Data

Several sources of data are used to document the trends described. The major source of data is a research study in progress entitled the National Adoption Study. It was funded by National Welfare Grants, Health and Welfare Canada, in October of 1990 and is directed by the authors. Included in this study are statistics on selected adoption trends provided to the researchers by the adoption coordinators for each of the provinces and territories. It also includes a national survey of approximately 350 adoption service providers in both the child welfare and private sectors. Finally, data that currently exist in the social-psychological literature have been critically reviewed with the proposed objectives in mind.

Goal of the Project

The document *What We Heard: Issues and Questions Raised During the Public Hearings*, produced by the Royal Commission on New Reproductive Technologies in 1991, singled out adoption as a particularly important non-technological alternative. Although adoption is not a complete solution to infertility, it may be an appropriate solution to childlessness for some couples. A distinction was made between "informed consent," as it is currently exercised within the medical profession, and "informed choice," which places medical procedures in the context of wider social choices such as childlessness, fostering, or adoption. This is an important distinction for the discussion of the adoption alternative, for if adoption is to be seriously and carefully considered by couples, then they must have information on all the factors that impinge upon that choice. It is the goal of this project to provide a picture of adoption that will serve as the basis upon which "informed choices" can be made.

Adoption in a Historical Legislative Context

Adoption as a means of family formation has roots that go back into antiquity. Perhaps the most famous of all ancient tales of adoption is the biblical story of Moses. Found by the handmaidens of the daughter of the Pharaoh, the infant Moses was taken into the palace as a prince of Egypt. In Greek mythology, the hero Hercules was adopted by Hera. Sophocles has Oedipus cry out, "I must pursue this trail to the end, till I have unravelled the mystery of my birth." Adoption practices were also detailed in the code of Hammurabi, a text of Babylonian law. In each of these examples of ancient adoption, the ties between the adoptee and biological relatives were severed. The child was considered for all intents and purposes to be the biological offspring of the adoptive parents. In fact, Hammurabi's code went so far as to prescribe that the tongue be cut out of an adoptee who mentioned biological origins other than those of the adoptive family, and that blindness was the punishment for searching for birth parents.

In the time of the Roman Empire, the statesman and essayist Cicero wrote, "Adoption of children should be permissible to those who are no longer capable of begetting children and who, when they were in their prime, put their capacity for parenthood to the test" (Presser 1972). For the adoptee of the early period of the Roman Empire, loyalty was exclusive to the adoptive family. However, 500 years into the modern era, the code of the emperor Justinian declared that adoptees had rights and responsibilities with both the birth and the adoptive families; they were allowed to inherit from both and in turn were responsible for the protection and well-being of each family.

Adoption in Eastern societies took on a different hue. In China, older males without an heir could claim the first-born son of a younger brother. The responsibility of the adoptive nephew was eventually to care for the ashes and the grave of the adoptive father, thus avoiding the "disturbance of the wandering spirit." Hindu law in India also allowed for adoption with the restriction that the adoptee be as similar as possible to the caste, colour, and social position of the adopting parents. The purpose of the adoption, much like those in other ancient settings, was to ensure that the adoptive parents had an heir to care for the well-being of kin and estate. In this way the continuation of the family was secure.

In North America, the Inuit have always practised a form of adoption. Childless couples within the kin circle are given a child by a fertile couple. The adoptee knows who the birth parents are. However, loyalty to either the birth or adoptive family is not considered an issue of importance, because the adoption is undertaken not in the interests of the adoptee or adoptive parents but as a means of expanding the strength and viability of the kin group. Hence, adoption serves the needs of the society more than those of its individual members.

The first provincial adoption statute in Canada was passed in New Brunswick in 1873. Unlike other Canadian legislation, this statute did not follow British laws, which did not deal with adoption until 1926. Instead, the New Brunswick legislation mirrored a Massachusetts statute of 1851. By today's standards, the New Brunswick statute was quite simple: all that was necessary to obtain an adoption was the acceptance by a court of a petition from the adoptive parents and a letter of consent from the birth parents. If the court was satisfied that the adopting parents were fit to raise and educate the child, the petition was accepted. Nova Scotia passed similar legislation in 1896. Between 1920 and 1930, the remaining provinces also passed statutes on adoption (MacDonald 1984).

This early legislation in Canada was grounded in the context of the indenturing system. Many children, who by today's standards should have been taken into care, became the indentured workers of farms and factories. Few or no restrictions were placed on the amount of labour that could be demanded of these children. Many children came from the slums of England in a program of immigration managed by the Dr. Bernardo Homes for Children (Garber 1985). For child activists, this exploitation of children was unacceptable. Intense lobbying resulted in amendments to these adoption laws, with the result being a better degree of protection than the indenture system could offer. In addition, adoption relieved the state of financial and protective responsibilities in the care of the children by shifting these responsibilities to the adoptive parents.

In the first half of this century adoption was considered a second-rate kind of family formation. The birth mother's pregnancy was seen to be the result of sexual impropriety and moral looseness. The infant, before adoption, bore the legal label "illegitimate" and was regarded by society as damaged goods. The infertile couple seeking to adopt, and more specifically the mother, were viewed as incomplete; biological motherhood was considered to be the ultimate fulfilment of the feminine role. In response to these hampering views, legal procedures were developed that were thought to be in the best interests of the adopting parents. The adoption was carried out in complete secrecy. Publicly, adoptive parents were presented as if they were the biological progenitors of the adoptee. This pretence was reflected in adoption policies such as the amendment of birth certificates to give adoptees the surname of the adopting parents. Adoption orders had the names of the birth parents removed. All records were sealed and were readily available only to the registrar of the office of vital statistics. Some adoption workers counselled parents never to mention the adoption. Others recommended that the child be told of the adoption but never be encouraged to think of having any "real" parents other than the adoptive ones. All of these tactics were used so that parents could proceed as if the child were their biological offspring.

This systematic denial of biological difference reflected in both legislation and social work practice failed to take into account the negative effects of secrecy experienced by the adoptive parents and their child (Kirk 1964, 1981). Kirk and McDaniel (1984) have argued that by adhering to a "principle of equivalence," adoptive parents were, paradoxically, less able to fulfil their hopes and expectations as parents. Communication with the child was hindered by the continual need to maintain the myth of consanguineous connection. The mysterious second family lurked in the background of family life. Even as an adult, the child was discouraged from probing too deeply into an understanding of a sense of self.

By the middle of this century, legislation was marked by a new belief that adoption should serve the best interests of the child. While this emphasis did little to change the secretive aspect of adoption, elaborate evidence had to be presented to the court that the child would be better served by the adopting parents than by either the biological parents or representatives of the child welfare system. If the child was old enough, his or her consent to the adoption was to be obtained. Because recognition of different biological origins was now considered to serve the best interests of the child, policies were developed to allow a degree of openness in the exchange of information between the adopting and birth parents. In addition, many provinces passed legislation allowing the establishment of adoption registries to facilitate the exchange of information and the possible reunion of adult adoptees and their birth families.

In many ways adoption in the last decade has maintained an idealized vision of family life that bears little resemblance to actual family experience. In screening applicants for the diminishing number of infant adoptions, adoption agencies seek families that meet this ideal. Specifically, applicants are to be living in a stable, loving, and heterosexual relationship. The income provider, usually male, is to be well educated and financially secure. The wife is to remain at home to care for the children. The age spread between the parents and child should be no more than 35 years. These idealized criteria do not match the realities of current family life: many couples are older before they attempt to become parents; the one-income, two-parent family represents less than one in five families; many children are being raised by single parents; and society is showing more tolerance for children being raised by homosexual couples. Thus, in pursuing an idealized vision of the family as the criterion for an infant adoption, service providers are in many ways out of step with the realities of current family life. As a result, adoptive applicants who do not meet these criteria are turning elsewhere to find children to adopt or have changed their understanding of what constitutes an acceptable adopted child.

As we shall detail in the section on the demographics of adoption, the possibility of being an adoptive parent became markedly more difficult over the past decade. Factors assumed to be contributing to the decrease in the availability of infants for adoption include greater accessibility to birth control, more liberal abortion legislation, and society's increased acceptance of single parenthood. As a result, new initiatives have been developed. Children in care who were once thought to be unadoptable because of age, race, or handicap are now being put forward as candidates for adoption. In many cases this has required the parallel formation of support services to aid parents throughout family development. Clearly, parents who adopt these hard-to-place children are able to hide neither their non-consanguineous connection to the child nor the fact that they may be infertile. It has been suggested that adoption professionals have changed their criteria for acceptable applicants in order to find homes for hard-to-place children. Single parents, foster parents, and those who need financial support to adopt are now considered. To date, there is no evidence to suggest that these changes in selection criteria have in any way negatively affected the children.

Another recent change in adoption as a result of the decreasing availability of infants has been a rise in the number of international adoptions. Reacting to the possibility that long waiting lists can be bypassed and that stringent criteria, especially age, can be ignored, many hundreds of prospective parents have flocked to other countries to seek a child. In the best of conditions these adoptions have been implemented through reputable international auspices and agents. In the worst of circumstances, vast sums of money have been exchanged in the quest to adopt an infant. While most foreign governments require some documentation that the adopting parents have secured a professionally assessed home study, there seem to be no attempts to match infant and parent professionally.

In choosing a foreign adoption, parents take several risks: the costs may be exorbitant; the prenatal history and current health of the child may not be known; and few social supports are available for parents and child when they return to Canada. Finally, although the media have portrayed international adoptions as a means of procuring a child of the same colour as the adopting parents, racial overtones in all likelihood play a diminished role (Serrill 1991). For the most part, couples pursuing an international adoption are simply seeking a more expeditious way to form a family. Considering the large number of children adopted from the developing countries of Asia and South America, it is hard to support the idea that these adoptions are motivated by same-colour considerations.

The final trend that distinguishes the past decade from other periods is the growth in private adoption services. As more and more birth mothers have turned to private agencies and practitioners to place their infants for adoption, there has been a dramatic shift in the delivery of infant adoption services. Motivated by the possibility of having more control over the decision made, put off by the "snatch-and-grab" reputation of child welfare facilities, and in some instances lured by the possibility of under-the-table financial remuneration, birth mothers have all but abandoned public agencies. Provinces have responded to this shift in different ways. Ontario encouraged the development of professional standards and licensing procedures. Others have preferred to treat it as a subcultural phenomenon that, barring unforeseen difficulties, is best ignored. In a few provinces, for example, Quebec and Newfoundland, private services have been outlawed. Interestingly, this has had no effect on the downward slide in the number of infants available through public adoption agencies. Finally, it is important to note that, with the switch to private services, infant adoptions have become less and less accessible to people who lack the money to procure private adoption services.

In summary, current legislation views adoption from the standpoint of the needs of the child rather than the needs of the adopting parents. Adults are considered, in law, to be able to adopt only if it can be demonstrated that the family serves the best interests of the child. Adoption laws do not recognize the rights of infertile individuals or any other adults to become adoptive parents. As a way of meeting the best interests of the adoptive parents, many couples have turned to international and private adoptions or have changed their criteria for adoption and have sought out hard-to-place children in the public domain.

Social-Psychological Issues for Infertile Couples Who Seek to Adopt

Infertile couples who choose adoption to gain a family encounter unique challenges. This section will explore the various contingencies that shape the adoption process. This includes discussions of

- the sociocultural context within which adoption decisions are made,
- the propensity of infertile couples to adopt,
- the transitional tasks experienced by couples through an adoption process, and

- the unique challenges of being an adoptive family following the experience of infertility.

Adoptive Parenthood in Sociocultural Context

Parenthood has taken on many new meanings in response to changes in the norms and structures of families. Once one could easily identify parents as spouses living together to create and raise their own biological children, but one must now take into account a wide variation in the parental role. In Canada, for example, the 1990 census shows that the traditional family (a single male wage earner and an at-home female spouse) declined from 63 percent of families in 1961 to 18 percent in 1986. As this would suggest, the vast majority of parents carry out their roles in non-traditional ways, within different contexts, and with different contingencies. Eichler (1988), for example, has documented the tremendous variation in family structure that has resulted from the disjunction of marital and parental roles, including step families, single-parent families, divorced families, childless families, and families with homosexual parents.

Although becoming an adoptive parent involves a set of experiences different from those of becoming a biological parent, each set occurs against the backdrop of common values and norms about what parenthood should be. Most central among these norms is the pro-natalist expectation that married couples have children (Blake 1974; Lasker and Borg 1987). Veevers (1980) elaborates on this pervasive cultural push toward parenthood when she says, "Parenthood is almost universally lauded as an intrinsically desirable social role." It is seen as a "moral obligation" that has its roots in both religious beliefs and cultural norms (Laurance 1982; Pohlman 1970). Davis suggests not only that there are coercive norms to have children, but also that couples are expected to acquire children and cope without assistance from the state or other institutions or individuals (Davis 1978).

This expectation for parenthood is so strong that there is much hesitancy to define a childless couple as a family. John Donne, preaching several centuries ago, stated that for "a couple to contract before that they will have no children makes it no marriage, but an adultery" (Bernard 1982, 55). Although perhaps severely stated by today's standards, the same principle still seems to hold true. For, to "become parents" is to "have a family," suggesting that to be married without children is not to be a family at all. In this sense, one could argue that identity as a family occurs when a couple begin to have children, rather than when they marry. Parenthood, not marriage, marks the critical transition into "family-hood."

For those couples whose family beliefs are shaped by normative cultural attitudes, the failure to become parents may be associated with a number of developmental consequences. One such consequence may be the compromising of adult status. Not having or rearing children eliminates the cultural definition of achieving "full" maturity. Hill and Aldous (1969, 923) point out that "parenthood rather than marriage appears to be the crucial role-transition point that marks the entrance into adult status in our society." As Blake (1974) explains, the pro-natalist pressure is so strong that parenthood is an explicit part of the definition of masculinity and femininity and is therefore seen as a necessary condition for adequately carrying out adult sex roles. Furthermore, infertility can be seen to precipitate a reorganization of self in order to cope with the lost ideal of biological parenthood and the corresponding desire for immortality (Kraft et al. 1980, 623). It is from this perspective that infertility can be seen as a "life crisis" that affects the marriage relationship, individual self-esteem, and the abilities of individuals to function, to communicate, and to feel normal (Bresnick 1981; Bresnick and Taymor 1979; Goodman and Rothman 1984; Pfeffer and Woolett 1983; Mai et al. 1972).

Of course, not all couples would experience infertility as a developmental block, but may see the crisis as an opportunity for the development of adult status through other challenges and relationships. In light of the increasing diversification of family structures (Eichler 1988), it is arguable that these other developmental opportunities take on greater salience and legitimacy.

Nevertheless, parenthood continues to play an important role in the way that families define themselves in our culture. As one indication of this, 95 percent of newly married couples anticipate that they will have children at some point in their lives (Glick 1977). For many couples, becoming parents, and thus becoming families, is non-problematic because they can have biological children. For other couples, however, taking on the family identity is blocked by an inability to bear biological children. As a consequence of a fertility problem, some couples cannot have a family when they set out to do so. With parenthood blocked by infertility, couples find themselves caught in a tension between their own desire to have children, the expectations of family and friends that they do so, and their powerlessness to overcome infertility.

Although much of the focus in the literature on involuntary childlessness is on the couple, gender plays a major role in the experiences of infertility, childlessness, and adoption. Without exception, the literature points to the greater salience of the parenthood identity for women than for men. Research into the perceived difficulty of childlessness for men and for women unanimously concludes that it is a more difficult experience for women (Bierkens 1975; Daly 1987; Humphrey and MacKenzie 1967; Link and Darling 1986; Van Keep and Schmidt-Elmendorff 1975; Veevers 1980). Furthermore, there are inequalities between men and women with respect to the diagnosis and treatment of fertility problems, and there are fundamental differences in the ways that men and women respond to the crisis of infertility in their relationship (Lasker and Borg 1987).

Although the chances for biological parenthood diminish in the face of infertility, for many couples parenthood itself continues to be an important and desirable role. In light of this, couples begin to examine alternative ways to become parents. Although advances in reproductive technology have increased the available options, adoption continues to be one of the main alternatives for becoming parents. Choosing adoption, however, necessarily involves a redefinition of what it means to be a parent. Couples who choose adoption must let go of the physical, hereditary, or biological aspects of parenthood in favour of the social aspects of the parenting experience.

Deeply embedded within this redefinition of parenthood is the cultural importance of "blood ties." Terms like "kinship," "consanguinity," "procreation," "generational linkages," and "lineage" have a taken-for-granted biological element. Blood ties in the parent-child relationship give it an obdurate quality unlike any other affiliation. The blood tie is "indissoluble and of a mystical nature that transcends legal or other kinship arrangements" (Miall 1987, 35). Seen in this light, the blood tie is central to the redefinition of parenthood to accommodate adoption. One implication of the absence of the blood tie is that adoptive relationships within our culture tend to be stigmatized. Based on the notion that adoptive relationships are "less authentic" and thereby elicit negative informal social sanctions, adoptive parent status is seen as a "discreditable attribute" (Miall 1986, 1987).

These stigmatizing responses are consistent with a set of negative cultural values about adoption itself. Historically, adoption is linked to the shame of an "illegitimate" or out-of-wedlock pregnancy. The children were social outcasts or "orphans," whose eventual placement was shrouded in secrecy to protect the "legitimate" family from the original disgrace. Although adoption practice has become more open since then, some of these early values about the "outcast" nature of adopted children have continued. For example, adoptees are still referred to as "second best" or "coming from bad blood." Miall (1987) identifies three general attitudes toward adoption as perceived by adoptive parents themselves: adoption is second best because of the absence of the biological tie; adopted children are second rate because of the absence of the genetic tie; and adoptive parents are not "real" parents.

Consistent with these cultural attitudes, adoptive parents are often seen as benevolent or altruistic caretakers who bring an unwanted child into their home. This reflects early beliefs about the charitable nature of social assistance. Although children's interests continue to be at the forefront of adoption service delivery, greater emphasis is now being put on the assessment of adoptive parent needs and expectations as a necessary component of placement. Nevertheless, public reaction continues to emphasize the altruistic aspects of adopting a child. The resulting bind for adoptive parents is that, although they are seen as benevolent in their willingness to adopt a child of different biological origin, they are also susceptible to the stigmatizing responses of people who have difficulty accepting the "difference" of the adoptive relationship.

To understand the specific challenges that are encountered by couples who seek to adopt, it is necessary to keep in mind the cultural context that gives meaning to adoptive parenthood. As the above discussion suggests, pro-natalist values are an important backdrop for understanding the motivation for adoptive parenthood. These values reinforce the importance of children for individual development and marital completion. Blood ties are an important dimension of parenthood, resulting in a unique challenge for adoptive parents who must somehow reconcile the absence of this biological link and manage the ensuing stigmatizing responses. Finally, social attitudes toward adoption result in a dramatically different set of preparations for adoptive parenthood than those involved in becoming biological parents. These preparation needs are discussed fully in the section entitled "Transitional Tasks in the Adoption Process."

The Propensity of Infertile Couples to Adopt

It is generally believed that the demand for adoption by infertile couples is very high. Media reports of long or closed waiting lists at adoption agencies, "black market" babies, and extravagant efforts to adopt children internationally reinforce this perception. Unfortunately, there are few reliable data to substantiate the actual extent of this demand.

Some reports, based on clinical estimates, have focussed on the number of infertile couples who seek to adopt. For example, Humphrey and MacKenzie (1967) estimated that approximately 30 percent of couples attending an infertility clinic would adopt children. Consistent with these results, Burgwyn (1981) suggests that one in four infertile couples in the United States seek to adopt. A more recent estimate, by the National Committee for Adoption, says that 37 percent of infertile couples will seek to adopt (National Committee for Adoption 1989).

Recent studies in the United States based on national samples offer more precise insight into the number of women who adopt children. As Poston and Cullen (1989) have pointed out, adoption is a relatively rare event, with only 2.3 percent of ever-married white women in the United States between the ages of 15 and 44 having adopted a child. Based on an analysis of national survey data in 1976, Bachrach (1983) calculated that among non-contraceptively sterile women with no live births, the rate of adopting ranged from 17.5 percent for women 15 to 29 years to 45.8 percent for those 30 to 44 years.

While these studies provide information about the characteristics of women who adopt, they give little insight into the real demand for adoption. Studies based on national samples of U.S. women indicate that about one out of every two infertile women seek to adopt. In one of the earliest studies, Bonham (1977) reported that 48 percent of women who projected being unable to have children would seek to adopt a child. Poston and

Cullen (1989) found that the propensity to adopt is 55 percent among non-contraceptively sterile women and almost 65 percent among subfecund women. Based on 1988 data, Bachrach et al. (1991) concluded that among childless, non-fecund women who had been treated for infertility, 47 percent had taken steps toward adoption. Data suggest that women seeking to adopt are typically infertile, married, and of higher socioeconomic status (Bachrach 1983; Bachrach et al. 1991; Bonham 1977).

One of the most useful ways of measuring the demand for adoption is to look at the ratio of women seeking to adopt to the number of non-relative adoptions for any particular year. Bachrach and colleagues calculated an adoption demand ratio of 3.3 seeking women for every non-relative adoption (Bachrach et al. 1991). This ratio is roughly compatible with waiting periods of "at least two years" as suggested by the National Committee for Adoption (1984).

Not all provinces keep records of the number of infertile couples who are seeking to adopt. In the absence of these Canadian data, one can only conjecture about the degree of similarity between the U.S. figures and the Canadian experience. Although the culture of parenthood may be similar in many respects, differences in demographic composition, service delivery, and government policy might result in different figures for the Canadian population. (See "Waiting Period," under "Accessibility of Public and Private Adoption," below.)

Transitional Tasks in the Adoption Process

Becoming an adoptive parent involves a set of preparatory experiences different from those encountered in becoming a biological parent (Kirk 1981). Foremost among these experiences are coming to terms with the difference of the adoptive relationship, and gaining support and legitimation for the new role identity. A couple may begin by entertaining the idea of adoption, fantasizing about themselves as adoptive parents, soliciting support from others, and taking concrete steps to become legitimated as adoptive parents. Unlike biologically formed families, who begin with symbiosis and are expected to move toward individuation, the adoptive family begins by experiencing distance but is expected to move toward closeness (Elbow 1986).

Like the loss of control they encounter in dealing with infertility, taking steps to become adoptive parents also takes away control. Couples surrender control to doctors in the infertility investigation, and to the official agents in the adoption process. Seeking parenthood is no longer the relatively simple matter of getting pregnant and having a child, but instead involves the social and emotional preparation for the difference of adoption along with applications, meetings, interviews, and other evaluation procedures that are designed to judge their eligibility to become parents.

There appear to be two dimensions to adoption, which Kent and Richie (1976) have referred to as "legal adoption" and "emotional adoption." Legal adoption brings into play the influence and decisions of a variety of community institutions. These institutional influences are embodied in the work of lawyers, judges, physicians, clergy, and social workers who, in varying degrees of directness, affect the adoption process (Katz 1964). Emotional adoption, by contrast, concerns the couples' subjective experience of adoption, which begins with the psychological preparation for adoptive parenthood and continues into adoptive parenthood as couples continue to seek to "resolve their loss [of a biological child] and make their wholehearted commitment to the [adopted] child" (Kent and Richie 1976, 520). As the distinction between legal and emotional adoption suggests, there are both formal and informal aspects to the adoption process: one that focusses on the legal and procedural aspects, the other that focusses on the social-psychological preparation for adoptive parenthood.   The discussion that follows focusses on the typical transitional tasks that can be expected in these formal and informal domains.

Informal Tasks

Although there are numerous socialization guidelines for how one should be a biological parent, there are considerably fewer guidelines for the process necessary to become an adoptive parent. On the socialization of parents to the adoptive parenthood role, Pringle (1967) points out that it is a fallacy to assume that adoptive parenthood is no different from biological parenthood when in fact it is "manifestly different" in the biological, social, and emotional domains. Similarly, Kirk (1964) suggests that adoptive parents are role-handicapped by the contradiction between the "culturally promised events" associated with biological parenthood and their "personal encounters" with adoption as a "very different reality." Furthermore, this alternative reality is mirrored in a set of distinctly different attitudes and values about adoptive parenthood among the reference groups with which they interact. From this perspective, the difference of adoption is present in both their subjective experience of making the transition to adoptive parenthood and the social context within which the transition is made. The informal transitional tasks for adoptive parenthood can be examined with respect to the following categories: coming to terms with the loss of biological parenthood; social-psychological and emotional preparations for adoption; and disclosing adoption plans to significant others.

Coming to Terms with the Loss of Biological Parenthood
The importance of grieving the inability to bear one's own child is widely recognized in the clinical literature as part of the preparation to become adoptive parents (Castle 1982; Kent and Richie 1976; Kraft et al. 1980; Krugman 1967; McNamara 1975; Sorosky et al. 1978). Grieving the loss of biological parenthood includes coming to terms with the sense of

personal failure and letting go of the fantasized child of their own making. In addition, it involves working through the loss of an ideal self, the restitution of a damaged body image, and an assessment of the importance of parenthood (Winkler et al. 1988).

Although the resolution of infertility issues is central to the process of preparing for adoption, there are a number of factors that come into play that complicate the relationship between infertility resolution and adoption readiness. Central among these is the question of what it means to "resolve" infertility. "Infertility resolution" is typically portrayed in the literature as having an end point. A number of works suggest that infertility resolution involves a progression through a set of identifiable periods or stages beginning with the shock of the initial awareness and ending with some form of resolution (Hertz 1982; Mazor 1979; Menning 1977; Renne 1977; Shapiro 1982). However, other literature suggests that the tension between infertility and the desire for biological parenthood is an ongoing experience that may not have a specific end point. As Kraft et al. (1980) point out, a "complete" or "final" resolution of infertility is not absolute, for the issue continues to reverberate and can be revived even though it may essentially be worked through. Likewise, Zaslove (1978, 2) suggests that some couples may experience "*chronic* depression, frustration, guilt, anger, feelings of isolation, alienation and inadequacy" (emphasis added). Rosenfeld and Mitchell (1979) say that alienation and isolation may be *prevailing* symptoms of infertility. Matthews and Martin Matthews (1986) add that infertility as a biological condition gets transformed into the ongoing social condition of involuntary childlessness. All these researchers suggest that issues of infertility resolution and biological parenthood identity may continue well into the adoption process.

From this perspective, infertility and adoption are interpenetrating processes. Recent research by Daly (1990) suggests that there are two distinct patterns in the way that infertile couples perceive the relationship between the two processes: sequential and concurrent. Out of 68 infertile couples who were considering adoption, two-thirds perceived the relationship between infertility resolution and adoption readiness in a sequential manner. They had a primary commitment to biological parenthood, and only when this was impossible to fulfil did they commit themselves to adoptive parenthood. These couples experienced the relationship between infertility resolution and adoption readiness as a linear, step-by-step progression whereby an end to infertility concerns had to be reached before they made the necessary adjustments to adoptive parenthood. Couples varied, however, in how they defined the end to infertility concerns. Some described this end as the completion of all infertility tests and treatments, while others described it as an affective process with reference to feelings of grief or resignation. In this respect, the "resolution" of infertility occurred within medical and affective domains.

By contrast, 28 percent of the couples experienced infertility resolution and adoption readiness in a concurrent manner. For these couples, it was unnecessary to resolve infertility before feeling ready for adoption. Rather, there was a bifurcating commitment to both biological and adoptive parenthood. In this sense, there was a continual reverberation between biological parenthood and adoptive parenthood, insofar as they continued to hope for a biological child while at the same time increasingly committing themselves as potential adoptive parents.   For these couples, the commitment to parenthood, regardless of whether it was biological or adoptive, seemed to be of paramount importance. Becoming a parent or having the parenting experience superseded the genetic or adoptive dimensions. As a result, infertility treatments and adoption took on equal importance as ways of achieving the goal of a child.

A key factor that may interfere with the resolution of infertility is the uncertainty often associated with medical diagnoses. Among the couples who have a fertility problem identified, relatively few are ever told by their physicians that they will *never* conceive.   Rather, they live with the uncertainty of having a *reduced chance* of ever conceiving. Infertility is thus an ambiguous loss that can be a barrier to moving ahead with an alternative such as adoption. Similar to other ambiguous losses, such as having children go missing from families, infertility leaves couples not knowing whether to mourn or be optimistic, brave or resigned; the "facts" around their loss are not clear; they do not have conventional rituals available to them to facilitate the mourning process; and they may be overwhelmed by guilt or shame wondering whether or not they are responsible (Boss 1991; Lloyd and Zogg 1986).   Without a clearly identifiable loss and with no obvious end to the struggle, resolution of infertility is often difficult to achieve (Lasker and Borg 1987).

Due to the ambiguity of the loss, couples typically equivocate when making their decision to give up on biological parenthood identity (Daly 1988). Many infertile couples set a deadline for when they will go no further in the testing and treatment process, but this has a way of being renegotiated when the end is reached. These vacillations give the process of relinquishing biological parenthood a reverberating quality. However, as the strains that accompany either years of unsuccessful testing or the failure of a major treatment become too great for the desired outcome of a biological child, couples turn to adoption as one option for realizing the identity of parenthood.

Social-Psychological and Emotional Preparations for Adoption

Perhaps one of the most fundamental features of coming to terms with adoptive parenthood as an identity is to fantasize about being an adoptive parent. Schutz (1973) has emphasized the importance of fantasizing as the foundation for any project of action. For infertile couples, this means visualizing the "little stranger" coming into their lives. This process raises questions about their ability to form an attachment with a child not of their own making. Biological parenthood is rooted in a familiar, taken-for-granted reality, but adoption presents contingencies that are unpredictable.

These may be expressed as concerns about the child's medical background, the care of the fetus during pregnancy, what the biological parents are like (i.e., is the child from "bad blood"?), and the child's genetic characteristics.

As a result of these concerns, many couples anticipate they might not be able to commit themselves as fully to the adoptive parenthood identity as they would to the biological parenthood identity. An infertile woman described this difference in terms of bonding: "With adopted kids, there is more of [a] chance that they will turn out bad. My friend adopted, and they turned out bad. I don't think there would be the same closeness. I don't think I would go all the way with bonding" (Daly 1988, 59).

Adoptive parenthood is also perceived to be a more tenuous identity than biological parenthood because of an uncertainty about whether the biological mother will change her mind about adoption. "The insecurity of not knowing whether or not the [biological] parents will show up on your doorstep" can be a barrier to a full commitment to adoptive parenthood (Daly 1988, 59). Couples considering adoption often refer to the biological parents as the "real" parents, thus removing themselves from the possibility of occupying the "real" parental role. This same anxiety is expressed in terms of the child's need to search for the "real" parents when he or she reaches a certain age. Underlying this anxiety is the fear that the adoptive parents will be abandoned when the children reconnect with these "real" parents.

Another challenge encountered by infertile couples in their efforts to identify with adoptive parenthood is coming to a consensus within the marriage on their readiness for adoption. Adoptive parenthood is a jointly constructed identity; disagreement between spouses may prevent their identification with adoption. Most important here is the reluctance on the part of one spouse to push the other spouse too hard, thereby risking resistance. One infertile man explained: "We're still at the discussion stage. I haven't fully investigated it [i.e., adoption] yet. If we are going to do it then we are going to do it together, and she isn't ready yet. I don't want to pressure her. She has to come to it when she is ready. And there is no point in me pushing, because then she might enter into it unwillingly" (Daly 1988, 57-58).

Media presentations of adoption also create problems in the preparation for adoptive parenthood. Infertile couples report that adoptive parenthood is usually portrayed in a negative light (Daly 1989b). Specifically, the popular press tends to focus on and glamourize cases of successful search where the adoptee finds and reunites with a birth parent. Similarly, popular television dramatizations focus on the unstable aspects of adoptive relationships. A common theme in these programs is the search for and happy reunion with birth parents; another theme is the birth mother's quest to regain custody of a child she relinquished for adoption. As one woman succinctly described it, "on TV, adoptees are always stepped on and they always seek their birth parents." These programs, often conveying false information about the birth mother's legal access to the child, make couples more apprehensive about adoption for fear that the child could be snatched away by the biological mother.

Disclosing Adoption Plans to Significant Others

As couples take on a new role identity of adoptive parenthood, they turn to significant others for support and legitimation (McCall and Simmons 1978). Consistent with the greater importance of parenthood to women, there is a tendency for women to have to account for their childlessness more often than men (Daly 1987; Van Keep and Schmidt-Elmendorff 1975). Perhaps most critical in this process of gaining support from family, friends, and the potential grandparents are the decisions about what to say about adoption plans.

The revelation of adoption plans is a significant transitional task, for it announces the couple's intentions to pursue a different kind of parenthood. For some couples, there is a reluctance to disclose adoption plans because such disclosure is an admission of their own reproductive failure. Furthermore, it may serve as a catalyst for negative reactions from family and friends (Miall 1987).

This reluctance to talk about adoption is consistent with the growing sense of social isolation reported by many infertile couples (Bierkens 1975). Due to the stigmatizing nature of both infertility and adoption, social isolation is a common experience. For example, infertile couples report a desire to avoid social situations that are associated with children, with the consequence that they decrease their opportunities to interact with others and gain sources of needed social support (Link and Darling 1986). Similarly, infertile couples report a feeling of "being left behind or set apart from their peers," which also contributes to their sense of isolation (Daly 1989b).

In spite of this isolation and the reluctance to say anything about adoption to others, when couples do disclose their adoption plans, they typically find that others are supportive. In one study, when 74 infertile couples were asked how others reacted when they told them about adoption, over three-quarters said that people were positive and supportive (Daly 1987). Adoption appears to be the appropriate means for meeting pro-natalist expectations. As one woman explained, "they expect us to adopt because we have been married for so long. Like we have our house and car. But people then expect you to have kids. So people are happy when we say we have adoption as an alternative" (Daly 1987). Although there is evidence that childlessness and actual adoptive parenthood elicit stigmatic responses (Miall 1986), it would seem that anticipated adoptive parenthood does not suffer this same stigma.

Disclosure of adoption plans to significant others is also a way of trying on the anticipated new identity of adoptive parenthood. As one woman described it, "Sometimes I tell people about adoption to see what their reaction is. I want to see how they respond. I knew that there were some negative ideas. It's part of the preparation. If they have something crummy to say [i.e., about adoption], I want to hear it now before I have a child" (Daly 1988).

Formal Tasks

The loss of control over the timing of parenthood is perhaps one of the most demanding adjustments facing couples who pursue adoption. Already having confronted the loss of control over their own fertility, couples are faced with the task of waiting and depending on others in order to become adoptive parents. The formal process of adopting a child is filled with risks and uncertainties: waiting lists are long; emotional and monetary costs are often high; the fear of rejection is strong; and there is a lack of clarity about what adoptive parents should do and how they should act.

The dependence of couples on adoption professionals reinforces feelings of loss of control. In the minds of couples, agency staff are powerful, not only because they control the adoption process, but also because they judge the couple's adequacy as parents. One infertile woman described how her experience with the adoption agency had affected her feelings about the adoption process: "it has opened my eyes to the frustration of going through the process. You are at their beck and call when *they* decide that the match is made. You have no control. You have to *submit* yourself to the process" (Daly 1989a). A further indication of this powerlessness is the language that couples use to describe the formal adoption procedure. As one man put it, "It's like having a drill instructor walk into your environment." Said another, "This stranger walks in and has power over you." Others said they felt "judged," "interrogated," "on trial," or "fine-combed," or that someone was "going to play God with us" (Daly 1987). As part of this powerlessness, couples express concerns about "failing" at parenthood again by being rejected by the adoption officials. These responses to the adoption evaluation are consistent with Joe's (1979) observations that many infertile couples respond to the evaluation with fear or rage at having to prove their fitness for parenthood.

In light of the prevailing attitude that the adoption agency exists to judge couples and not to help them, couples respond to the formal adoption process in two distinct ways. According to Goffman's (1959) distinction between front-stage and back-stage behaviour, couples stage a public impression to the agency that they will make excellent parents, while in their private disclosures to each other they express anger and resentment at having to prove themselves worthy to the agency. One man said that his feelings of resentment stemmed from the unfairness of the process: "I resent being tested and prodded and being asked my feelings. People who have to adopt, and I understand the reason for it, people who suffer infertility have to lay bare their soul whereas those who have biological children don't have to do anything to show they are good parents. The system is unfair" (Daly 1987). Compounding the sense of unfairness is the prospect of ultimately being turned down by the agency due to the scarcity of adoptable babies.

In keeping with their sense of powerlessness, many couples express confusion about what to expect from the adoption agency and what is expected of them in return. As a result, aimlessness is characteristic of the formal process of becoming an adoptive parent. One man expressed his disappointment at having no direction in preparing for adoptive parenthood: "I really wish that there was something that could help you to prepare for adoption. We went into it all just not knowing what to expect" (Daly 1987). This uncertainty reinforces feelings of loss of control. As one man explained, the only certainty in an otherwise obscure process was that it would be a long wait: "I am really very vague about the whole process and what you have to go through — like I've never been through it before, eh? I don't know what to expect — what you have to do — what is involved in the home study and what you have to do — legally and things like that. They [the agency] just don't tell you what to expect except that it is a long wait" (Daly 1987). This uncertainty is also manifested in the absence of appropriate role models for adoptive parents (Brodzinsky 1987; DiGiulio 1987). Although most adults approach biological parenthood with a reasonable idea of what to expect, most prospective adoptive couples do not have any close relatives or friends who can provide them with a realistic perspective on the adoption experience.

Paradoxically, although the formal adoption process is perceived as involving a long wait, there is also a perception that there is a lack of preparation time for becoming adoptive parents. Unlike having a biological child where there is a nine-month period to get ready for parenthood, the preparation for adoptive parenthood is perceived as occurring between the call from the agency that there is a child and the arrival of the baby, which is usually a period of only two or three days (Daly 1987). This perception can be attributed to the uncertainty of whether the adoption will occur, and, if so, its exact timing (DiGiulio 1987; Levy-Shiff et al. 1990). These uncertainties are manifested in a reluctance to invest in an adoption until it is a reality, resulting in a cautious and inert preparatory stance.

The abruptness of adoption creates difficulties in taking on the role identity of parent when the child does arrive. Couples in the adoption waiting period have expressed concerns about being distant or disconnected from the child who enters the family with such abruptness (Daly 1987). This concern is compounded by the fact that the parental status of the adoptive parents is not fully secured when the baby arrives, for there is always the possibility that the child will be taken away during the probation period (Levy-Shiff et al. 1991). The abruptness of adoption can also create some very practical problems of preparation. It is difficult to change busy, independent lifestyles at short notice. Because most wives and husbands are in the paid labour force, arranging for parental leave or physically preparing the home for the arrival of the adopted child on such short notice may prove awkward.

Challenges of Being an Adoptive Family Following Infertility

The experience of adoption presents parents and children with a unique set of family development tasks. Some have argued that infertile couples who adopt face additional stresses in becoming parents when compared to biological families (Brodzinsky 1987). At the same time, it has been argued that infertile couples may have more resources from which to draw in coping with the additional stresses of adoption. For example, due to the delays of infertility, adoptive parents are usually older than biological parents, and are therefore likely to be more skilled at dealing with life stresses (Brodzinsky and Huffman 1988). Related to this, adopting couples have usually been married longer, which may facilitate the adjustment that is required with the adoption (Levy-Shiff et al. 1990).

In one of the few comparative studies that examined differences in the transition to parenthood between 52 biological parent couples and 52 adoptive parent couples, the researchers found that adoptive parents were as well adjusted as biological parents and in some instances were better adjusted (Levy-Shiff et al. 1990, 1991). This was contrary to the expectation that adoptive parents would experience short-term adverse effects because of the unique hurdles and stresses of adoption. For example, adoptive couples scored higher on measures of marital satisfaction, which can be attributed not only to the longer duration of the marriage, but also to being together through the stresses and upheavals associated with infertility and adoption. This stronger marital bond is consistent with research that has found that the crisis of infertility appears to have fostered more empathy and sensitivity between spouses (Kraft et al. 1980). Similar trends in the positive adjustment of adoptive parents in the early years of the adoptive family life cycle are found in other research (Hoopes 1982; Singer et al. 1985).

Several explanations have been offered for the better functioning of adoptive parents at this early stage. One is that they experience a kind of "honeymoon" phase resulting from the long deprivation of parental experience, which makes them more appreciative of the gratifications of parenthood (Levy-Shiff et al. 1991). Another possible explanation is that their better functioning may reflect their efforts to deny the difference of adoption by reassuring themselves and others that their experience of parenting does not differ from that of biological experiences (Kirk 1981; Brodzinsky 1990).

One of the ongoing developmental challenges for adoptive families is to manage the difference of adoption. In his classic work on the way that couples deal with this difference, Kirk (1964) identifies two patterns of coping. The first pattern is called *rejection-of-difference* and is characterized by the effort on the part of adoptive parents to deny the additional tasks, challenges, and conflicts that are encountered in the adoptive family. In their effort to emulate biological families as closely as possible, they disclose as little information as possible and discourage discussion about adoption. The second pattern is referred to as *acknowledgment-of-difference*, which involves openly dealing with differences of adoption. In these families, parents allow and encourage their children to explore the differences that they experience by virtue of their adoptive status. Kirk suggests that although these patterns are not mutually exclusive, the acknowledgment-of-difference pattern is much more beneficial for positive adjustment in adoptive families.

In keeping with Kirk's idea of acknowledging the difference, Hajal and Rosenberg (1991) have suggested that the basic developmental issue for adoptive families is to establish the "metafamily," which includes the "ghosts" of the biological parents and, by extension, their families and bloodlines. These biological links for the adopted child constitute a kind of "super-extended family system." Although these members are not necessarily present physically, "their shadows hover over" and inevitably affect the established bonds and relationships in the adoptive family. One of the implications of acknowledging adoption is that the image of the biological parents is introduced into the family system, thereby threatening the exclusiveness of the relationship between the adoptive parents and the child (DiGiulio 1987).

Managing the differences of adoption occurs in different forms throughout the family life cycle. From the early discussions of the adoption — when the child makes few distinctions between the processes of birth and adoption (Brodzinsky et al. 1984) — to the disclosure of identifying information and reunion, adoptive families face a continuing number of unique challenges. What appears to be of paramount importance in dealing with these challenges is the availability of the information and the willingness on the part of adoptive parents to share it with their adopted child.

In the next section, this theme is developed more fully by examining the implications of adoptive difference for the identity of those who do not have a biological link with their parents. Specifically, there is an examination of how adoption and reproductive technologies, where there is either a partial or no genetic link to the parents, affect the development of the child's identity.

Adoptive Identity and New Reproductive Technologies

Adoptions usually take one of two forms: the adopted child has no genetic relationship to either of the adopting parents; or, as in step-parent adoption, the child is the genetic offspring of one but not the other parent. For the most part, offspring of NRTs have a parallel genetic relationship to their social parents. With therapeutic donor insemination, ovum donation with insemination by husband, and surrogate motherhood with insemination by the social father, the offspring share half of the genetic material with one of the parents. In the case of combining the husband's sperm with that of at least one more donor, this procedure requires subsequent genetic analysis to determine the genetic source of the offspring. It is only with *in vitro* fertilization (IVF), using the couple's ovum and sperm, that the child has a full genetic relationship to the social parents. Given the striking parallel to the genetic relationship of adopted children and their parents, Bell (1986) has referred to the pregnancies of NRTs as "adoptive" pregnancies.

However, the similarities do not stop at the level of genetics. Those choosing to use these technologies, as for their adoptive counterparts, must determine how they wish to manage the public identities of themselves and their children. We will deal with several related issues in turn.

The Creation of the Origins Narrative

Adoption practice has been guided over the latter half of this century by a determination to serve the "best interests of the child." At one time this meant that the child was to be treated as the consanguineous offspring of the adoptive parents. Similarities between child and parent were to be stressed. Differences were to be played down. The adoption story was to be told, but with as little information about the biological origins of the child as possible. Many parents considered it best never to mention the adoption, hoping that they would thus obliterate not only the social stigma of their own infertility but also the "damaged goods" identity of the adoptive child. This quest for maintaining the myth of equivalence between adoptive and biological families was strongly attacked by Kirk (1964, 1981), who argued that by encouraging silence and ignoring differences, family communication would always be strained by the need to maintain consistency. Secrets were simply too difficult to keep. Too many people knew of the origins of the child. Too many extended family members had to join into the ruse to make it work, at least on a surface level. And as typically happened, at some point the myth of consanguinity was destroyed by an inadvertent word or an unintended piece of shared information.

Fortunately, Kirk's analysis has been taken seriously. Today, adoptive parents are counselled to be far more open about the adoption story. They are encouraged to tell the child how it was that the birth mother came to place the child with the adopted parents. They are urged to retell the story in more elaborated fashion as the child develops new cognitive capacities to understand the meaning of adoption (Brodzinsky et al. 1984). Paradoxically, by sharing the story with the child and hence with their extended social milieu, the adoptive couple are relieved of that part of their role handicap that is maintained by silence. They do not have to live up to a conception of family that does not match their history or current experience. They can nurture the uniqueness of their child without viewing differences between themselves and the child as the result of a flawed parenting style.

How have parents of NRT offspring responded to the challenge of controlling the narrative of family origin? For the most part, the strategies employed are similar to those used by parents favouring adoptive secrecy. Many infertile couples are counselled not to tell anyone of the steps they have taken to have a child that shares some or no genetic connection to them (Andrews 1984). There are reports that even obstetricians, who were not involved in the impregnation procedures but who subsequently delivered the infant, may be unaware of the genetic status of the infant. Like the adoption situation, however, secrecy comes with a price. By holding to the myth that the parents are the sole genetic source for the child, the parents must always remain on guard to control information concerning the child's origins. Temperamental, physical, and cognitive differences between child and parent must be ignored so as not to give away the secret. The genetically non-related parent's personal concerns about a sense of completeness cannot be dealt with since, in the narrative, this parent must be thought of as a biological parent. Hence, the couple remain out of balance as one parent must always be presented fraudulently in the family narrative. When strains emerge in the normal course of family life, especially around child management, it is at the intersection of created family myths that communication breaks down. Judging by the adoption literature, it is better for all members of the family to be cognizant of the origins of its constituents than to hide behind a narrative that one day will be exposed as false.

Should the Child Be Told?

Today, almost all adoptive parents tell their children that they have been adopted. While professionals have differed as to the timing of the telling of the adoption story, most parents start before the child is old enough to understand even the rudiments of the events leading to entrance into the family (Brodzinsky et al. 1984; Schechter et al. 1964). This early rehearsal eases the parents' transition from achieving parenthood to being able to share information openly with the child.

The consensus in the NRT literature is not to tell the child but to attempt to preserve the "best interests of the parents." Generally this is based on the belief that since most NRT pregnancies appear to outsiders to be like any other normal pregnancy following impregnation, there is no need to destroy the myth of the couple's fertility. Furthermore, many in the NRT field hold that telling the child will only stimulate fantasies about the non-present genetic parent. This, in turn, is assumed to weaken the bond between the child and the social parent and eventually to lead to a search for the biological parent (Andrews 1984).

Again, judging by the adoption literature, such an approach is ill advised. Kirk (1981) has presented evidence suggesting that even when adoptees are not told that they come from a different genetic background, many of them sense that they are out of step with their adoptive families.

For some, the eventual knowledge that they were adopted helps them to come to terms with this sense of being an outsider. To the extent that children of NRTs may not share genetically mediated interests, temperament, and style with the parent, they, too, are prone to this sense of not really being part of the family. Interestingly, adoptees who differ temperamentally from their adoptive parents, but are aware that the parents acknowledge the difference as the result of non-shared genetic background and the child's adoptive status, feel a much closer bond to the adoptive parents (Sobol and Cardiff 1983). This suggests that for NRT offspring, information about the circumstances that led to the birth of the child should not be withheld.

What exactly is available to tell NRT offspring of their biological heritage? For the most part, very little. Annas (1980) has found that less than two-thirds of physicians involved with NRTs kept records on children born through artificial insemination and only a third kept records of the sperm donors themselves. Regardless of record keeping, since many women have been impregnated with sperm from multiple sources, it is unlikely that such records would shed much light on the genetic origins of the child. Unfortunately, because of this paucity of accurate records, offspring of NRTs are shut off from genetic, medical, and psychological information that could help them to form an important part of their sense of self.

We know that many adoptees who have little or no information about their origins feel as if their life stories began at chapter two. Being unable to account for how they came to be adopted, they develop a sense of uncompleted identity or lack of "personal gestalt" (Sobol and Cardiff 1983). Subsequent searching for biological roots becomes one of the primary foci of adult life (Sorosky et al. 1978). For many, the search is undertaken not to establish a relationship with birth parents but to come to understand their beginnings, to see who they look like, and to assure the birth parent that the adoption had a favourable outcome (Schechter and Bertocci 1990; Sobol and Cardiff 1983). It is anticipated that children of NRTs, once they learn of the technological procedures that led to their beginnings, will also want to know more of their biological roots. However, if records are not kept, if routes to personal information are obstructed, then they will literally have no means of forming a sense of personal gestalt other than to block out of their lives any consideration of their genetic origins. This is a great psychological price to ask of those interested in their beginnings. However, if adequate records were kept and procedures followed that would allow access to information, it is anticipated that many of the concerns around identity could be avoided.

Finally, it should be noted that offspring of NRTs, like their adoptive counterparts, will in all likelihood differentiate between their social parents who raised them and their biological parent(s) who gave them a genetic heritage. Their personal loyalty will be to their social parents, who need not fear the adoptee's desire to know. Summarizing the search and reunion literature, Schechter and Bertocci (1990) concluded that a search for roots drew adoptive parents and children closer together. It is anticipated that the same result will occur for those born through NRTs.

In summary, issues of identity for the offspring of NRTs mirror those of adoptees and their parents. By following current adoption practices for managing issues of identity, it is expected that several pitfalls may be avoided. Parents of NRT offspring will have more difficulty controlling secrecy than facing openness. Their children have a need to know of their biological origins in order to complete a sense of identity. Without such knowledge, the past will ever remain a present concern.

Demographics of Adoption in Canada

In March of 1991, provincial and territorial adoption coordinators were asked to supply 1981-1990 adoption statistics for the following variables:

- total number of children placed for adoption for each year from 1981 to 1990;

- the number of domestic adoptions for each year from 1981 to 1990;

- the number of international adoptions for each year from 1981 to 1990 by country of origin;

- the number of *relative* (e.g., by a grandparent, aunt, etc.) adoptions for each year from 1981 to 1990;

- the number of *step-parent* adoptions for each year from 1981 to 1990;

- the number of domestic children placed for adoption with individuals other than relatives or step-parents for each year from 1981 to 1990 by age;

- the number of domestic special needs children placed for adoption with individuals other than relatives or step-parents for each year from 1981 to 1990, indicating where possible the various categories used to define special needs children;

- the number of public or ministry agency placements for each year from 1981 to 1990;

- the number of private agency placements for each year from 1981 to 1990;

- the number of adoption placements by independent private practitioners for each year from 1981 to 1990;

- the number of Native adoptions for each year from 1981 to 1990;

- the number of adoption disruptions for each year from 1981 to 1990 (disruption is defined as all placements that end with the return of the child to the agency, whether before or after the adoption finalization);

- the number of subsidized adoptions for each year from 1981 to 1990;

- the number of homes awaiting placement for each year from 1981 to 1990; and

- the number of homes awaiting home studies for each year from 1981 to 1990.

Since many of the provinces did not maintain records for several of the categories, it was possible to generate statistics only for the variables considered below. Coordinators also provided explanations of record-keeping procedures and definitions of data categories.

Statistics for live births and abortions came from Statistics Canada annual reports. Employment and Immigration Canada provided information on the number of children brought into Canada from other countries who were subsequently adopted.

Throughout this discussion of demographics, public adoptions will refer to all adoptions that were facilitated through provincial ministerial offices and agencies or through other agencies, at arm's length to the ministry, whose funding came from provincial governmental sources. Private adoptions, on the other hand, are those facilitated by individuals and agencies that do not receive direct funding or frontline supervision from provincial ministries.

Caveats Concerning the Accuracy of the Data

In attempting to establish a clear demographic picture of the adoption scene in Canada, it is first necessary to begin with a series of caveats concerning the validity of the statistics available in the public domain.

Record keeping of adoption information remains at the provincial level in the hands of the ministries responsible for the facilitation of adoptions. As the ministries' mandates are service and not research, it is rare to find complete record keeping over any substantial period of time. Furthermore, whether statistics are gathered at the provincial ministry level or remain the responsibility of regional offices seems to affect the trustworthiness of the figures. In general, ministry officials believed that figures that they personally collected were more valid than those gathered in the field without direct ministry supervision.

Another problem in gathering adoption data is that there has been no attempt to coordinate the categories of adoption information across the country. It becomes problematic to combine or compare information on the provinces when not all of them use the same definitions for coding the data.

Some provinces have chosen to collect adoption figures not only for adoption in the public domain but also for private adoptions that do not fall directly under the mandate or supervision of the provincial ministry. In other provinces, adoptions in the private domain continue without the possibility of provincial ministry scrutiny. In these cases, it is difficult to determine the extent to which adoption has been used as a means of family formation. As a result, it has been necessary to estimate various pieces of information concerning adoption from the trends that have emerged in other provinces. While this is a somewhat risky undertaking, we have been struck by the overall uniformity in the adoption trends that have emerged. This consistency across provinces with comparable information leads us to believe that the estimates are valid. However, in those cases where it has not been possible to provide estimates, this has been noted.

Demand for Adoptable Children

There are no precise data available for determining exactly how many individuals and couples are seeking to adopt a child. In the private domain, no records are kept of waiting lists for adoption. In the public domain, figures were available only for seven provinces. The totals for these provinces from 1982 to 1990 are presented in Table 1.

In 1982, there were 9 666 applicants in various stages of waiting for a child to adopt in the public domain in all provinces, excluding New Brunswick, Nova Scotia, Ontario, and the territories. By 1986, this figure had risen by 32.1 percent to 14 229. However, from 1987 (12 774) to 1990 (9 272) there was a steady decrease in the number of applicants who chose to avail themselves of this service. In fact, the figures for the end of the decade are lower, both absolutely and in proportion to the population, than they were at the beginning. Caution, however, must be taken before concluding that demand for adoptable children has truly decreased. In all likelihood this decrease in the number of applicants seeking a child reflects a turning toward private and international adoption services as applicants become aware that demand far outstrips the quantity of children available for adoption in the public domain.

While no exact data on the number of applicants using private facilities are available, the National Adoption Study's survey of private practitioners and agencies identified 3 302 applicants who were seeking to adopt in 1990 through 146 private auspices. Unfortunately, there is no way to determine exactly what proportion of those seeking to adopt through the private domain this figure represents. Furthermore, there were no means available for estimating how many of these applicants were also pursuing an adoption in the public domain.

Finally, discussions with private individuals and groups that facilitate international adoptions have yielded estimates of those pursuing international adoptions to be in the 2 000 to 5 000 range. Again, no information is available to determine the degree of overlap with other waiting list categories. At the very least, it can be concluded that, if adoptable children are available, there is no shortage of prospective adoptive parent applicants.

Total Domestic Adoptions

The number of Canadian-born children placed in adoptive homes has declined steadily over the past decade (Table 2). In 1981, approximately 5 376 children were adopted. In 1990, only 2 836 were placed. This represents a 47.3 percent drop in the use of domestic adoption as a means of family formation.

Public Adoptions

A majority of domestic adoptions are still facilitated through the public domain. However, it is clear that the number of public adoptions has fallen quite dramatically over the decade (Figure 1). In 1981, 82.6 percent of all domestic adoptions were through public agencies. By 1990, this had fallen to 61.0 percent. In absolute terms, however, the decline is even more dramatic. In 1981, 4 441 children were placed through public agencies. In 1990, only 1 731 followed the same route. This represents a decline of 61.2 percent.

Private Adoptions

The picture for adoptions carried out in the private domain is the inverse of the public one. At the beginning of the decade, only 17.4 percent of all domestic adoptions were private. By 1990, this had risen to 39.0 percent. Interestingly, the total number of private adoptions per year has wavered only slightly across the decade, with the average number being 1 071. In other words, although the absolute number of private adoptions has remained constant, relative to public adoptions they have risen dramatically.

Domestic Adoptions of Children Under the Age of One Year

The number of children less than one year of age (infants) who have been placed for adoption by public agencies has dropped from a high of 2 736 in 1981 to a low of 698 in 1990 (Table 3). This represents a 74.5 percent decrease over the decade. On the other hand, private adoption of infants has remained relatively steady (mean of 955 per year) with a slight peak in 1988 (1 102). Comparing the two routes for facilitating the adoption of infants, it is clear that public agency adoptions have fallen off substantially (Figure 2). At the beginning of the decade, 77.7 percent of all domestic infant adoptions were undertaken by public agencies. By the end of the decade, the percentage had fallen to 41.1 percent. This trend is mirrored in the percentages of the caseload that infant adoptions represent in the two adoption delivery systems: in the public domain, infant adoptions dropped from 61.6 percent of all public adoptions in 1981 to 40.3 percent in 1990; in the private domain, infant adoptions ranged from 82.6 percent to 94.6 percent across the decade. Thus, the private domain has clearly taken over the adoption of very young children.

Decline in Infant Adoptions

To understand fully the dramatic drop in the adoption of infants in the past decade, it is necessary to consider this decline within the context of decisions about responses to a pregnancy. Although it has been often assumed that the dramatic fall in adoption figures has primarily been a result of increased access to abortion, this assumption is wrong.

From 1981 to 1989, the number of unmarried women below the age of 25 who became pregnant rose from 68 755 to 77 210 (Table 4). This cohort represents the pool from which the vast majority of those who place an infant for adoption are to be found. Across the decade, the number of these young women who chose abortion as a response to the pregnancy steadily declined (Figure 3). In 1981, nearly half (48.8 percent) of all these pregnancies ended in abortion. By 1989, the percentage had fallen to 37.9. At the same time, the percentage of these pregnancies that resulted in the placing of the infant for adoption showed a somewhat less dramatic decline from 5.1 in 1981 to 2.2 in 1989. Clearly, the abortion rate was declining far faster than the adoption rate. Interestingly, the most striking change in alternative responses to the pregnancy was to be found in the percentage of pregnancies that resulted in the birth mother or a non-adopting surrogate raising the infant. In 1981, 46.1 percent of young single women chose to raise their infant. In 1989, this figure had risen to 59.9 percent, a gain of almost 14 percentage points. Hence, the decline in adoption is in all likelihood unaffected by the abortion rate but instead is closely linked to the greater likelihood of choosing to become a single mother.

This trend is amplified when adoption rates are considered in terms of the percentage of live births within the same cohort (Figure 4). The 1981 figures indicate that 10.0 percent of children born to unmarried women under 25 years of age were placed for adoption. This figure dropped to 3.6 percent by 1989. Thus, whether considered as a percentage of pregnancies or of live births, the adoption rate has dropped steadily across the decade.

Alternatives to Adopting an Infant: The Hard-to-Place Child

If prospective adoptive parents are finding it increasingly difficult to find an infant to adopt, one alternative is to adopt a child labelled "hard to place." Children who fit this category may display any of the following characteristics: over one year of age; physically, emotionally, or cognitively challenged; possessing a racial or ethnic minority status; and having a previous foster or adoptive placement history that has been shown to be related to future adoption disruption. Unfortunately, provincial records are not consistently kept according to these characteristics. However, given that the child's age at the time of adoption placement is correlated with all of these factors, those children over one year old at placement will be considered for the present analysis to be hard to place.

The adoption of hard-to-place children follows the same downward trend as the other indices of adoption (Table 5). In 1981, 1 855 children above one year of age were placed for adoption. By 1990, this figure had fallen 38.7 percent to 1 138. The vast majority of these adoptions were facilitated in the public rather than the private domain (Figure 5). The range of public hard-to-place adoptions across the decade was 88.9 percent to 95.7 percent of all hard-to-place adoptions. In terms of the impact on publicly facilitated caseloads, adoptions of older children comprised 38.4 percent of all public adoptions in 1981. This rose in a linear fashion to 59.7 percent by 1990 (Figure 6).

Privately facilitated adoption of children above one year of age has shown no consistent trend across the decade. In 1983, it reached a peak of 11.1 percent of all older adoptions. In 1986, it dropped to 4.3 percent, while in 1990, 9.2 percent of all adoptions of older children were facilitated privately. Given these wide changes in percentage across the decade, in absolute terms there have been no substantial changes in the actual number of older children adopted through private facilities. Finally, the percentage of private adoptions of older children as a function of all private adoptions displayed no consistent trend across the decade, the range being 5.4 to 17.4 percent.

Native Adoptions

It is difficult to determine how many Native children have been adopted across the decade, as record keeping by the provinces and territories has been haphazard, with information rarely being available for the complete decade. As well, some provinces have chosen not to keep records of the number of adoptions of Native children or of the cultural groups who adopt these children. Hence, trends must be inferred from the scattered information available (Table 6).

Overall, there seems to have been a decrease in the number of Native children who have been adopted through public facilities. Reported figures for the latter half of the decade indicate a drop from a high of 428 in 1986 to a low of 201 in 1990. Since not all provinces have kept accounts of the number of adoptions of Native children, these figures should be considered only suggestive of a downward trend.

Who is adopting Native children? The answer depends on the province in which they are adopted and the Native group to which the children belong. In Manitoba, where there are seven status Indian public agencies, between 70 and 100 percent of all status Indian children adopted were placed with at least one parent who was also a status Indian. On the other hand, an average of only 26.3 percent of Métis children were placed with a culturally similar adoptive parent. In the Northwest Territories, on average,

23.7 percent of Native children placed by public facilities found their way to a home with at least one Native parent. However, this figure rises dramatically when custom adoptions are considered. Custom adoptions take place within the Native community but are not facilitated by public agencies or officials. They follow the rules and customs of the Native community. They are recorded at the territorial office to allow the adoptive family to receive family and educational benefits. When added to other Native adoptions facilitated by the territories, the average number of culturally similar placements rises to 77.7 percent. In Ontario, across the decade, 29.4 percent of status placements and 11.4 percent of non-status placements were in homes with at least one culturally similar adoptive parent. The difference in the two groups' placements in all likelihood reflects the fact that there are three status placement facilities in the province. Finally, Quebec figures are available only for Inuit adoptions. Across the decade, between 83.3 and 93.4 percent of all Inuit adoptions followed custom traditions. As an indication of the strength of custom adoptions as a means of family formation, between 16.1 and 32.2 percent of all births in Inuit communities were placed as custom adoptions.

It would seem that custom adoption procedures, where allowed by law or practised without legislative authorization, are the primary means by which Native people are able to ensure the continued enculturalization of their adopted children. Use of Native-controlled social service agencies also increases the likelihood that the child will be raised in a home with at least one Native parent. However, non-Native service facilities, for the most part, place Native children in non-Native homes. While the National Adoption Study survey indicated that these service providers are aware of the need to sensitize adopting parents to the child's Native origins, there has been no evidence to date that speaks to the success of these efforts.

International Adoptions

There are two kinds of international adoptions in Canada. In the first, children are brought into Canada where the adoption is subsequently finalized. Unfortunately, few of these adoptions are recorded as international adoptions; instead, most are grouped with other domestic adoptions. In the second and more common type, children are adopted by Canadian citizens in the child's home country and then brought into Canada. It is difficult to determine exactly how many of these children have come into Canada, since record keeping for this group of adoptees began at the federal level only in late 1991. However, one province, Quebec, assuming its own control of immigration into the province, has kept accurate records since 1982 (Table 7).

No consistent trends for international adoptions appear across the decade. The range is between 123 in 1982 and 592 for the first eight months of 1991. Some countries, such as Bolivia, Guatemala, India, and Peru, have been a steady but not an overwhelming source of children. In

1986, 74 children were adopted in Korea. That figure dropped to one in 1991. Haiti has also had fluctuations in the number of adoptions. In 1983, 169 children were adopted; in 1986, 5; and in 1991, 83. Major adoption initiatives have begun in the past year in China (176) and Romania (155). In this latter case, foreign adoptions have been halted since July 1991 so that the country can establish more formal and controlled procedures for facilitating an international adoption. As well, Mexico (45) and Taiwan (20) have been countries of some adoption activity in 1991.

Since figures for the last four months of 1991 were not available, an estimate for the year was determined based on the assumptions that there would be no further Romanian adoptions and that the rate of adoption would not change for the last four months. We thus anticipate approximately 816 Quebec international adoptions for 1991. While it is not possible to determine how representative the Quebec figures are for Canada as a whole, an estimate was made based on the conservative assumption that Quebec's international adoptions represented one-third of all international adoptions. If these assumptions are correct, there will be at least 2 448 international adoptions for the entire country in 1991. If the same number of domestic infant adoptions occur in 1991 as in 1990 (1 698), then there will be approximately 800 more international than domestic adoptions in 1991. If this estimate is within acceptable bounds of accuracy, then international adoptions have become the most common means of adopting an infant for Canadians.

Adoption Alternatives Available to Infertile Couples

Infertile couples who wish to adopt have three main alternatives: public, private, and international adoption. Since these different kinds of adoption do not have universal meanings across the country, definitions are warranted. For the sake of consistency, we define *public adoption* as an adoption that is facilitated by a public welfare agency or ministry facility where no fees are charged to the adoptive couple. A *private adoption* is facilitated by a non-government agency or private practitioner who typically charges the prospective adoptive couple a fee for the service. *International adoptions* can be coordinated by a public welfare agency, a private third-party practitioner, or, in some instances, the couple themselves.

The focus of this section is on the implications of public and private adoptions. Following a brief overview of traditional assumptions about the role of the state in adoption, the discussion will focus on data collected from a national survey of adoption service provision. These data are part of the National Adoption Study funded by National Welfare Grants, Health and Welfare Canada, in 1990. Questionnaires were sent to service providers working in public and private adoption agencies, and to practitioners who had some involvement in the facilitation of a private adoption. The analysis is based on the responses of 202 public service agencies, 130 private practitioners, and 16 private adoption agencies. In this analysis, private practitioners and private agencies are analyzed together.

Although international adoptions appear to be on the increase, record keeping is poor; as a result, few data are available. Nevertheless, there will be a brief discussion of motivations for international adoption and an overview of key issues involved in attempting to adopt a child from outside of the country.

Assumptions About the Role of the State

Current adoption practice in Canada is rooted in a philosophy of child welfare. This represents a shift from the historical emphasis on the protection of adoptive parents' rights. Now, children whose biological parents are unable or unwilling to care for them are perceived to be in need of protection. As a result, most publicly funded agencies are mandated to place the needs of the adoptable child in the forefront. The principle of the best interests of the child is embodied in the laws governing adoption placements for most provinces in Canada. However, as private adoptions account for an increasing proportion of all adoptions, the traditional focus on the best interests of the child is called into question. As prospective adoptive parents become the paying consumers of adoption services, there is the potential in practice for the needs of the couple to supersede the needs of the child. In particular, concerns have been expressed in practice about the poor preparation and selection of adoptive parents and the possible exploitation of birth mothers in private adoptions (MacDonald 1984).

The central question of whose interests are being served is part of a larger question about the degree of formal control over the adoption process. At one extreme is the almost complete government control in the provincially supported public welfare agency. At the other extreme is the almost complete absence of government control where an independent practitioner coordinates and facilitates an adoption, with no government involvement save for the signing of final documents. As this range of formal involvement would suggest, there is tremendous variation in the way that the interests of the child, the parents, and the state are served.

There has been considerable debate among researchers and within the field of child welfare about the relative merits of public and private adoptions. Although there are few reliable data available that support the success of one over the other, it appears that each has certain advantages (Segal 1982). Public adoptions have a professional staff who are experienced in assessment, special adoption problems, and placement; there is usually a larger pool of adoptive homes from which to select; records are kept of the child's medical and social histories, which can then be made available to adoptive parents; alternative resources are available in the event of an adoption disruption; and, finally, there is an ongoing availability of counselling services for all parties in the adoption. Private adoptions also have a number of advantages: the birth mother can avoid agency stigmatization; in light of fewer policy restrictions, birth parents and adoptive parents can have more control over how the adoption placement is handled; the process is less bureaucratic; and there is an opportunity to avoid counselling if it is undesired.

Variation in the amount of government control is also evident in international adoptions. While some international adoptions are coordinated through public agencies, others may involve a prospective couple going to the source country to facilitate the adoption themselves. Again, serious questions arise with respect to the importance of state involvement in adoption and the protection of rights for all parties concerned.

The degree of state control over adoption is of central importance in the consideration of public and private adoptions. Stemming from this are numerous ramifications for prospective adoptive couples. In the section that follows, private and public adoptions are analyzed in terms of the following: characteristics of prospective adoptive parents, birth parents, and adoptable children; restrictions on accessibility; and the kinds of adoption services that are available to birth and adoptive parents. The central focus of this discussion is how these factors affect the adoption alternatives available to infertile couples.

Adoptive Applicant Profile

The first step for understanding the differences between public and private adoptions is to examine the profile of the adoptive applicants who use the service. The characteristics considered are age, education, marital status, adoptive status, religious background, fertility status, and prior parenting experience.

As part of the National Adoption Study, service providers in both the public and private domains were asked to identify the most typical characteristics of the men and women who approached them to adopt an infant. No significant differences (using a Pearson Chi-square analysis, $p < 0.01$) between public and private adoptions were found for marital status, adoptive status, religious background, race, or the presence of a fertility problem. Therefore, for both public and private adoptions, 98 percent of people who adopted were married and not adopted.[2] About two-thirds (66 percent in public; 62 percent in private) were Protestant, while 30 percent in public and 39 percent in private were Catholic. Approximately 95 percent of the applicants were Caucasian. The only significant difference to emerge was for Native applicants, virtually all of whom sought to adopt through a public agency. Although there were also no significant differences with respect to the presence of infertility, approximately three-quarters in both the public and private domains were infertile. Given the shortage of adoptable children, one might have expected the proportion of those with infertility to be higher, especially in the public domain.

For age, education, and parenting experience, there were significant differences between public and private adoptions.

Age

For men and women, the typical age range for both public and private adoptions was 31 to 35. However, there was a significant difference between public and private at the higher age categories. Whereas 25 percent of men in public agencies were in the 36-40 year category, 41 percent of men in private adoptions were in this age range ($p < 0.001$). Similarly for women, 8 percent in the public sector compared to 22 percent in the private sector were in the 36-40 year range ($p < 0.001$). The difference is significant ($p < 0.05$) again in the over-40 category for men, with only 0.5 percent in the public domain and 5 percent in the private domain. Women were less typical in the over-40 age category. Hence, the typical age profile for both men and women is higher in the private sector. Although public agencies can no longer discriminate on the basis of age as a result of the *Canadian Charter of Rights and Freedoms*, it appears that there is a perception that this restriction continues to exist.

Education

The most pronounced difference between the profiles of those adopting in the public and private domains was in their education. For both women and men, one-fifth in the public domain had a university degree compared to nearly two-thirds in the private domain ($p < 0.001$). Since education is a predictor of socioeconomic status, these figures strongly suggest class differences between those who pursue private adoption and those who pursue public adoption. This may be attributable to a number of factors. Paramount among these is the ability to pay the fees that are typically associated with private adoption. Another possibility is that couples of higher socioeconomic status are more comfortable approaching the professionals who typically coordinate private adoptions.

Prior Parenting Experience

Although most adoptive applicants have no parenting experience, whether adopting publicly or privately, significantly more of those adopting through a public agency had some parenting experience. In public agencies, 17 percent were biological parents compared to 5 percent in private adoptions ($p < 0.001$). In the public domain, 18 percent were prior adoptive parents compared to 8 percent in the private domain ($p < 0.01$). In public adoptions, 10 percent had been foster parents, while less than 1 percent of those in private adoptions had been foster parents ($p < 0.01$).

In summary, applicants who pursue adoption in the private sphere tend to be older, better educated, and without prior parenting experience.

Women Who Place for Adoption

Although emphasis has been placed on involving the father in decisions about pregnancy resolution, it is the young pregnant woman who carries the primary responsibility for the decision to place a child for adoption. For that reason, this section will focus on the experiences of young women who place a baby for adoption. Two areas are explored: the reasons why a young woman voluntarily places a child for adoption, and a comparison of the characteristics of young women who place a child for adoption in the public and private domains.

Reasons

When service providers were asked to give the reasons why young women voluntarily place their children for adoption, the most prevalent reason given was that they were too young to parent. Although not statistically significant, 53 percent of the public service providers compared to 46 percent of the private service providers identified age as the major reason. The second most prevalent reason was that they were financially unable to parent, with 20 percent in the public agencies compared to 34 percent in the private agencies citing this as a reason. Again, this difference was not statistically significant.

Characteristics

The profile of young women who place for adoption was very similar in the public and private domains. About three-quarters (75 percent in public; 73 percent in private) were between 15 and 19 years of age. Only 4 percent in public and 2 percent in private were under the age of 15. Approximately one-half (47 percent in public and 46 percent in private) were attending high school, while 45 percent in public and 39 percent in private were not attending school at all. Almost half (46 percent in public; 48 percent in private) were Protestant, 27 percent in public and 32 percent in private were Catholic, and 18 percent in public compared to 11 percent in private had no religious affiliation. Two-thirds (66 percent in public; 65 percent in private) were living at home with their parents when the pregnancy was discovered.

In both the public and private sectors, women who placed a child for adoption exhibited some unusual characteristics. While adoptive status is relatively rare in the general population (less than 3 percent) (Dickson et al. 1990; Kotsopoulos et al. 1988), 11 percent of birth mothers in this sample were adopted themselves. One possible explanation for the relatively high proportion of birth mothers who were adopted themselves is that they were seeking to understand and normalize the fact that they were placed for adoption through the process of placing a child themselves. Moreover, 12 percent of the birth mothers in this sample had already placed a child for adoption. The repetition of the placement experience could be attributed to the need to reopen the unresolved process of grief associated with the ambiguous loss of the first adoption placement.

Birth mothers tended to be late in approaching adoption professionals for help in placing their babies. Approximately one-half of birth mothers contacted the adoption service in the third trimester, while one-third contacted it in the second trimester.

Significant differences were found between public and private adoptions for the race of the birth mother. While 94 percent of birth mothers in private adoptions were Caucasian, 81 percent in public adoptions were Caucasian (p < 0.001). More Native birth mothers (17 percent) placed their children through public adoption agencies than through private facilities (6 percent) (p < 0.01). There was a small but significant difference between public and private adoptions in terms of marital status. While virtually all birth mothers in private adoptions were single, 96 percent of birth mothers in public adoptions were single, with the rest being divorced or common-law. There were also small differences with respect to a diagnosed medical problem. Five percent of birth mothers in the public agencies, compared to less than 1 percent in the private agencies, had a diagnosed medical problem (p < 0.05). Significant differences were found for employment status before the pregnancy, with 38 percent of birth mothers using private adoption services being employed, while only 17 percent of those in the public agencies were employed (p < 0.001). Although it is difficult to explain this difference, one possible reason is that their employment status may represent greater autonomy, which would be compatible with the greater sense of control they could exercise in a private adoption.

These data suggest that birth mothers who place a child for adoption in both the private and public domains are typically single, white, Protestant teenagers over the age of 15 who are living at home and attending high school. The few significant differences to emerge suggest that birth mothers in private adoptions were even more homogeneous with respect to this profile. Birth mothers who were employed before the pregnancy tended to choose private adoption. Birth mothers who were non-white, of a marital status other than single, and who had a diagnosed medical problem used public adoption services. One could speculate that the wider range of services that are typically available in public agencies would be better able to serve some of the idiosyncratic needs arising from these adoptions.

Profile of Adoptable Children

The kinds of children who are placed for public adoption are radically different from those in private adoptions. While almost all private adoptions involve the placement of healthy infants, most public agency adoptions involve the placement of a special needs child. In public adoptions, only 42 percent of children placed are infants (less than one year of age) without special needs. By contrast, 91 percent of adoptions in the private domain are healthy infants. The majority of children placed through public agencies have special needs: 50 percent of all placements are children older than one year of age, with the remaining 8 percent being placements of children who are less than one year of age but who have special needs.

Accessibility of Public and Private Adoption

The different structures and organizations of public and private adoptions suggest that there is variation in the accessibility of service. This section focusses on the factors that enhance or restrict access to public and private adoptions for prospective adoptive couples.

Cost

Public adoptions do not involve fees for adoptive couples. Although there may be small charges such as a court registration fee, these are nominal. Ability to pay fees is therefore the critical factor in the use of private adoption. There is tremendous variation in the fees that are charged to adopting couples. In private adoption agencies, for example, the average cost of an adoption is $3 684, ranging from a low of $2 500 to a high of $6 000. For adoptions facilitated by private practitioners, the average fees are approximately $3 100, based on the average lawyer's fee of $2 100 and a social work fee of $1 000. These figures can go much higher depending on whether the adoptive couples agree to pay for additional services such as pre- and post-adoption counselling for birth parents, home study updates, or other birth parent expenses.

The costs associated with adopting a child through private services are clearly restrictive for those with limited financial means. This restriction is consistent with the finding reported earlier that there is a higher proportion of better educated couples in the adoptive couple profile of private adoptions.

Waiting Period

The average number of applicants on a waiting list in 1991 was 59 couples in public agencies compared with 25 couples for private adoptions. The average waiting period to adopt a child was approximately two years (22.5 months) for a private adoption and almost six years (70.3 months) for an adoption through a public agency. When the total number of applicants waiting to adopt is compared with the number of adoptions facilitated, of all kinds, there is a "demand" ratio of 3.2 applicants per adoption in the public sphere and 2.7 applicants per adoption in the private sphere. When the number of applicants is considered in relation to infant adoptions only, the "demand" ratio rises to 7.7 applicants per infant adoption in the public sphere and 3 applicants per infant adoption in the private sphere. These figures are consistent with the decreasing number of infants that are available for adoption in the public domain and the relatively steady availability of infants in the private domain. Furthermore, waiting lists were closed in 12 percent of public agencies and 9 percent of private agencies. These figures suggest that the length of time that it takes to adopt through a public agency, coupled with the prospect that the list may be closed, is prohibitive for some couples.

Eligibility Criteria

Public and private service providers were asked to provide information on the importance of various criteria used to determine an adult's eligibility to adopt an infant. With few exceptions, these criteria were not different in public and private adoptions. Nine out of 10 service providers in both the public and private domains ranked the following criteria as important or very important: marriage stability; motivation to parent; problem-solving ability; adaptability; warmth and nurturance; and understanding of adoption. Approximately three-quarters of both indicated that the health of parents was important or very important. About one-half indicated that sexual orientation was important or very important. Criteria that were not considered to be as important included parents' education, income, and employment; religion; presence of a fertility problem; and presence of other children in the family.

Significant differences were found for only two eligibility criteria. Religion, although not ranked as an important criterion overall, was more important in the selection of adoptive couples in the private (21 percent) than the public domain (11 percent). Coping with infertility also had more importance as a criterion for private service providers. Ninety-four percent of private service providers, compared to 76 percent of public service providers, ranked this criterion as important.

Selection Guidelines

Service providers were also asked to rank the factors that they considered important when they had more than one eligible adoptive applicant to choose from. One of the most striking differences to emerge here was the heavier emphasis that was placed on birth mother expectations by private adoption practitioners. For example, while 37 percent of public adoption service providers ranked birth parent expectations as very important, 69 percent of private service providers ranked them as very important (p < 0.001). Surprisingly, there were no significant differences between public and private adoption service providers for adoptive parent expectations. While public adoption agencies appear to give roughly equal weight to birth parent and adoptive parent expectations (37 percent and 40 percent respectively), private adoption practitioners appear to place much more emphasis on birth parent expectations when compared to adoptive parent expectations (69 percent and 48 percent respectively). This runs contrary to the argument that since adoptive parents are the paying consumers in private adoption, their expectations take precedence over those of the birth parents.

Significant differences (p < 0.05) were also found between public and private service providers on a number of other items used in the selection of adoptive parents. Religion, marital status, occupation, and hobbies or interests received more emphasis from private service providers. These may mirror the greater emphasis given to birth parent expectations in the private domain. Only temperament received more emphasis from public service providers.

Restrictions on Placement

Service providers were asked whether there were specific circumstances under which they would have reservations about placing a child for adoption. Only minor concerns were expressed about placing an infant with parents of a different religion and placing an infant where both parents were working full time.

The strongest restriction on adoption placement was sexual orientation. There was a significant difference ($p < 0.05$) between service groups, with 87 percent of private adoption practitioners compared to 78 percent of public practitioners expressing reservations about placing an infant with a homosexual parent. Forty-four percent of private service providers and 25 percent of public agencies would not place an infant with a homosexual parent under any circumstances. About one-half (43 percent of public; 53 percent of private) of all service providers expressed concerns about placing a child with a single parent. Approximately one-third (34 percent public; 30 percent private) would have reservations about placing an infant with parents of a different race. Only 1 percent of public service providers and 3 percent of private service providers would absolutely not place a child with parents of a different race. Finally, there was a significant difference ($p < 0.05$) for placements with parents over the age of 40, with 34 percent of public service providers compared to 22 percent of private practitioners having reservations about placing an infant with such parents.

When restrictions on placement were examined with respect to a special needs child, there was a general tendency for these restrictions to soften.[3] For example, although 25 percent of public service providers said they would not place an infant with a homosexual parent, this dropped to 18 percent when the child had special needs. Reservations about placing a child with a single parent dropped by half (from 43 percent to 22 percent) when the child had special needs. Similarly, there was a drop from 34 percent to 21 percent of public service providers who had reservations about placing a child with parents of a different race when the child had special needs. Finally, there was a similar drop regarding the placement of a child with parents over 40 years of age. Whereas 34 percent had reservations about placing an infant, only 20 percent had reservations about placing a special needs child.

The data above suggest that there are a number of formal and informal policies in practice that can restrict access to adoption for prospective adoptive parents. Although the *Canadian Charter of Rights and Freedoms* and provincial human rights codes explicitly prohibit discrimination on the basis of sexual orientation and age, it would appear that these restrictions, and others, are common in practice. Homosexuals, single parents, and parents over 40 have considerable difficulty adopting an infant in either a public or private adoption. Their chances of adopting a special needs child are better, but still limited.

Overall, it appears that cost and the waiting period are the key factors when comparing public and private adoptions. While private adoptions appear to be more accessible in terms of the waiting period, they are accessible only to those who can afford to pay for the full costs of the adoption.

Services Available

An issue of importance for the choice of public or private adoption is the availability of various services for both birth parents and adoptive parents. In general, public service providers indicate more services available to both sets of parents. For example, 32 percent of public compared to 21 percent of private service providers offer support groups for new adoptive parents. Sixty-six percent of public compared to 47 percent of private service providers offer short-term support services for the birth parents after the placement. There was one exception to this trend: 27 percent of private compared to 19 percent of public service providers offer long-term birth parent support services after placement. The degree to which these differences play a role in either the accessibility or the success of the adoption would be purely speculative. The differences do, however, suggest that more structured support is available in public adoption, should it be needed.

Openness in adoption has been a major issue affecting adoption practice in recent years. Openness is perhaps best conceptualized on a continuum ranging from the full disclosure of identifying information to the tight restriction of both identifying and non-identifying information between birth parents and prospective adoptive parents. To examine the degree of openness in public and private adoption, service providers were asked whether they had ever facilitated a fully open adoption where birth parents and prospective adoptive parents meet before the placement with the exchange of identifying information. Twice as many private practitioners (41 percent) as public service providers (20 percent) had ever facilitated such an adoption. In a more moderate openness scenario, where birth parents and adoptive parents exchange information anonymously through the service provider, private practitioners were again more likely to be involved. While 62 percent of private adoption practitioners had ever facilitated an adoption like this, 55 percent of public adoption providers had done so.

When service providers were asked whether they would like to change the degree of openness in their adoption practice, 67 percent of private adoption practitioners indicated that they would not change the degree of openness, while 29 percent said they would increase the degree of openness $(p < 0.001)$. Public service providers were exactly the opposite, with only

34 percent not wanting to change the degree of openness and 64 percent wanting to increase the degree of openness (p < 0.001). Both public and private service providers believe that open adoptions, where the birth parents and adoptive parents have met, are likely to be more successful. Although not significantly different, 79 percent of public providers of adoption compared to 70 percent of private providers of adoption rate open adoptions as more successful than closed adoptions where little information has been exchanged.

These figures suggest a movement toward greater openness in adoption practice. Consistent with the fact that private service providers are more frequently using open arrangements is their general satisfaction with the degree of openness. For public service providers, while there is a belief in the success of openness and a desire to move toward more openness, they are relatively slow in moving toward this goal. The movement toward greater openness has been spawned by the recognition that information about the adoption is important for an adoptee's sense of identity (Sachdev 1984; Sobol and Cardiff 1983) and the birth parents' experience of loss (Sobol and Daly 1992). Unfortunately, the research base upon which to make these decisions is sadly lacking. As Demick and Wapner (1988) suggest in their review of open and closed adoptions, there is an extensive body of literature focussing on the negative outcomes of closed adoptions, but little empirical literature that attests to the effectiveness of open adoptions. Hence, the trend toward more open adoptions is based largely on positive clinical impressions, rather than well-documented research. A recent Canadian study suggests that although all members of the adoption triangle tend to favour the release of identifying information, there is a strong undercurrent of fear and suspicion within the triad about the loss of privacy, unwanted intrusion, and disruption of relationships (Sachdev 1989).

The differences reported here in the degree of openness have at least two possible implications for prospective adoptive parents. On the one hand, prospective adoptive parents might welcome the move toward more openness for the advantages that it brings to them. For example, it can provide them with more information about the social and medical histories of the birth mother; it can help solidify the "phantom" image of the birth parents; and it can facilitate the acknowledgment of difference that Kirk has emphasized as important for healthy adoption adjustment (Kirk 1981). On the other hand, greater openness can also be perceived as a threat by adoptive parents. Concerns about the birth mother interfering with their lives or "showing up on their doorstep" suggest that openness can also be perceived and potentially experienced as intrusive, rather than adaptive.

Issues in International Adoptions

Private practitioners reported that in 17 percent of the adoptions that they facilitated, the children came from countries outside of Canada. On the other hand, 4 percent of public adoptions were international. Given the large number of international adoptions that were estimated to have occurred in the past year and the fact that international adoptions are estimated to outnumber domestic infant adoptions three to two, it must be assumed that a majority of international adoptions are not being facilitated by licensed individuals or agencies but instead by private groups or individuals.

When service providers were asked to comment on the motivation of parents in pursuing an international adoption, 9 out of 10 indicated that the desire to avoid the delay of an infant domestic adoption was a motivator. Wanting a child of the same skin tone and wanting one of the same ethnic background were not considered to be strong motivators. Similarly, adopting internationally for altruistic reasons was not a strong motivator.

International adoptions provide unique challenges to the adoptive family. The child may have experienced poor pre- and post-natal conditions, resulting in the possibility of future physical or cognitive disabilities. In some instances, as a consequence of inadequate record keeping, adoptive parents are unprepared for the onset of genetically mediated diseases. For many children who do not share a racial background similar to that of the adoptive parents or the surrounding community, an identity crisis much like that experienced by children of domestic transracial adoptions can be expected. The primary feature is a profound sense of alienation from both the parents' and the child's racial groups. Thus, the child is faced with the challenge of coming to terms with two identities: one is racial, the other adoptive. Clinical reactions may include anger, depression, and aggressive behaviour on the part of the adoptive child and guilt, confusion, and rejection by parents.

Given that international adoptions yield some unique challenges for the adoptive family, what services are available to meet their needs? To answer this question it is necessary to differentiate between service providers who do and those who do not facilitate international adoptions. Virtually no adoption practitioners provide services for problems related to international adoptions that they did not facilitate. On the other hand, those who facilitate international adoptions also provide follow-up services: psychological and educational assessments (public, 7 percent; private, 10 percent); family counselling within the first year of the adoption (public, 41 percent; private, 49 percent); and family counselling after the first year of the adoption (public, 18 percent; private, 20 percent). They differ, however, on the provision of disruption resolution services. While 38 percent of the public international facilitators offer this service, only 9 percent of the private practitioners do so. Given the increased likelihood of international adoptions being disrupted, there seems to be a serious shortage of appropriate backup services in the private domain.

Summary and Conclusions

Making an informed choice about adoption requires attentiveness to a wide range of issues. Individual and cultural values play key roles in determining the acceptability of adoption as a viable alternative. Historical changes in the meaning of adoptive relationships have had an impact on the interpersonal experience of adoption, the delivery of adoption services, and adoption legislation and policy. Recent social-psychological research has provided insight into some of the unique and predictable tasks that are encountered when becoming adoptive parents. Identity has emerged as a central focus in the adoption literature, with the accessibility of information about biological heritage being a key to healthy adoption adjustment. Changing social conditions have influenced the availability of adoption alternatives including traditional adoptions facilitated by the state, private adoptions, and international adoptions.

The major findings of this report can be summarized as follows:

- Early adoption legislation stressed the best interests of the parents. However, for the past 40 years, the best interests of the child have marked adoption legislation and policy.

- Implementation policies reinforce a model of the family that is characterized by a married, heterosexual couple.

- Those seeking adoptable children have turned to private and international adoptions to better meet the best interests of the parents.

- Infertile couples continue to encounter strong cultural pressures to have children. Women typically experience this pressure more acutely than men.

- Based on figures from the United States, approximately one out of two infertile women will seek to adopt a child.

- Culture continues to place a strong emphasis on "blood ties" for defining families. As a result, adoptive parenthood is often experienced as "second best," suggesting that it is stigmatizing and discrediting.

- Informally, the transition to adoptive parenthood involves coming to terms with several issues: the loss of biological parenthood; fantasizing both about the anticipated child and about themselves in the role of adoptive parents; coming to some negotiated state of readiness within the couple; and disclosing adoption plans to friends and family members as a way of gaining social support.

- Formally, becoming adoptive parents requires going through an adoption assessment that is typically perceived as intrusive and that reinforces a sense of loss of control and powerlessness.

Although the formal adoption process involves a long wait, this waiting period is not seen as useful preparation time for adoptive parenthood.

- When infertile couples form an adoptive family, they encounter the unique challenge of acknowledging that they are different but not deficient in relation to biological families.

- In spite of these unique challenges, adoptive parents are as well adjusted as biological parents, or better, in the early stages of family development.

- The social parents and offspring of NRTs where a donor is involved face many of the same identity challenges that adoptive children and their parents encounter.

- By openly acknowledging that the social parent of a child conceived through NRTs does not share a genetic connection to the child, the necessity of maintaining a false narrative of the child's origins and such a falsehood's negative side-effects are lessened.

- Better genetic record keeping is necessary if children of NRTs are to be able to use genetic information to establish a more complete sense of identity.

- The typical adoptive applicant is Caucasian, married, Protestant, and between 31 and 35 years of age, with at least a high school diploma and no prior parenting experience. Those who pursue adoption in the private sphere tend to be older and better educated.

- The typical woman who places her child for adoption is Caucasian, single, Protestant, and between 15 and 19 years of age; she attends high school, and lives at home with her parents. The main reasons for placing the child for adoption are that the birth mother is too young or is financially unable to parent.

- The typical adoptable child in the public domain has special needs (over the age of one, physically or mentally challenged, or both). In private adoptions, the typical adoptable child is a healthy infant.

- Adopting a child privately happens faster but costs more than a public adoption. Couples who adopt privately wait an average of two years compared to six years for public adoptions and can expect to pay between $3 000 and $4 000 on average.

- The most important eligibility criteria for adopting a child, as identified by public and private service providers, are marriage stability; motivation to parent; problem-solving ability; adaptability; warmth and nurturance; and understanding of adoption. The criteria that are not considered to be important include parents' education, income, and employment; religion; the presence of a fertility problem; and presence of other children in the family.

- Some adoptive applicants would have a difficult time adopting an infant in Canada. Homosexuals would encounter the greatest difficulty when trying to adopt. There are also attitude and policy restrictions on placement for single persons, people of a different race, and people who are over 40 years of age.

- Public and private service providers agree that open adoptions are more likely to be successful.

- Adoptions in the private domain are more open than those in the public domain.

- The major motivation for couples who pursue international adoptions is to avoid the long wait for a domestic adoption.

- In 1990, 2 836 domestic adoption placements were made in Canada. For every infant who is placed for adoption in the public sphere, it is estimated that there are approximately eight available applicants. In the private sphere, there are approximately three available applicants for every infant placed.

- While adoptions in the public domain have dropped 47.3 percent over the past decade, there has been little change in the number of private adoptions during the same period. In 1981, private adoptions accounted for 17.4 percent of all domestic adoptions. This figure rose to 39.0 percent by 1990. More than half of all infant adoptions are currently through private facilities.

- There is no evidence to indicate that the fall in the number of infants available for adoption is related to the rate of abortion. Instead, the decline is directly related to the increase in the number of single women who have chosen to raise their child.

- Most adoptions of hard-to-place children now take place in the public domain. For people seeking to adopt a child but who do not meet the traditional guidelines for acceptance, the adoption of hard-to-place children is an option that public facilities are increasingly supporting.

- It is estimated that there are three international adoptions for every two domestic infant adoptions in Canada.

These findings suggest that the availability of adoption as an alternative has changed dramatically in recent years. Adoption continues to be a viable option for some infertile couples; however, the manner in which one goes about exploring these options is more complex and varied than ever before. Where once adoption was a matter of approaching an agency in order to choose a child, now couples must investigate a range of options including public versus private, hard-to-place versus infant, and international versus domestic. For many infertile couples who find their way through this maze of possibilities, their quest to form a family succeeds through the eventual adoption of a child. For others, age, finances, sexual orientation, and marital status may keep adoption just out of reach.

Appendix 1*

* The National Adoption Study, University of Guelph, 1992, is the source for all data appearing in these tables.

Table 1. Demand for Adoptable Children in the Public Domain*

	1982	1983	1984	1985	1986	1987	1988	1989	1990
Number of applicants on reported waiting list	9 666	8 873	13 221	14 844	14 229	12 774	11 331	11 254	9 272

* Except for New Brunswick, Nova Scotia, Northwest Territories, Ontario, and Yukon.

Table 2. Public and Private Domestic Adoptions

	1981	1982	1983	1984	1985	1986	1987	1988	1989	1990
Total domestic (n)	5 376	5 050	4 995	4 576	4 516	3 701	3 692	3 358	2 868	2 836
Total private (n)	935	976	1 097	1 041	1 044	1 115	1 118	1 196	1 086	1 105
Private adoptions as a % of total	17.4	19.3	22.0	22.7	23.1	30.1	30.3	35.6	37.9	39.0
Total public (n)	4 441	4 074	3 898	3 535	3 472	2 586	2 574	2 162	1 782	1 731
Public adoptions as a % of total	82.6	80.7	78.0	77.3	76.9	69.9	69.7	64.4	62.1	61.0

Table 3. Domestic Adoption of Children Under the Age of One Year

	1981	1982	1983	1984	1985	1986	1987	1988	1989	1990
Total infant adoptions (n)	3 521	3 338	3 276	2 898	2 930	2 317	2 221	2 062	1 730	1 698
Public infant adoptions (n)	2 736	2 518	2 370	1 987	1 979	1 262	1 181	960	747	698
Public infant adoptions as a % of all infant adoptions	77.7	75.4	72.3	68.6	67.5	54.5	53.2	46.6	43.2	41.1
Public infant adoptions as a % of all public adoptions	61.6	61.8	60.8	56.2	57.0	48.8	45.9	44.4	41.9	40.3
Private infant adoptions (n)	785	820	906	911	951	1 055	1 040	1 102	983	1 000
Private infant adoptions as a % of all infant adoptions	22.3	24.6	27.7	31.4	32.5	45.5	46.8	53.4	56.8	58.9
Private infant adoptions as a % of all private adoptions	n.a.	84.0	82.6	87.5	91.1	94.6	93.0	92.1	90.5	n.a.

Table 4. Responses to a Pregnancy by Unmarried Women Under 25 Years of Age

	1981	1982	1983	1984	1985	1986	1987	1988	1989	1990
Number of abortions	33 577	33 607	32 140*	30 673	29 564	29 247*	28 929	27 802	29 246	n.a.
Number of births	35 178	38 180	38 262	39 131	40 120	41 317	42 038	44 518	47 964	n.a.
Number of adoptions of infants <1 year**	3 521	3 338	3 276	2 898	2 930	2 317	2 221	2 062	1 730	1 698
% of pregnancies resulting in adoption	5.1	4.6	4.7	4.2	4.2	3.3	3.1	2.9	2.2	n.a.
% of pregnancies resulting in abortion	48.8	46.8	45.7	43.9	42.4	41.4	40.8	38.4	37.9	n.a.
% of pregnancies, mother raises child	46.1	48.6	49.6	51.9	53.4	55.3	56.1	58.7	59.9	n.a.
% of pregnancies brought to gestation	51.2	53.2	54.3	56.1	57.6	58.6	59.2	61.6	62.1	n.a.
% of live births placed for adoption	10.0	8.7	8.6	7.4	7.3	5.6	5.3	4.6	3.6	n.a.
% of live births, mother raises child	90.0	91.3	91.4	92.6	92.7	94.4	94.7	95.4	96.4	n.a.

* Estimate based on an average of the previous and subsequent years' figures.

** Estimate based on percentage of ward adoptions in provinces reporting age figures plus 90 percent of private figures. This latter number reflects Ontario's average number of infant adoptions in the private domain over the decade.

Table 5. Public and Private Domestic Adoptions of Children over the Age of One Year

	1981	1982	1983	1984	1985	1986	1987	1988	1989	1990
Total older adoptions (n)	1 855	1 712	1 719	1 678	1 586	1 384	1 471	1 296	1 138	1 138
Public older adoptions (n)	1 705	1 556	1 528	1 548	1 493	1 324	1 393	1 202	1 035	1 033
Public older adoptions as a % of all older adoptions	91.9	90.9	88.9	92.3	94.1	95.7	94.7	92.7	90.9	90.8
Public older adoptions as a % of all public adoptions	38.4	38.2	39.2	43.8	43.0	51.2	54.1	55.6	58.1	59.7
Private older adoptions (n)	150	156	191	130	93	60	78	94	103	105
Private older adoptions as a % of all older adoptions	8.1	9.1	11.1	7.7	5.9	4.3	5.3	7.3	9.1	9.2
Private older adoptions as a % of all private adoptions	n.a.	16.0	17.4	12.5	8.9	5.4	7.0	7.9	9.5	n.a.

Table 6. Reported Native Adoptions

	1981	1982	1983	1984	1985	1986	1987	1988	1989	1990
Total Native public adoptions	260	419	473	366	373	428	436	369	265	201*
Manitoba — culturally similar status Indian placements as a % of all status placements	39.5	70.0	78.4	88.2	90.0	100	85.7	100	80.0	78.3
Manitoba — culturally similar Métis placements as a % of all Métis placements	14.3	13.0	40.0	19.2	50.0	10.7	12.5	27.3	46.2	30.0
NWT — culturally similar Native placements (excluding custom adoptions) as a % of all Native placements	n.a.	n.a.	n.a.	41.2	n.a.	34.6	14.3	25.0	16.7	10.5
NWT — culturally similar Native placements (including custom adoptions) as a % of all Native placements	n.a.	n.a.	n.a.	n.a.	n.a.	59.5	75.3	89.9	87.0	77.0
Ontario — culturally similar status placements as a % of all status placements	n.a.	6.0	9.1	39.5	35.5	41.7	34.5	33.3	45.2	20.0
Ontario — culturally similar non-status placements as a % of all non-status placements	n.a.	5.7	0.0	13.6	13.3	30.3	17.2	0.0	22.2	0.0
Quebec — Inuit adoptions following custom traditions as a % of all Inuit placements	83.3	93.4	89.5	86.2	89.4	86.7	92.9	83.3	n.a.	n.a.
Quebec — Inuit custom adoptions as a % of all Inuit births	17.5	30.9	25.1	24.5	32.2	25.6	30.9	16.1	n.a.	n.a.

* Does not include Quebec Inuit adoptions.

Table 7. Quebec International Adoptions

	1982*	1983	1984	1985	1986	1987	1988	1989	1991**
Antigua	0	0	0	0	0	0	1	0	0
Argentina	0	0	0	0	0	0	0	2	0
Bangladesh	0	0	0	0	0	1	0	2	0
Barbados	0	0	0	0	0	0	0	0	3
Bolivia	4	15	7	9	4	2	3	7	4
Brazil	6	15	5	1	0	2	1	4	4
Burkina Faso	0	0	0	0	0	2	0	0	0
Chile	12	8	3	10	3	1	0	4	7
China	0	2	1	1	0	0	3	24	176
Columbia	2	10	15	14	16	5	19	18	8
Costa Rica	0	0	0	6	3	7	4	6	1
Dominican Republic	19	15	26	49	11	2	1	7	6
Dominique	0	0	0	0	1	0	0	0	0
El Salvador	0	1	0	0	0	0	1	0	19
Ecuador	0	0	1	0	0	0	1	0	0
Ethiopia	0	0	1	0	1	0	1	0	0
Grenada	0	0	1	0	0	0	0	0	0
Guatemala	11	16	27	20	10	11	5	10	9
Guyana	0	0	0	2	0	0	2	2	0
Haiti	28	169	68	77	5	9	44	68	83
Honduras	11	8	0	0	2	8	0	1	3
India	1	11	3	6	1	8	15	15	8
Italy	0	1	0	0	0	0	0	0	0

Table 7. *(cont'd)*

	1982*	1983	1984	1985	1986	1987	1988	1989	1991**
Jamaica	0	1	0	2	3	2	0	3	1
Japan	0	0	0	0	0	0	0	2	0
Korea	9	31	42	30	74	67	43	15	1
Libya	1	0	3	1	0	0	4	0	4
Macau	5	8	3	1	2	1	0	0	0
Madagascar	0	0	0	2	2	2	4	1	0
Mali	0	0	0	0	1	0	0	0	1
Mauritius	0	0	0	1	0	0	0	0	0
Mexico	0	1	1	0	0	12	33	43	45
Montserrat	0	0	0	0	0	0	1	0	0
Morocco	0	0	0	0	1	0	0	0	4
Pakistan	0	0	0	0	0	0	1	1	0
Panama	1	2	0	0	0	0	0	0	0
Paraguay	1	0	0	0	0	0	0	0	0
Peru	3	1	9	12	10	3	7	10	13
Philippines	3	5	4	4	5	4	10	5	5
Poland	0	1	1	0	2	0	0	3	1
Portugal	0	0	0	2	1	2	0	1	0
Romania	0	0	0	0	0	0	0	0	155
Rwanda	3	0	0	3	0	0	0	0	5
Senegal	0	1	0	0	0	1	1	0	0
South Africa	0	0	0	0	0	2	0	0	0
Spain	0	0	0	0	1	0	1	0	0
Sri Lanka	0	1	0	0	0	0	1	1	0
St. Vincent & Grenadines	0	1	1	1	1	0	1	2	0
Switzerland	0	0	1	0	0	0	0	0	0
Taiwan	1	1	1	2	8	9	6	7	20
Thailand	0	2	0	0	0	1	1	8	5
Trinidad & Tobago	1	1	0	0	0	2	0	1	0

Tunisia	0	0	0	0	0	0	0	0	0
United States	1	1	3	4	3	0	2	4	1
Venezuela	0	0	0	0	1	0	0	0	0
Vietnam	0	0	0	0	1	1	1	1	0
West Germany	0	0	0	0	0	0	1	0	0
Zaire	0	0	0	0	0	0	0	3	0
TOTAL	123	329	227	260	171	167	218	281	592

* From 1 April of the year indicated to 30 March of the following year.

** From 1 January 1991 to 31 August 1991.

Note: Figures for 1990 were not available.

Appendix 2*

*   The National Adoption Study, University of Guelph, 1992, is the source for all data appearing in these tables.

Figure 1. Public and Private Domestic Adoptions as a Percentage of All Domestic Adoptions

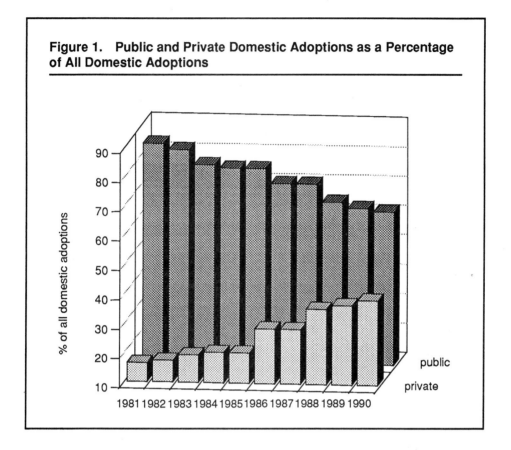

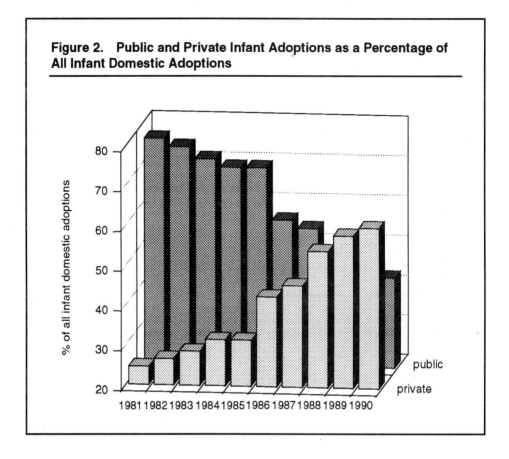

Figure 2.   Public and Private Infant Adoptions as a Percentage of All Infant Domestic Adoptions

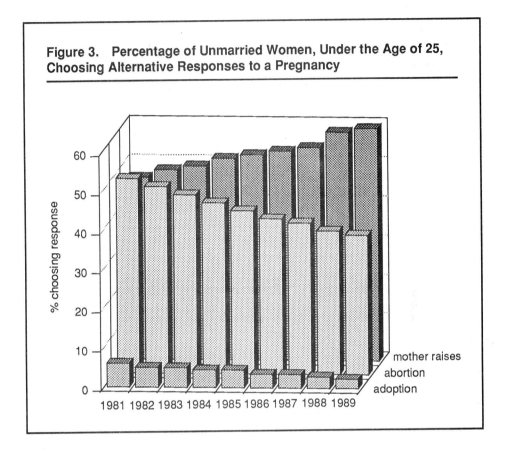

Figure 3.   Percentage of Unmarried Women, Under the Age of 25, Choosing Alternative Responses to a Pregnancy

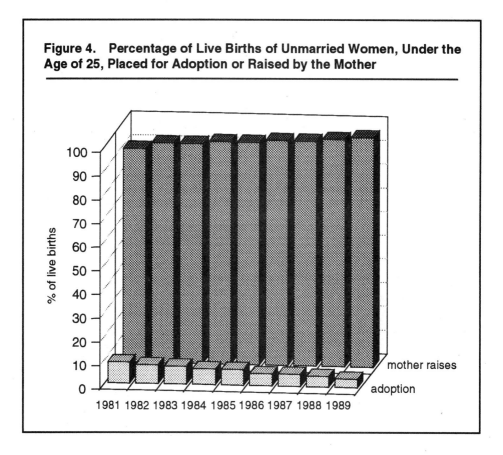

Figure 4.   Percentage of Live Births of Unmarried Women, Under the Age of 25, Placed for Adoption or Raised by the Mother

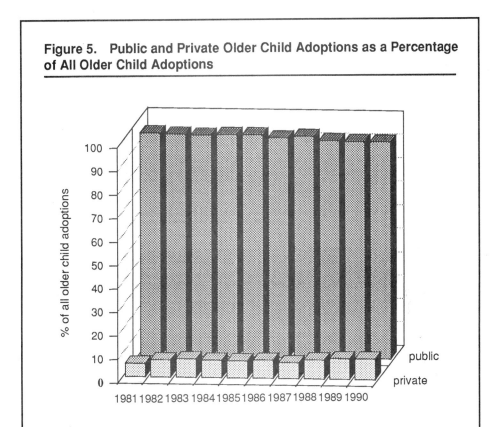

Figure 5. Public and Private Older Child Adoptions as a Percentage of All Older Child Adoptions

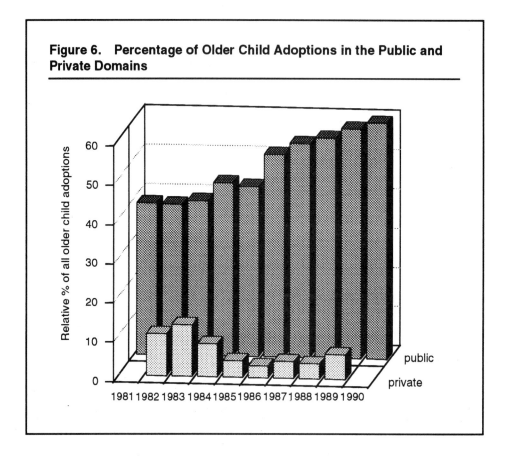

Figure 6. Percentage of Older Child Adoptions in the Public and Private Domains

Notes

1. Since adoption services are legislated and administered by the provinces and territories, data are collected for different purposes and with different categories in each of the provinces. This makes interprovincial comparisons difficult and creates unique challenges for constructing federal trends.   A discussion of the methodological differences of each of the provinces underscores some of the difficulties in tracing these federal trends. Nevertheless, national trends can be identified, but within the limitations imposed by the idiosyncrasies of the provincial data.

2. Throughout this section, all percentages are rounded off to the nearest whole number.

3. Since private practitioners do very few placements of special needs children, data are reported for public practitioners only.

Bibliography

Andrews, L.B. 1984. *New Conceptions: A Consumer's Guide to the Newest Infertility Treatments, Including In Vitro Fertilization, Artificial Insemination, and Surrogate Motherhood.* New York: St. Martin's Press.

Annas, G.J. 1980. "Fathers Anonymous: Beyond the Best Interests of the Sperm Donor." *Family Law Quarterly* 14: 1-13.

Bachrach, C.A. 1983. "Adoption as a Means of Family Formation: Data from the National Survey of Family Growth." *Journal of Marriage and the Family* 45: 859-65.

—. 1986. "Adoption Plans, Adopted Children, and Adoptive Mothers." *Journal of Marriage and the Family* 48: 243-53.

Bachrach, C.A., K.A. London, and P.L. Maza. 1991. "On the Path to Adoption: Adoption Seeking in the United States, 1988." *Journal of Marriage and the Family* 53: 705-18.

Bell, C.J. 1986. "Adoptive Pregnancy: Legal and Social Work Issues." *Child Welfare* 65: 421-36.

Bernard, J. 1982. *The Future of Marriage.* New Haven: Yale University Press.

Bierkens, B.P. 1975. "Childlessness from a Psychological Point of View." *Bulletin of the Menninger Clinic* 39: 177-82.

Blake, J. 1974. "Coercive Pronatalism and American Population Policy." In *The Family: Its Structure & Functions.* 2d ed., ed. R.L. Coser. New York: St. Martin's Press.

Bonham, G.S. 1977. "Who Adopts: The Relationship of Adoption and Social-Demographic Characteristics of Women." *Journal of Marriage and the Family* 39: 295-308.

Boss, P. 1991. "Ambiguous Loss." In *Living Beyond Loss: Death in the Family,* ed. F. Walsh and M. McGoldrick. New York: Norton.

Bresnick, E.R. 1981. "A Holistic Approach to the Treatment of the Crisis of Infertility." *Journal of Marital and Family Therapy* 7: 181-88.

Bresnick, E., and M.L. Taymor. 1979. "The Role of Counseling in Infertility." *Fertility and Sterility* 32: 154-56.

Brodzinsky, D.M. 1987. "Adjustment to Adoption: A Psychosocial Perspective." *Clinical Psychology Review* 7: 25-47.

—. 1990. "A Stress and Coping Model of Adoption Adjustment." In *The Psychology of Adoption*, ed. D.M. Brodzinsky and M.D. Schechter. New York: Oxford University Press.

Brodzinsky, D.M., and L. Huffman. 1988. "Transition to Adoptive Parenthood." *Marriage & Family Review* 12: 267-86.

Brodzinsky, D.M., L.M. Singer, and A.M. Braff. 1984. "Children's Understanding of Adoption." *Child Development* 55: 869-78.

Burgwyn, D. 1981. *Marriage Without Children*. New York: Harper and Row.

Castle, R.E. 1982. "When Adoption Fails." *Royal Society of Health Journal* 102 (February): 9-10.

Daly, K.J. 1987. "Becoming Adoptive Parents: Shifts in Identity from Biological Parenthood to Adoptive Parenthood Among Infertile Couples." Ph.D. dissertation, McMaster University.

—. 1988. "Reshaped Parenthood Identity: The Transition to Adoptive Parenthood." *Journal of Contemporary Ethnography* 17: 40-66.

—. 1989a. "Anger Among Prospective Adoptive Parents: Structural Determinants and Management Strategies." *Clinical Sociology Review* 7: 80-96.

—. 1989b. "Preparation Needs of Infertile Couples Who Seek to Adopt." *Canadian Journal of Community Mental Health* 8: 111-21.

—. 1990. "Infertility Resolution and Adoption Readiness." *Families in Society: The Journal of Contemporary Human Services* 71: 483-92.

Davis, N.J. 1978. "The Political Economy of Reproduction: An Analysis of Childlessness and Single-Child Fertility Among U.S. Women." Ph.D. dissertation, University of Wisconsin.

Demick, J., and S. Wapner. 1988. "Open and Closed Adoption: A Developmental Conceptualization." *Family Process* 27: 229-49.

Dickson, L.R., W.M. Heffron, and C. Parker. 1990. "Children from Disrupted and Adoptive Homes on an Inpatient Unit." *American Journal of Orthopsychiatry* 60: 594-602.

DiGiulio, J.F. 1987. "Assuming the Adoptive Parent Role." *Social Casework: The Journal of Contemporary Social Work* 68: 561-65.

Eichler, M. 1988. *Families in Canada Today: Recent Changes and Their Policy*. 2d ed. Toronto: Gage.

Elbow, M. 1986. "From Caregiving to Parenting: Family Formation with Adopted Older Children." *Social Work* 31: 366-70.

Erikson, E.H. 1963. *Childhood and Society*. 2d ed. New York: Norton.

Garber, R. 1985. *Disclosure of Adoption Information: The Report of the Special Commissioner, Ralph Garber, D.S.W., Dean of the Faculty of Social Work, University of Toronto, to the Honourable John Sweeney, Minister of Community and Social Services, Government of Ontario.* Toronto: Ontario Ministry of Community and Social Services.

Glick, P.C. 1977. "Updating the Life Cycle of the Family." *Journal of Marriage and the Family* 39: 5-13.

Goffman, E. 1959. *The Presentation of Self in Everyday Life.* New York: Doubleday.

Goodman K., and B. Rothman. 1984. "Group Work in Infertility Treatment." *Social Work with Groups* 7 (Spring): 79-97.

Hajal, F., and E.B. Rosenberg. 1991. "The Family Life Cycle in Adoptive Families." *American Journal of Orthopsychiatry* 61: 78-85.

Hertz, D.G. 1982. "Infertility and the Physician-Patient Relationship: A Biopsychosocial Challenge." *General Hospital Psychiatry* 4 (July): 95-101.

Hill, R., and J. Aldous. 1969. "Socialization for Marriage and Parenthood." In *Handbook of Socialization Theory and Research,* ed. D.A. Goslin. Chicago: Rand-McNally.

Hoopes, J.L. 1982. *Prediction in Child Development: A Longitudinal Study of Adoptive and Nonadoptive Families — The Delaware Family Study.* New York: Child Welfare League of America.

Humphrey, M., and K.M. MacKenzie. 1967. "Infertility and Adoption. Follow-up of 216 Couples Attending a Hospital Clinic." *British Journal of Preventive and Social Medicine* 21: 90-96.

Joe, B.E. 1979. *Public Policies Toward Adoption.* Washington, DC: Urban Institute.

Katz, S.N. 1964. "Community Decision-Makers and the Promotion of Values in the Adoption of Children." *Social Service Review* 38(1): 26-41.

Kent, K.G., and J.L. Richie. 1976. "Adoption as an Issue in Casework with Adoptive Parents." *Journal of the American Academy of Child Psychiatry* 15: 510-22.

Kirk, H.D. 1964. *Shared Fate: A Theory of Adoption and Mental Health.* New York: Free Press of Glencoe.

—. 1981. *Adoptive Kinship: A Modern Institution in Need of Reform.* Toronto: Butterworths.

Kirk, H.D., and S.A. McDaniel. 1984. "Adoption Policy in Great Britain and North America." *Journal of Social Policy* 13 (Pt. 1): 75-84.

Kotsopoulos, S., et al. 1988. "Psychiatric Disorders in Adopted Children: A Controlled Study." *American Journal of Orthopsychiatry* 58: 608-12.

Kraft, A.D., et al. 1980. "The Psychological Dimensions of Infertility." *American Journal of Orthopsychiatry* 50: 618-28.

Krugman, D.C. 1967. "Differences in the Relation of Parents and Children to Adoption." *Child Welfare* 46: 267-71.

Lasker, J.N., and S. Borg. 1987. *In Search of Parenthood: Coping with Infertility and High-Tech Conception.* Boston: Beacon Press.

Laurance, J. 1982. "The Moral Pressure to Have Children." *New Society* (5 August): 216-18.

Levy-Shiff, R., O. Bar, and D. Har-Even. 1990. "Psychological Adjustment of Adoptive Parents-to-Be." *American Journal of Orthopsychiatry* 60: 258-67.

Levy-Shiff, R., I. Goldschmidt, and D. Har-Even. 1991. "Transition to Parenthood in Adoptive Families." *Developmental Psychology* 27: 131-40.

Link, P.W., and C.A. Darling. 1986. "Couples Undergoing Treatment for Infertility: Dimensions of Life Satisfaction." *Journal of Sex and Marital Therapy* 12: 46-59.

Lloyd, G.M., and C. Zogg. 1986. "Missing Children." In *Parental Loss of a Child*, ed. T.A. Rando. Champaign: Research Press.

McCall, G.J., and J.L. Simmons. 1978. *Identities and Interactions: An Examination of Human Association in Everyday Life*. Rev. ed. New York: Free Press.

MacDonald, J.A. 1984. "Canadian Adoption Legislation: An Overview." In *Adoption: Current Issues and Trends*, ed. P. Sachdev. Toronto: Butterworths.

McNamara, J. 1975. *The Adoption Adviser*. New York: Hawthorn Books.

Mai, F.M., R.N. Munday, and E.E. Rump. 1972. "Psychiatric Interview Comparisons Between Infertile and Fertile Couples." *Psychosomatic Medicine* 34: 431-40.

Matthews, R., and A. Martin Matthews. 1986. "Infertility and Involuntary Childlessness: The Transition to Nonparenthood." *Journal of Marriage and the Family* 48: 641-49.

Mazor, M.D. 1979. "Barren Couples." *Psychology Today* 12 (May): 101ff.

Menning, B.E. 1977. *Infertility: A Guide for the Childless Couple*. Englewood Cliffs: Prentice-Hall.

Miall, C.E. 1986. "The Stigma of Involuntary Childlessness." *Social Problems* 33: 268-82.

—. 1987. "The Stigma of Adoptive Parent Status: Perceptions of Community Attitudes Toward Adoption and the Experience of Informal Social Sanctioning." *Family Relations* 36 (January): 34-39.

National Committee for Adoption. 1984. *Adoption Facts Summary, 1984*. Washington, DC: National Committee for Adoption.

—. 1989. *Adoption Factbook: United States Data, Issues, Regulations and Resources*. Washington, DC: National Committee for Adoption.

Pfeffer, N., and A. Woolett. 1983. *The Experience of Infertility*. London: Virago Press.

Pohlman, E. 1970. "Childlessness, Intentional and Unintentional." *Journal of Nervous and Mental Disease* 151(July): 2-12.

Poston, D.L., and R.M. Cullen. 1989. "Propensity of White Women in the United States to Adopt Children." *Social Biology* 36 (Fall-Winter): 167-85.

Presser, S.B. 1972. "The Historical Background of the American Law of Adoption." *Journal of Family Law* 11: 443-516.

Pringle, M.L.K. 1967. *Adoption Facts and Fallacies: A Review of Research in the United States, Canada and Great Britain Between 1948 and 1965*. London: Longmans.

Ram, B. 1990. *New Trends in the Family: Demographic Facts and Features*. Ottawa: Statistics Canada.

Renne, D. 1977. "'There's Always Adoption': The Infertility Problem." *Child Welfare* 56: 465-70.

Rosenfeld, D.L., and E. Mitchell. 1979. "Treating the Emotional Aspects of Infertility: Counseling Services in an Infertility Clinic." *American Journal of Obstetrics and Gynecology* 135: 177-80.

Sachdev, P. 1984. "Unlocking the Adoption Files: A Social and Legal Dilemma." In *Adoption: Current Issues and Trends*, ed. P. Sachdev. Toronto: Butterworths.

—. 1989. *Unlocking the Adoption Files*. Lexington: Lexington Books.

Schechter, M.D., and D. Bertocci. 1990. "The Meaning of the Search." In *The Psychology of Adoption*, ed. D.M. Brodzinsky and M.D. Schechter. New York: Oxford University Press.

Schechter, M.D., et al. 1964. "Emotional Problems in the Adoptee." *Archives of General Psychiatry* 10 (February): 109-18.

Schutz, A. 1973. *Collected Papers: I: The Problem of Social Reality*. 4th ed. The Hague: Martinus Nijhoff.

Segal, B. 1982. *Private Adoption: A Background Paper on Assessment of Applicants*. Toronto: Ontario Ministry of Community and Social Services.

Serrill, M.S. 1991. "Wrapping the Earth in Family Ties." *Time* 138 (4 November): 52-57, 59.

Shapiro, C.H. 1982. "The Impact of Infertility on the Marital Relationship." *Social Casework: The Journal of Contemporary Social Work* 63: 387-93.

Singer, L.M., et al. 1985. "Mother-Infant Attachment in Adoptive Families." *Child Development* 56: 1543-51.

Sobol, M.P., and J. Cardiff. 1983. "A Sociopsychological Investigation of Adult Adoptees' Search for Birth Parents." *Family Relations* 32: 477-83.

Sobol, M.P., and K. Daly. 1992. "The Adoption Alternative for Pregnant Adolescents: Decision Making, Consequences, and Policy Implications." *Journal of Social Issues* 48: 143-61.

Sorosky, A.D., A. Baran, and R. Pannor. 1978. *The Adoption Triangle: The Effects of the Sealed Record on Adoptees, Birth Parents, and Adoptive Parents*. Garden City: Anchor Press.

Van Keep, P.A., and H. Schmidt-Elmendorff. 1975. "Involuntary Childlessness." *Journal of Biosocial Science* 7: 37-48.

Veevers, J.E. 1980. *Childless by Choice*. Toronto: Butterworths.

Winkler, R.C., et al. 1988. *Clinical Practice in Adoption*. New York: Pergamon.

Zaslove, H.K. 1978. "Infertility as a Life Event." *Journal of Human Stress* 4 (September): 2.

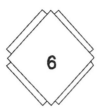

6

Annotated Bibliography on the Prevalence of Infertility

Michael R.P. de la Roche

Executive Summary

Fifty-three papers documenting the prevalence of infertility in Canada and other industrialized countries are summarized in this annotated bibliography. The papers were identified through searches of relevant data bases. A total of 320 citations were identified from the years 1980-1991, and all titles indicating analyses of prevalence or incidence of infertility were reviewed.

Each annotation sets out whether the data in the study are primary or secondary, the research design, population characteristics, and when and where the research was carried out, as well as how infertility was defined and what the findings of the study were. In addition to information on the prevalence or incidence of infertility, the annotations include, where available, the source of the physiological breakdown causing the infertility — the female partner, the male partner, both partners, or unexplained infertility — and information on the nature of the physiological breakdown — for example, tubal, cervical, or ovulatory problems in women, varicocele or impotence in men.

This paper was completed for the Royal Commission on New Reproductive Technologies in June 1992.

Introduction

Rates of infertility are useful in giving a sense of the magnitude of the problem of infertility. The main objective of this annotated bibliography is to document published data on the prevalence of infertility among the population of Canada and other industrialized countries. Where available in the literature, information is also included on the breakdown of physiological factors associated with diagnosed infertile couples and originating from the female, the male, both partners, and unexplained sources, and on the breakdown of female physiological factors (e.g., tubal, cervical, or ovulatory) and male physiological factors (e.g., varicocele or impotence).

For each article reviewed, information is presented under two headings: "source" and "infertility data." Under "source," the source of the data used in the article is provided — that is, primary or secondary sources, along with the research design (e.g., case-control study, retrospective study, cohort study, or descriptive research), population characteristics (multinational, national, regional, health centre based), the country in which the research was carried out, and, when appropriate and available, the year the data were collected. Under "infertility data," information is provided on the definition of infertility, sample size, characteristics of the sample population, infertility prevalence, and causes of infertility.

It is important to underline that not only do definitions of infertility vary but also not all authors use the same definitions or the same methods to calculate prevalence and incidence. Thus, it is important to emphasize that not all infertility prevalence data are comparable. As a guide, the following definitions of prevalence and incidence as they are generally used in epidemiological discussions are provided.

The dichotomous measurement of a disease state is called prevalence, i.e., prevalence is the presence of a disease at a hypothetical point in time. The dichotomous measurement of a change in disease status is called incidence, i.e., incidence is the development of a change in disease during a given period. (See the discussion in MacMahon and Pugh 1970, Chapter 5.)

Prevalence as defined above is also called "point prevalence." "Lifetime prevalence" is also commonly used and includes any person who has lived through an episode of infertility during his or her reproductive years; lifetime prevalence rates are, of course, higher than point prevalence rates. In most cases, infertility prevalence is calculated for married and cohabiting women.

Methodology

A review of the literature was accomplished by first using MEDLINE, a medical literature databank, to identify articles published since 1980 in world medical journals and other publications. The initial search parameter used was "infertility" combined with female, male, incidence, prevalence, and epidemiology. A total of 104 citations were identified using MEDLINE for the years 1986-1991, of which 37 were subsequently reviewed. A further search using "trends" as a title word combined with "infertility" and beginning with literature published from 1980 to 1991 produced an additional 103 references. Of these, 26 were ultimately reviewed.

The EMBASE data base was also reviewed; it identified 29 additional references, of which five were reviewed. The PSYCHINFO, BIOBUSINESS, PASCAL, FEDERAL RESEARCH IN PROGRESS, NIOSH SCISEARCH, and SOCIAL SCISEARCH data bases were also queried, and this identified another 47 papers, of which 12 were appropriate for evaluation. To limit duplication, a MEDLINE search was performed in conjunction with these searches and all papers that were also identified in the MEDLINE search were selected out.

As a result of these searches, a total of 283 citations were identified, of which 80 were selected for review. Only those titles indicating prevalence or incidence of infertility analyses were reviewed. Publications written in either official language were included.

Animal studies, condition- or disease-specific papers, letters to the editor, and treatment or intervention papers were excluded from the review process. Reference lists of papers included in the study were also reviewed and an additional 37 citations were subsequently identified that met the criteria for being included in the study. In all, 117 papers were reviewed. Of the papers reviewed, 64 were not included in the end as they addressed issues outlined above as exclusion criteria, leaving 53 papers for inclusion here.

Of the papers included here, 29 were based upon "primary" sources (i.e., sources that described original research) and 23 were "secondary" sources in that they used research or statistics obtained elsewhere or reviewed current literature. One paper was an editorial and as such presented opinions based upon the "current thought" of the time.

Annotated Articles

Anderson, K. 1989. "Infertility: The Silent Crisis." *Canada's Mental Health* 37 (March): 9-12.

Source: Secondary sources, various data sources, United States

Infertility Data:
The author quotes Unruh and McGrath (1985) as stating that one-sixth of couples (16.7%) experience infertility (lifetime prevalence). She cites Link and Darling (1986) as giving 10% as the point prevalence. She also credits Blank (1985) as giving 18% as the prevalence for Americans between the ages of 22 and 40 years. The author outlines some of the reasons for "increased infertility" and deals primarily with socioeconomic and psychosocial effects of infertility on couples and individuals.

Aral, S.O., and W. Cates, Jr. 1983. "The Increasing Concern with Infertility: Why Now?" *JAMA* 250: 2327-31.

Source: Secondary sources, national survey, United States, 1976

Infertility Data:
The authors, quoting the National Disease and Therapeutic Index, state that the number of infertile females is on the rise.
They make no comment regarding whether there are, in fact, more visits for infertility (Table 1), whether records are more accurate, or whether patients are more readily seeking medical care. The authors provide figures for "currently married American couples" in 1976 (Mosher 1982b) (Table 2).

Table 1. Visits for Infertility

Year	Visits for infertility	Infertility (per 100 000 visits)
1968	609 660	69.5
1972	953 327	92.7
1976	922 607	95.6
1980	897 547	101.9

Table 2. Infertility by Age, 1976

Age	Percent Infertile
15-19	2.1
20-24	6.4
25-29	9.0
30-34	10.3
35-39	12.5
40-44	15.9

Four reasons are given for increasing concern:

1. there are more infertile women in the population;

2. more infertile couples are seeking infertility services;

3. more physicians are interested in infertility; and

4. the social milieu is more conducive toward promoting infertility services.

The authors suggest five factors that contribute to the absolute increase in infertile couples in the United States to 1980:

1. baby-boomers having gone beyond their primary reproductive ages;

2. increases in age-specific rates of infertility among the baby-boom generation (they examine fertility rates and attribute decline to infertility);

3. delays in childbearing until late reproductive years;

4. use of oral contraceptives — once discontinued, there is a longer period of time before conception can occur than with the use of other contraceptives; and

5. "condensing" effect — by delaying childbearing, couples have condensed the period of desired fertility into a shorter period of time.

Baird, D.D., and A.J. Wilcox. 1985. "Cigarette Smoking Associated with Delayed Conception." *JAMA* 253: 2979-83.

Source: Primary sources, pregnancy class based data, United States, 1983

Infertility Data:

Subjects of this study were volunteers canvassed from early pregnancy classes in the Minneapolis area during the latter half of 1983. Subjects were asked to participate in a 15-minute telephone questionnaire if they had stopped using birth control prior to conceiving. Subjects had to be between 18 and 40 years of age. Seven hundred and sixty-two females volunteered for the study, of which 84 were excluded.

Of those excluded, 1 was less than 18 years of age; 23 were using birth control at the time of conception; 35 were not married throughout the contraception period; 9 had taken fertility drugs; 13 had not conceived within 24 months of trying; and 3 were excluded because of incomplete data.

Six hundred and seventy-eight females were ultimately included in the analysis, 31% of whom were primigravida. Twenty percent of the group were "smokers" (women who smoked at least one cigarette per day during the first month of pregnancy were considered to be smokers).

Findings:

- 38% of non-smokers conceived during their first cycle
- 28% of smokers conceived during their first cycle
- 98% of non-smokers had conceived within 12 cycles (90% within six cycles)
- 92% of smokers had conceived within 12 cycles (76% within six cycles)
- The pregnancy rate per menstrual cycle for smokers was 72% of the rate of non-smokers. The authors feel that impaired fertility among smokers has biological plausibility. No comment is made regarding the 13 females excluded from the study who had not conceived after 24 months of trying.

Balakrishnan, T.R., K.J. Krótki, and E. Lapierre-Adamcyk. 1985. "Contraceptive Use in Canada, 1984." *Family Planning Perspectives* 17: 209-15.

Source: Primary sources, national survey, Canada, 1984

Infertility Data:

The authors use data from the 1984 Canadian Fertility Survey to analyze contraceptive use in Canada. The survey used a two-stage probability process to select an eligible sample population. In the end, 5 315 women aged 18-49 years were interviewed by telephone. As part of determining contraceptive use among women exposed to pregnancy, the authors give figures for all women and for currently married women who are not contraceptively sterile (Table 1).

Table 1. Contraceptive Use

Status	Percentage not contraceptively sterile
All women (n = 5 315)	7.0
Currently married (n = 3 283)	8.7
Never married (n = 1 430)	1.5
Cohabiting (n = 289)	1.4*
Not cohabiting (n = 1 141)	1.7
Previously married (n = 601)	10.6
Cohabiting (n = 162)	11.2
Not cohabiting (n = 439)	10.2

* Relative standard of error of 0.30 or more.

Barrett, J.C. 1986. "The Estimation of Natural Sterility." *Genus* 42 (3-4): 23-31.

Source: Secondary sources, Ireland, Census of Ireland 1911 data

Infertility Data:
Based upon Census of Ireland 1911 data, the author simulated the reproductive histories of 10 000 females married at age 22.5 years. Primary infertility was calculated to be 4.8% and secondary infertility to be 0.36% for ages 20-24. He concludes that up to the age of 30, fertility is relatively constant; however, after age 35, fertility decreases with age.

Belsey, M.A. 1984. "Infertility: Prevalence, Etiology, and Natural History." In *Perinatal Epidemiology*, ed. M.B. Bracken. New York: Oxford University Press.

Source: Secondary sources, multinational review

Infertility Data:

The article reviews various definitions of infertility. World Health Organization (WHO) (1975) definitions of infertility are as follows:

> *Primary infertility:* The woman has never conceived despite cohabitation and exposure to pregnancy for a period of two years.

> *Secondary infertility:* The woman has previously conceived, but is subsequently unable to conceive, despite cohabitation and exposure to pregnancy for a period of two years; if the woman has breast-fed a previous infant then exposure to pregnancy should be calculated from the end of the period of lactational amenorrhoea.

Primary infertility varies from 1.0% to 1.5% for married women 35-39 years of age in Thailand (World Fertility Survey 1977) and Korea (Korean Institute for Family Planning 1971) to 13-23% for women of similar age in urban areas of Colombia (Estrada et al. 1972) and one urban area of New Guinea (Ring and Scragg 1973). Secondary infertility (women who had only "one child ever born" in countries where the average family size is normally well above two children) for women 35-39 years of age and married for 10-19 years in Pakistan and Thailand was 4.0% and 5.1% respectively (World Fertility Survey 1977). The author quotes Ussing and Schmidt (1972) when stating a Canadian figure of 7% primary infertility in married women 35-39 years of age. He quotes Gunaratne (1979) when stating that the male factor relating to infertility (excluding Africa) is implicated in 20-30% of couples seeking treatment for infertility. The author relates a number of factors that affect infertility, such as frequency of intercourse (Table 1), sexually transmitted disease, ignorance of human physiology, and other infective or contaminating factors. One study revealed, for example, that 40% of the women thought that ovulation took place during menstruation.

Table 1. Frequency of Intercourse and Its Effect on Conception

Average frequency of intercourse per week	Number of cases	Percent conceptions in less than six months
<1	24	16.7
1 but <2	109	32.1
2 but <3	123	46.3
3 but <4	100	51.0
≥4	72	83.3

Source: J. Macleod and R.Z. Gold, as cited in Behrman and Kistner (1975).

Bendvold, E. 1989. "Semen Quality in Norwegian Men Over a 20-Year Period." *International Journal of Fertility* 34: 401-404.

Source: Primary sources, hospital-based data, Norway, 1966 and 1986

Infertility Data:
The author quotes Mosher and Pratt (1985) when stating that "it is generally accepted that some 15% of couples are infertile." He examined the semen quality of 135 randomly selected men in 1966 and 148 men in 1986 (method of selection and randomization not specified) and found that the semen quality had decreased from the 1966 group to the 1986 group. Percent sperm with a "normal morphology" decreased from 60% in 1966 to 41% in 1986. The author goes on to discuss the causes and implications of infertility.

Bergström, S. 1990. "Genital Infections and Reproductive Health: Infertility and Morbidity of Mother and Child in Developing Countries." *Scandinavian Journal of Infectious Diseases* (Suppl. 69): 99-105.

Source: Secondary sources, Africa, 1974 and 1976

Infertility Data:
The author quotes Belsey (1976) when stating that "childlessness at the end of reproductive age affects up to 30% of women in some African countries." He quotes Modawi (1976) and Adadevoh (1974) as stating that in some regional areas figures can be as high as 50%. The author relates the incidence of various genital infections to the prevalence of infertility.

Bongaarts, J. 1982. "Infertility After Age 30: A False Alarm." *Family Planning Perspectives* 14: 75-78.

Source: Secondary sources, multinational, seventeenth, eighteenth, and twentieth centuries

Infertility Data:
The author reviews the literature concerning conception delays, drawing from specific examples from the CECOS (Fédération des centres d'étude et de conservation des œufs et du sperme humains) et al. (1982) study in France and the study of Vessey et al. (1978) in England. He

proposes that "infertility estimates based on 12 months of exposure greatly exaggerate the risk of ultimate involuntary childlessness inherent in voluntary postponement of childbearing." The author selects historical data on infertility from groups that either did not have contraception available or did not practise birth control to establish historical infertility rates (Table 1).

Table 1. Estimated Percentage of Women Permanently Infertile (with Present Husband)*

Age group	Percent infertile		
	25 historical populations	Hutterites	Average
20-24	5.3	3.0	4.1
25-29	5.8	5.3	5.5
30-34	9.8	9.0	9.4
35-39	17.5	22.0	19.7

* In a study of 25 historical populations (17th and 18th century France) and in a group of Hutterite women (first half of the 20th century in the United States and Canada).

Boyd, R.L. 1989. "Racial Differences in Childlessness: A Centennial Review." *Sociological Perspectives* 32: 183-99.

Source: Secondary sources, United States, 1910, 1940-1980 census data

Infertility Data:

This article is a retrospective review of fertility and infertility among white and black women in the United States from the nineteenth century to the present.

The author examines childlessness by race (Tables 1 and 2), labour force status, and level of education. He draws some conclusions regarding causes of childlessness among differing social and ethnic groups.

Table 1. White Women (Ever Married), Percent Childless

Year	Age group					
	15-19	20-24	25-29	30-34	35-39	40-44
1975	58.4	45.1	21.7	9.0	5.3	6.5
1970	53.7	37.7	16.1	8.1	7.0	8.1
1965	49.5	28.7	11.8	7.0	8.1	10.2
1960	46.0	25.0	12.3	9.7	10.2	13.0
1950	55.4	34.0	20.1	15.8	17.5	18.9
1940	50.8	36.8	27.3	20.7	17.4	15.6

Source: U.S. Bureau of the Census, 1943, 1955, 1969, 1974, and 1976.

Table 2. Black Women (Ever Married), Percent Childless

Year	Age group					
	15-19	20-24	25-29	30-34	35-39	40-44
1975	35.5	20.5	16.2	8.3	6.4	11.4
1970	31.0	20.8	12.3	9.1	9.8	13.0
1965	38.9	22.4	10.5	8.5	13.3	17.8
1960	25.3	17.0	14.2	15.8	20.0	24.7
1950	38.1	28.6	29.6	30.2	31.9	29.6
1940	41.6	35.3	32.0	29.0	26.8	23.8

Source: U.S. Bureau of the Census, 1943, 1955, 1969, 1974, and 1976.

Bryant, H. 1990. "The Infertility Dilemma: Reproductive Technologies and Prevention." Ottawa: Canadian Advisory Council on the Status of Women.

Source: Secondary sources, multinational review with emphasis on U.S. figures

Infertility Data:

This article is essentially a literature review of papers pertaining to fertility and infertility. The author examines the causes, trends, therapeutic interventions, and controversies that exist. She quotes Tietze et al. (1950) as stating that for 1 727 pregnant women, 91.2% of the pregnancies occurred within the first year of attempting to conceive and

4.5% within the second year. She quotes Mosher (1985) and Mosher and Pratt (1987) as giving infertility rates of almost 14% and stating that 2.4 million married couples in the United States were infertile in 1982 and that infertility in females 19-24 years of age has increased from 3.6% in 1965 to 10.6% in 1982. The author quotes Balakrishnan et al. (1985) as indicating a total infertility rate of less than 7.0% based on data from the 1984 Fecundity Survey in Canada. The causes of infertility and success of intervention methods are also assessed.

For three clinical studies that were reviewed, the breakdown of infertility for couples is as follows:

Male factor:	18-30%
Female factor:	
Tubal defects	12-20%
Ovulation defects	15-30%
Endometriosis	3-25%
Unexplained infertility	3-30%

Cates, W., T.M.M. Farley, and P.J. Rowe. 1985. "Worldwide Patterns of Infertility: Is Africa Different?" *Lancet* (14 September): 596-98.

Source: Primary sources, World Health Organization (WHO) multinational study, infertility clinic based data, 1979-1984

Infertility Data:

A total of 5 600 couples were involved in this study. Eligibility criteria consisted of being infertile for a period of at least 12 months. The study focussed on various causes of infertility among countries. Prevalence and incidence data were not emphasized. Statistics on primary and secondary infertility were compiled (Table 1).

Table 1. Primary and Secondary Infertility in Various Countries (as a Percentage of Total Infertility)

Type of infertility	Developed countries	Developing countries			
		Africa	Asia	Latin America	East Mediterranean
Primary (%)	71	48	77	60	84
Secondary (%)	29	52	23	40	16

Clark, R.L., and B. Keefe. 1989. "Infertility: Imaging of the Female." *Urologic Radiology* 11: 233-37.

Source: Secondary sources, United States

Infertility Data:

Infertility is defined as failure to conceive after one year of unprotected intercourse. This definition is based on the "monthly fecundability of 20 to 25% of normal couples, which results in 95% of sexual partners conceiving in 13 months" (no sources given). A pregnancy rate of 16% is achieved over six months if coital frequency is less than once per week (no sources given). If coital frequency is greater than three times per week, the pregnancy rate increases to 83% (no sources given). Fifteen percent of couples or one in seven marriages experience some form of infertility problem (no sources given). The author relates infertility rates to increases in sexually trans-mitted diseases and delays in childbearing. The article focusses on investigative procedures. Medical factors that individually cause infertility are outlined and their estimated rate of incidence is given.

Table 1. Medical Factors Causing Infertility (%)

Factor	Incidence
Central or ovulatory factor	15
Mucous or cervical factor	10
Uterine/endometrial factor	5
Tubal factor	10
Peritoneal factor	20
Male factor	30
Other	10

Dubin, L., and R.D. Amelar. 1980. "A Plea for a More Scientific Approach in the Treatment of Male Infertility." *Fertility and Sterility* 34: 74-75.

Source: Secondary sources, United States, 1971

Infertility Data:

The authors state that in 30% of infertility cases, the male is "mainly" responsible, and that in another 20% of cases, the male represents a "definite contributing factor." Semen analysis is the basic tool of analysis.

In many cases, the cause of male infertility is "multi-factorial." Varicocele can often be the cause of low sperm counts; 85% of varicoceles occur on the left side and in 15% of cases the problem is bilateral.

Ducot, B., and A. Spira. 1988. "Utilisation de la notion de fécondabilité dans le pronostic de l'infécondité." *Journal de Gynécologie obstétrique et Biologie de la Reproduction* 17: 461-66.

Source: Secondary sources, France

Infertility Data:

The authors state that approximately 4% of couples who want a child do not have one by the end of their reproductive years and that an estimated 15% of couples are unable to achieve a pregnancy at some time. The authors divide couples with fertility problems into two groups: those that for one reason or another are "sterile" (biologically unable to conceive) and those that simply have a reduced capacity (transient or otherwise) to conceive. They go on to propose a method of estimating the probability of conception given various fertility rates (the number of conceptions per "cycle").

Ebomoyi, E., and O.O. Adetoro. 1990. "Socio-Biological Factors Influencing Infertility in a Rural Nigerian Community." *International Journal of Gynecology and Obstetrics* 33: 41-47.

Source: Primary sources, regional survey, Nigeria, 1985

Infertility Data:

The authors examined a rural Nigerian community in which there were 1 626 females of reproductive age. Eight hundred and thirteen women were contacted (using random sampling), of which 749 agreed to participate. Infertility was defined as being exposed to pregnancy for more than two years without being able to conceive. Findings are presented in Table 1.

Table 1. Infertility Among Women in a Nigerian Community

Age group	Number*	Number infertile	Percent infertile
15-19	55	6	10
20-24	84	41	49
25-29	171	108	63
30-34	161	82	51
35-39	90	51	57
40+	78	58	74
Total	639	346	54

* Women who had previously conceived.

Subjects with missing data were excluded from the above data. Overall, 97 (13.0%) of the 749 women had been married for more than two years but were unable to conceive (i.e., primary infertility); 346 (54.1%) of the 639 women suffered from secondary infertility.

Greenhall, E., and M. Vessey. 1990. "The Prevalence of Subfertility: A Review of the Current Confusion and a Report of Two New Studies." *Fertility and Sterility* 54: 978-83.

Source: Primary sources, clinic-based data, United Kingdom

Infertility Data:
Two studies were carried out, one involving a general practice (872 patients) and one in a hospital (702 patients). Questionnaires were sent to each patient.

Definitions:
Subfertility: 12 months of "regular" (not defined) intercourse without conceiving or more than two consecutive natural miscarriages or stillbirths
"Resolved" subfertility: as defined above, but eventually resulting in conception
Primary infertility: never having conceived
Secondary infertility: having previously conceived, followed by a period of infertility as defined above under subfertility

General Practice Study:
This study involved females between the ages of 25 and 44 years who were registered with a four-partner practice in Oxford, United Kingdom.

One thousand two hundred and four women were identified as being within this age range, but 332 were not at their recorded addresses. The remaining 872 women were sent a questionnaire. Six hundred and eighty-three (78%) responded, of which 178 (26.1%) exhibited unresolved subfertility. Of these 178 women, 117 were subsequently interviewed. Of the other 504 original respondents, 102 exhibited resolved infertility; 67 of these women replied to an additional detailed questionnaire.

Findings:

Unresolved primary subfertility	23/674	3.4%
Resolved primary subfertility	49/674	7.3%
Unresolved secondary subfertility	43/561	7.7%
Resolved secondary subfertility	55/561	9.8%
Any primary subfertility	72/674	10.7%
Any secondary subfertility	91/561	16.2%
Any episode of subfertility	138/674	20.5%

Hospital Study:

This study consisted of "ever-married women" who sought treatment for breast cancer at any one of eight different hospitals in London and Oxford over a period of four years. The women ranged from 25 to 45 years of age. Of the 702 females participating in the study, 95 were identified as experiencing primary infertility and 108 were identified as experiencing secondary infertility.

Findings (Age-Corrected):

Unresolved primary subfertility	19/650
Resolved primary subfertility	76/650
Unresolved secondary subfertility	32/532
Resolved secondary subfertility	81/532
Any primary subfertility	95/650
Any secondary subfertility	108/532
Any episode of subfertility	181/650

Combined Data:

(a) Of the combined groups, 3.3% experienced unresolved primary infertility and 10%, resolved primary infertility.

(b)   About 24% of all women attempting to conceive have an episode of subfertility during their lifetime.

(c)   About 13% of women will experience this episode of infertility when attempting to conceive their first child.

(d)   About 18% of women will experience difficulty when attempting to conceive subsequent children.

(e)   Three percent of women are involuntarily childless.

(f)   Six percent of parous women are unable to conceive as many children as they would like.

The article also reports on various other studies: childlessness figures from census data vary from 6% to 15% in long-standing marriages in the United Kingdom, Canada, and the United States; an overall rate of "impaired fecundity" of 8.2% occurred in the United States in 1982; in the United Kingdom, a general household survey yielded a subfertility rate of 4% in 1983; a combined primary and secondary resolved infertility rate of 19% was obtained from pooled data from 12 separate studies carried out in the United States involving 9 500 pregnancies; a similar rate of 17% was obtained from the examination of 1 452 pregnancies in the United Kingdom, but a much lower rate of 5.4% came from the examination of 5 880 Israeli births; different retrospective studies yield similar rates for unresolved primary subfertility of between 2.4% and 5.9%, the rates for unresolved secondary subfertility range from 4.2% to 7.2%, and those for resolved subfertility of any type range from 22% to 24%; and the proportion of women who have experienced any type of subfertility ranges from 14.1% to 28%.

Hirsch, M.B., and W.D. Mosher. 1987. "Characteristics of Infertile Women in the United States and Their Use of Infertility Services." *Fertility and Sterility* 47: 618-25.

Source: Primary sources, national surveys, United States, 1976 and 1982

Infertility Data:
The authors quote Mosher (1985) when stating that 8.5% of all currently married couples in which the wife is 15-44 years of age were infertile in 1982. Data sources for this article were derived primarily from Cycles II and III of the National Survey of Family Growth conducted in 1976 and 1982. Infertility is defined as couples who were living together, were not practising any form of birth control, and had not conceived for at least 12 months. Data from the 1982 survey are based on interviews with 7 969 women aged 15-44 years, of whom 3 551 (44.6%) were currently married.

Data from the 1976 survey are based upon interviews with 8 611 women, of which 6 482 (75.3%) were currently married. Criteria for inclusion in the survey were not specified. The two groups of currently marrried women were combined, totalling 10 033, and then those couples that were surgically sterile (either the female or her partner) were excluded, leaving a final group of 6 961 couples. One thousand one hundred and six couples (15.9%) fulfilled the criteria of being infertile and 5 855 were fecund. Of the infertile couples, 299 (4.3%) fell into the primary infertility category and 807 (11.6%) into the secondary infertility category. The article goes on to discuss the socioeconomic factors associated with these rates of infertility and the causes of infertility.

Högberg, U., and S. Åkerman. 1990. "Reproductive Pattern Among Women in 19th Century Sweden." *Journal of Biosocial Science* 22: 13-18.

Source: Secondary sources, Central Bureau of Statistics data, Sweden, nineteenth century

Infertility Data:

   The authors examined demographic data from church records in seven Swedish parishes during the nineteenth century. They looked at all married females (4 722). The fertility rate at the time was 4.1%. The authors made the following assumptions: women married to have children; married females who by the age of 50 years were without children were considered to be infertile; married women with only one child by the age of 50 were considered to be subfertile. Of the 4 722 married women, only 999 could be traced as being alive at the age of 50. Findings are presented in Table 1.

Table 1. Infertility Among Women in 19th-Century Sweden

Date of marriage	Number of married women	Infertility		Subfertility		Total	
		n	%	n	%	n	%
1810-1870	999	75	7.5	61	6.1	136	13.6

Howe, G., et al. 1985. "Effects of Age, Cigarette Smoking, and Other Factors on Fertility: Findings in a Large Prospective Study." *British Medical Journal* 290: 1697-1700

Source: Primary sources, prospective contraceptive study, United Kingdom, 1968-1983

Infertility Data:

Data for this study were derived from the Oxford Family Planning Association contraceptive study. Subjects were recruited between 1968 and 1974 and were followed until 1983 (the average follow-up period was 11.5 years). The study group consisted of white married females between the ages of 25 and 39 years. A total of 17 032 women participated in the study. There were 6 199 episodes when a female stopped practising birth control and, subsequently, was at risk of becoming pregnant. Infertility was not specifically defined in the article.

The authors consider that there is a "strong association" between smoking and fertility, and the dose-response relationship illustrated in Table 1 supports this view. The authors also looked at the number of females who remained undelivered at various times after they stopped practising contraception, by age and parity (Table 2).

Table 1. Estimated Proportions (%) of Women Remaining Undelivered

| Cigarettes per day | Months after stopping contraception | | | | | |
	12	18	24	36	48	60
Never smoked	41.0	18.7	12.5	7.8	6.2	5.4
Ex-smoker	41.3	19.0	12.8	8.0	6.3	5.5
1-5	41.1	18.8	12.6	7.9	6.2	5.4
6-10	42.3	19.8	13.5	8.5	6.8	6.0
11-15	43.8	21.1	14.5	9.3	7.5	6.6
16-20	50.4	27.4	20.0	13.8	11.5	10.4
21+	50.9	27.9	20.5	14.2	11.9	10.7

Table 2. Estimated Proportions (%) of Women Remaining Undelivered of a Live Birth or Stillbirth After Stopping Contraception, by Age

(i) Nulliparous women

Age	Months after stopping contraception					
	12	18	24	36	48	60
25-27	50.3	23.1	14.4	9.8	7.3	5.9
28-29	53.6	26.3	17.1	12.0	9.2	7.5
30-31	58.6	31.9	22.0	16.2	12.8	10.8
32-33	60.3	33.8	23.8	17.8	19.3	12.2
34-35	69.6	45.9	35.6	28.8	24.5	21.8
36-37	73.1	51.0	41.0	37.1	29.6	26.8

(ii) Parous women

Age	Months after stopping contraception					
	12	18	24	36	48	60
25-27	38.7	14.7	8.5	4.2	2.8	2.5
28-29	34.9	12.0	6.6	3.0	1.9	1.8
30-31	38.8	14.7	8.6	4.2	2.8	2.6
32-33	43.0	18.1	11.1	5.9	4.1	3.8
34-35	45.0	19.8	12.5	6.8	4.8	4.5
36-37	39.7	15.5	9.1	4.6	3.1	2.8
38-39	55.9	30.6	21.8	13.9	10.8	10.1
40+	64.5	40.9	31.6	22.5	18.5	17.7

Hull, M.G.R., et al. 1985. "Population Study of Causes, Treatment, and Outcome of Infertility." *British Medical Journal* 291: 1693-97.

Source: Primary sources, retrospective study, infertility clinic based data, United Kingdom, 1982-1983

Infertility Data:

The authors defined infertility as the inability to achieve any pregnancy (including a miscarriage) for at least 12 months. They examined those couples who attended an infertility clinic in a single health district in England "during part of 1982 and 1983." The total population in the area was approximately 393 000. The total number of couples who attended the clinic was 708, of which 472 were from the immediate area. Of the total population, 84 100 were females between the ages of 15 and 44 years. The authors calculated the "lifetime incidence" of infertility by first determining that the average number of females in each age bracket was 2 803. Then they calculated the "lifetime incidence" rate by dividing the number of couples from the immediate area by the number of females in each age bracket, giving a value of 17%. Although not stated in the article, this calculation assumes that the number of females in each age bracket is constant and that all couples experiencing infertility problems during the study period attended the clinic. Fifty-nine percent were classified as having primary infertility, 29% had a child prior to attending the clinic, and 11% had undergone previous therapeutic termination of a pregnancy; the remaining 1% was not accounted for in the article. The article went on to examine some of the causes of infertility in the study group.

For the 472 couples examined at the health district infertility clinic, the final diagnostic classification breakdown is as follows:

Ovulatory failure	21%
Tubal damage	14%
Endometriosis	6%
Mucous defect/dysfunction	3%
Sperm defect/dysfunction	24%
Other male infertility	2%
Coital/suspected coital failure	6%
Unexplained	28%
Others	11%

The total adds up to 115% because some couples experienced more than a single cause.

Johnson, G., et al. 1987. "Infertile or Childless by Choice? A Multipractice Survey of Women Aged 35 and 50." *British Medical Journal* 294: 804-806.

Source: Primary sources, retrospective study, clinic-based data, United Kingdom, women born in 1935 and 1950

Infertility Data:

The population used in this study was derived from the patients of 10 general practitioners. The combined patient list totalled 1 369, of which 748 women were born in 1950 and 621 were born in 1935. Complete data were available for 617 of those women born in 1950 and for 533 of those born in 1935. Eighty-eight of those women born in 1950 and 41 of those born in 1935 were childless. Of these women, 68 of those born in 1950 and 17 of those born in 1935 were childless by choice. The remaining childless women fulfilled the criteria of being infertile. Infertility rates, therefore, are as follows:

    1950 cohort: 3.3%
    1935 cohort: 4.5%

The authors found no increase in involuntary childlessness between the two cohorts, but an increase in voluntary childlessness was observed.

Kistner, R.W. 1979. "Endometriosis and Infertility." *Clinical Obstetrics and Gynecology* 22: 101-19.

Source: Secondary sources, United States

Infertility Data:

The author states that the "usual incidence of infertility [approximates] 15%." In those women with endometriosis, the incidence of infertility "approximates 30-40%." The author goes on to provide some of the factors that influence the pregnancy rate among those women with endometriosis as well as to discuss some of the treatments available and their ultimate success rates.

Li, Y., et al. 1990. "Infertility in a Rural Area of Jiangsu Province: An Epidemiological Survey." *International Journal of Fertility* 35: 347-49.

Source: Primary sources, regional survey, China, 1986

Infertility Data:

The authors used a random stratified multi-stage and probability sampling procedure to identify 2 884 couples for interview from 272 villages in Jiangsu province. Of these, 2 593 couples responded and were subsequently interviewed. Complete data were available on 2 578 couples (Table 1). Infertility was defined as an inability to conceive over a period of at least two years. Overall, the infertility rate was 5%.

Table 1. Effect of Smoking and Drinking on Fertility

Groups	Number of couples	Infertile	
		n	%
Neither smoker nor drinker	2 462	118	4.8
Smoker only	47	7	14.9
Drinker only	29	2	6.9
Both smoker and drinker	13	2	15.4
Unknown	27	1	3.7
Total	2 578	130	5.0

The authors attribute the low incidence of infertility to a low incidence of sexually transmitted diseases and a high ratio of monogamous relationships.

Lodh, F. 1987. *Explaining Fertility Decline in the West (with Special Reference to Canada): A Critique of Research Results from Social Sciences.* Ottawa: Vanier Institute of the Family.

Source: Secondary sources, Canada and the United States

Infertility Data:

This paper reviews the multidimensional aspects of fertility rates in Canada. Infertility is defined as one year of unprotected coitus without conception. The author quotes Armitage (1986) as stating that 10% of Canadian couples are subject to medical infertility; of the 10% that are infertile, 90% will, "subsequent to medical intervention, conceive within two years." Lodh concludes that only 1% of Canadian couples, therefore, are involuntarily childless (no reference provided). The author also quotes Westoff (1986) and Burgwyn (1981) when stating that "15 or 16% of couples in the United States have difficulty conceiving or carrying a baby to term."

Marchbanks, P.A., et al. 1989. "Research on Infertility: Definition Makes a Difference." *American Journal of Epidemiology* 130: 259-67.

Source: Primary sources, retrospective study, control group of a cancer study, United States, 1980-1983

Infertility Data:

The authors quote Mosher (1985) when stating that infertility rates affect 10-15% of all couples in the United States. In this retrospective study, 5 698 females aged 20-54 years were "randomly" selected from the Cancer and Steroid Hormone Study control group. The sample was selected by random digit dialling in eight regions of the United States: the metropolitan regions of Atlanta, Detroit, San Francisco, and Seattle; the states of Connecticut, Iowa, and New Mexico; and the four urban counties of Utah. Of the 5 698 females selected, 4 754 (83.4%) participated, 678 (11.9%) refused, and 266 (4.7%) could not be located. Trained interviewers questioned each participant. The following definitions of infertility were used to split the participants into five groups (Table 1):

(a)   24 months of trying to conceive;

(b)   24 months of trying to conceive, physician consulted;

(c)   24 months of trying to conceive, physician consulted who diagnosed a problem with one or both partners;

(d)   12 months of unprotected intercourse; and

(e)   24 months of unprotected intercourse.

Table 1. Percentage of Population Defined as "Having a History of Infertility" by Definition and Age Group

		Definition				
		a	b	c	d	e
Age	Total n = 4 754	n = 764	n = 582	n = 321	n = 1 837	n = 1 285
20-29	5.8	2.5	2.2	3.7	3.5	2.7
30-39	21.6	21.6	22.3	25.2	20.3	17.9
40-44	16.4	16.5	16.0	14.6	15.2	14.4
45-49	26.1	24.7	24.2	24.3	28.1	28.2
50-54	30.1	34.7	35.2	32.1	32.9	36.9
Total	100.0	100.0	100.0	100.0	100.0	100.0

Findings:

   For all definitions, the highest proportion of women classified as being infertile occurred in the 20-29 age group (Table 2). Definition (d) reflected the highest prevalence of infertility (Table 3).

Table 2. Age at Infertility by Definition of Infertility (%)

	Age					
	<20	20-29	30-39	>39	Total	n
Physician diagnosis	7.6	73.8	18.2	0.4	100.0	236
Intercourse for 12 months	26.2	59.9	11.0	2.9	100.0	1 761
Intercourse for 24 months	15.7	61.7	17.9	4.7	100.0	1 220

Table 3. Prevalence of Infertility for Each Group

	Crude prevalence	Age-adjusted prevalence*
Tried for two years	16.1	12.5
Physician consultation	12.2	9.6
Physician diagnosis	6.8	6.1
Intercourse for 12 months	38.6	32.6
Intercourse for 24 months	27.0	20.6

*   There was a preponderance of older women in the study population.

Conclusion: The definition of infertility can affect prevalence rates.

Martin, T.E. 1989. "Infertility in a Large Royal Air Force General Practice." *Journal of the Royal Army Medical Corps* 135 (June): 68-75.

Source: Primary sources, clinic-based data, United Kingdom citizens in Germany, 1985-1988

Infertility Data:
The author quotes Hull et al. (1985) when stating that there is an annual incidence of infertility of 1.2 couples per 1 000 and that 17% of all couples seek medical advice for infertility at some point in their lives. The study examined couples who sought medical care at a United Kingdom military air base in Germany. The study included 56 couples who were attending a fertility clinic out of a population of 1 079 couples on the air base. The study involved those couples who had failed to achieve pregnancy after at least 12 months of unprotected intercourse. The subjects were females between the ages of 18 and 45 years. The author inferred that all couples experiencing problems conceiving attended his medical clinic, giving prevalence rates of 1.2%, 2.5%, and 3.6% for the dates 25 March 1987, 25 September 1987, and 25 March 1988, respectively. He inferred an overall prevalence of 3.6%. The primary infertility rate was calculated as 2.4% and the secondary infertility rate as 1.2%. The article addresses some of the causes of infertility among these couples as well as some of the successful methods currently used to treat infertile couples.

Menken, J., J. Trussell, and U. Larsen. 1976. "Age and Infertility." *Science* 233: 1389-94.

Source: Secondary sources, multinational

Infertility Data:
The authors reviewed the literature for infertility and subfecundity rates. They identified increasing infertility as a fundamental by-product of aging. When compared with females aged 20-24 years, fertility is reduced 6% on average for those females aged 25-29, 14% for those aged 30-34, and 31% for those aged 35-39. The authors identified confounding variables when calculating infertility rates. For example, 23% of women in rural English parishes who married between the ages of 20 and 24 failed to have a live birth within two years of marriage and 4.6% never had a child. They also examined three fertility surveys carried out in the United States: the National Fertility Survey of 1965 and the National Survey of Family Growth for 1976 and 1982. Infertility was defined as not conceiving within the previous year while not practising birth control. Infertility for wives aged 20-24 years was 3.6% in 1965, 6.7% in 1976, and 10.6% in 1982. Data from the three surveys are averaged in the table below.

Age	Impaired fecundity (%)*	Infertile (%)**
15-19		
20-24	10.8	7.0
25-29		8.9
30-34	25.2	14.6
35-39		21.9
40-44	55.1	28.7

* Impaired fecundity: The numerator is composed of those (i) who are surgically sterile for non-contraceptive reasons; (ii) who are non-surgically sterile; (iii) who are subfecund (self-reported difficulty in conceiving or delivering a child); and (iv) who failed to conceive in the previous three years while married and not using contraception. The denominator excludes those couples who are surgically sterile for contraceptive reasons.

** The numerator consists of those who failed to conceive in the previous year while married and not using contraception. The denominator excludes those couples who are surgically sterile for any reason.

Moghissi, K.S. 1979. "Current Concepts in Infertility." *Clinical Obstetrics and Gynecology* 22 (March): 9-10.

Source: Editorial, United States

Infertility Data:
The opening sentence of this editorial states that infertility affects approximately 10 to 15% of couples. The author states that one area of concern is that knowledge of the male reproductive process lags behind that of the female.

Mosher, W.D. 1982a. "Fertility and Family Planning in the 1970s: The National Survey of Family Growth." *Family Planning Perspectives* 14: 314-20.

Source: Primary sources, national surveys, United States, 1965-1976

Infertility Data:

Information was derived from Cycles I and II (1973 and 1976) of the National Survey of Family Growth (NSFG) and the National Fertility Survey (1965) in the United States. The author defines infertility as the inability to conceive after one year of unprotected intercourse.

Based upon 1976 NSFG data, the author states that about 56% of married couples (wife aged 15-44 years) were fecund, 29% were surgically sterile (19% for contraceptive reasons and 10% for non-contraceptive reasons), and 16% (4.3 million couples) had non-surgical fecundity problems. Of the 16%, 1.5 million had no births (primary infertility) or only one child (secondary infertility) and wanted to have children.

Both the 1965 National Fertility Survey and the 1976 National Survey of Family Growth indicate that about 1 in 10 couples in which the wife is 15-44 years of age is infertile. However, the proportion of infertile couples increased between 1965 and 1976 among couples aged 15-29 and decreased among couples aged 30-44. The author, quoting Mosher (1982b), relates the increase in infertility among younger couples to an increase in the number of cases of gonorrhoea reported in the United States between 1965 and 1975. The decrease in infertility among older couples is attributed to a decrease in syphilis and a masking of infertility due to dramatic increases in contraceptive sterilization.

Mosher, W.D. 1982b. "Infertility Trends Among U.S. Couples: 1965-1976." *Family Planning Perspectives* 14: 22-27.

Source: Primary sources, national surveys, United States, 1965 and 1976

Infertility Data:

Findings presented in this article are based upon data obtained from the 1965 National Fertility Study and the 1976 National Survey of Family Growth. Details on the study characteristics, sample population, method of collecting data, and criteria used to determine whether certain data should be included or excluded are not specified in the article. The author provides overall percentages for the prevalence of surgical infertility, and primary and secondary infertility by race, age, parity, and level of education for married women in the United States (Tables 1-3). Infertility is defined as failure to conceive after one or more years of marriage without contraception.

Findings:

Wives with the least amount of education are the most likely to be sterilized; as the wives become older, the incidence of sterility and infertility increases; and more couples were surgically sterile in 1976 than in 1965 (28% versus 16%).

Table 1. Currently Married Females

Age	Surgically sterile (%)		Infertile (%)		Fecund (%)		Total (%)
	1965	1976	1965	1976	1965	1976	
15-19	0.6	1.0	0.6	2.1	98.9	96.9	100
20-24	3.1	4.5	3.5	6.4	93.4	89.2	100
25-29	9.5	16.6	6.5	9.0	84.0	74.4	100
30-34	17.0	36.2	11.6	10.3	71.3	53.5	100
35-39	22.8	45.3	14.2	12.5	63.0	42.2	100
40-44	26.8	49.0	20.2	15.9	52.9	35.2	100
Total	15.8	28.2	11.2	10.3	73.0	61.6	100

Table 2. Currently Married White Females

Age	Surgically sterile (%)		Infertile (%)		Fecund (%)		Total (%)
	1965	1976	1965	1976	1965	1976	
15-19	0.6	0.8	0.6	2.0	98.7	97.3	100
20-24	3.1	4.5	3.4	5.6	93.4	89.9	100
25-29	9.1	17.1	6.1	8.4	84.8	74.5	100
30-34	17.2	37.8	10.8	9.5	72.0	52.7	100
35-39	22.8	45.9	13.4	11.4	63.8	42.7	100
40-44	26.7	50.2	18.5	14.6	54.8	35.2	100
Total	15.9	29.0	10.5	9.4	73.6	61.6	100

Table 3. Currently Married Black Females

Age	Surgically sterile (%)		Infertile (%)		Fecund (%)		Total (%)
	1965	1976	1965	1976	1965	1976	
15-19	0.0	3.5	0.0	3.7	100.0	92.8	100
20-24	3.4	5.5	3.4	15.4	93.1	79.1	100
25-29	12.0	13.5	7.1	11.2	80.9	75.4	100
30-34	13.5	20.0	15.7	18.1	70.8	62.0	100
35-39	21.5	37.8	24.4	23.3	54.1	38.9	100
40-44	27.3	40.3	39.0	28.8	33.7	30.9	100
Total	14.2	21.6	16.3	18.1	69.5	60.3	100

Mosher, W.D. 1985. "Reproductive Impairments in the United States, 1965-1982." *Demography* 22: 415-30.

Source: Primary sources, national survey, United States, 1982

Infertility Data:
   Findings presented in this article are based upon the results of Cycle III of the National Survey of Family Growth conducted by the National Center for Health Statistics between August 1982 and February 1983. Women aged 15-44 years were interviewed regardless of their marital status. Sample characteristics are as follows:

White women	4 577
Black women	3 201
Women of other races	191
Total	7 969
Married	3 300
Never married	3 500
Previously married	1 100
Total	7 900

Infertility is defined as experiencing difficulty in conceiving. Impaired fecundity is defined as experiencing difficulty in both conceiving and carrying a pregnancy to term.
   The author concludes that one in seven couples is infertile at age 30-34 years, increasing to one in five at age 35-39, and one in four at age 40-44. Also, the proportion of infertility at the given age ranges has not changed significantly since 1965 (Tables 1 and 2).

Table 1. Percentage of Currently Married Couples in Which the Wives Are 15 to 44 Years of Age

	Infertile		
Age	1965	1976	1982
15-44	11.2	10.3	8.5
15-19	0.6	2.1	2.1
20-24	3.5	6.4	9.7
25-29	6.5	9.0	7.0
30-34	11.6	10.3	7.7
35-39	14.2	12.5	10.3
40-44	20.2	15.9	9.0

Table 2. Percentage of Currently Married Couples, in Which the Wives Are 15 to 44 Years of Age, Who Are Infertile, Excluding Surgically Sterile

Age	Infertile		
	1965	1976	1982
15-44	13.3	14.3	13.9
15-19	0.6	2.1	2.1
20-24	3.6	6.7	10.6
25-29	7.2	10.8	8.7
30-34	14.0	16.1	13.6
35-39	18.4	22.8	24.6
40-44	27.7	31.1	27.2

Mosher, W.D. 1988. "Fecundity and Infertility in the United States." *American Journal of Public Health* 78: 181-82.

Source: Primary sources, national survey, United States, 1982

Infertility Data:
The article, quoting Mosher and Pratt (1987) extensively, states that 1 million couples in the United States experienced primary infertility in 1982, 1.4 million couples experience secondary infertility, and an estimated 4.5 million women (or couples) experience impaired fecundity (difficulty in both conceiving and carrying a pregnancy to term).

Infertility is defined as 12 months or more of unprotected intercourse without conception.

Data were obtained from the 1982 National Survey of Family Growth. The survey, based upon 7 969 interviews — "weighted" to achieve a representative group — is estimated to represent 54 million females. No medical exam/tests were conducted. The results are based upon a detailed questionnaire that includes a pregnancy history, a contraceptive history, a marital history, questions on sterilization and infertility, and a number of demographic questions (Table 1).

Table 1. Percentage of Married Women 25 to 44 Years of Age, Excluding Those Who Are Surgically Sterile, 1982

Age	Primary impaired fecundity	Secondary impaired fecundity	Spontaneous pregnancy loss
25-34	16.00	12.00	17.00
35-44	33.00	27.00	31.00

Mosher, W.D., and S.O. Aral. 1985. "Factors Related to Infertility in the United States, 1965-1976." *Sexually Transmitted Diseases* 12: 117-23.

Source: Primary sources, national surveys, United States, 1965, 1973, and 1976

Infertility Data:

Findings presented in this article are based upon data obtained from the 1965 National Fertility Study and the National Survey of Family Growth for 1973 and 1976. Details on the study characteristics, sample population, method of collecting data, and criteria used to determine whether certain data should be included or excluded are not specified in the article. Major emphasis is placed upon factors contributing toward the increase in infertility among young black females from 1965 to 1976. Findings are presented in Table 1.

Table 1. Percent Infertility for Currently Married Women 20-29 Years of Age

1965		1973		1976	
White (n = 1 292)	Black (n = 413)	White (n = 2 162)	Black (n = 926)	White (n = 2 075)	Black (n = 671)
4.8	5.2	5.3	8.5	7.2	13.1

Major reasons given for the increase in infertility among young black females are the younger age at which they are sexually active, the increased number of sexual partners, and the increased frequency of sexually transmitted diseases among the black cohort. Infertility among the white cohort was essentially unchanged from 1965 to 1976.

Mosher, W.D., and W.F. Pratt. 1987. *Fecundity, Infertility, and Reproductive Health in the United States, 1982.* Vital and Health Statistics: Data from the National Survey of Family Growth, Series 23, No. 14. Hyattsville: U.S. Department of Health and Human Services.

Source: Primary sources, national survey, United States, 1982

Infertility Data:
This periodic survey is used by a variety of authors (most notably Mosher) as a source of infertility data pertaining to the United States.

A couple is defined as being infertile if neither spouse is surgically sterile and if they have had at least 12 months of unprotected intercourse without pregnancy.

Impaired fecundity covers women who are classified as being non-surgically sterile, subfecund (experience difficulty in conceiving or carrying a pregnancy to term), or long-interval (during three years of continuous marriage, the woman did not use contraception and did not have a pregnancy).

The sample population consisted of 7 969 females between the ages of 15 and 44 years. The study was conducted between August 1982 and February 1983. Statistics obtained from the study group were extrapolated to represent the national population. The study group consisted of the following:

White women	4 577
Black women	3 201
Women of other races	191
Total	7 969

In this report, actual numbers were not presented. Instead, percentages were used to provide incidence and prevalence rates (Table 1-3). The results of this survey are also reported in a number of other articles.

Table 1. Percentage of Women 15 to 44 Years of Age with Impaired Fecundity, 1982

	All marital statuses		Currently married	
Age	All women	Not surgically sterile	All women	Not surgically sterile
15-44	8.4	11.3	10.8	17.7
15-19	2.1	2.1	6.1	6.1
20-24	6.4	6.7	9.2	10.0
25-29	10.6	12.5	10.0	12.5
30-34	9.3	14.8	9.4	16.7
35-39	13.0	27.9	14.3	34.1
40-44	11.0	28.2	11.6	34.8

Table 2. Percentage of Currently Married Women with Impaired Fecundity, Excluding Those Who Are Surgically Sterile, 1976 and 1982

Age	1976	1982
15-44	21.8	17.7
15-24	11.2	9.5
25-34	20.9	14.2
35-44	36.0	34.4

Table 3. Percent Distribution of Currently Married Women 15 to 44 Years of Age Considered Infertile, by Age Group

	Infertile					
	1965		1976		1982	
Age	(1)	(2)	(1)	(2)	(1)	(2)
15-44	11.2	13.3	10.3	14.3	8.5	13.9
15-19	0.6	0.6	2.1	2.1	2.1	2.1
20-24	3.5	3.6	6.4	6.7	9.7	10.6
25-29	6.5	7.2	9.0	10.8	7.0	8.7
30-34	11.6	14.0	10.3	16.1	7.7	13.6
35-39	14.2	18.4	12.5	22.8	10.3	24.6
40-44	20.2	27.7	15.9	31.1	9.0	27.2

(1) Including those who are surgically sterile.
(2) Excluding those who are surgically sterile.

Mosher, W.D., and W.F. Pratt. 1990. *Fecundity and Infertility in the United States, 1965-88*. Advance Data from Vital and Health Statistics of the National Center for Health Statistics, No. 192. Hyattsville: U.S. Department of Health and Human Services.

Source: Primary sources, national surveys, United States, 1965-1988

Infertility Data:

Data for 1976, 1982, and 1988 are from Cycles II, III, and IV of the National Survey of Family Growth (NSFG). Data for 1965 are from the National Fertility Study. The 1988 NSFG was based on personal interviews with a national sample of 8 450 women 15-44 years of age in the civilian, non-institutionalized population of the United States.

This report presents the first national estimates of trends (1982-1988) in the fecundity status of all women of reproductive age in the United States, regardless of marital status, and trends in the use of infertility services. It also updates earlier publications of National Surveys (1965, 1976, and 1982) describing trends in fecundity and infertility among married couples.

The authors define infertility as difficulty in conceiving after 12 months or more of intercourse without contraception. Impaired fecundity is defined as both difficulty in conceiving and difficulty (or danger) in carrying the pregnancy to term.

Based upon the 1982 and 1988 NSFG data, the authors make the following conclusions about trends in delayed childbearing and impaired fecundity in the United States for all women aged 15-44 (Table 1):

1. The number of women aged 25-44 who have had no births is increasing. The authors attribute this, in part, to the baby boom generation (born between 1946 and 1964).

2. The percentage of women with impaired fecundity dropped among childless women aged 25-34 and 35-44.

3. The increasing number of childless women in the age range of 25-44 years has increased the number of childless women who have impaired fecundity, despite the decline in the percentage who have impaired fecundity.

From 1964, 1976, 1982, and 1988 data on married couples, the authors conclude that the number of married couples with secondary infertility has declined from 2.5 million in 1965, to 1.4 million in 1982, to 1.3 million in 1988 (Table 2). Overall, from 1982 to 1988 there was virtually no change in the number of couples who were infertile.

Table 1. Number of Women 15-44 Years of Age and Percent Distribution by Fecundity Status, According to Parity, United States, 1988, 1982

Parity	No. of women (thousands)		Impaired fecundity (%)	
	1988	1982	1988	1982
All parities	57 900	54 099	8.4	8.4
Parity 0	25 129	22 941	8.8	8.4
Parity 1 or more	32 771	31 158	8.1	8.5

Table 2. Number of Currently Married Women 15-44 Years of Age Who Were Infertile by Parity, United States, 1988, 1982, 1965

Parity	No. of women (millions)		
	1988	1982	1965
All parities	2.3 (7.9%)	2.4 (8.5%)	3.0 (11.2%)
Parity 0	1.0 (18.5%)	1.0 (19.6%)	0.5 (14.5%)
Parity 1 or more	1.3 (5.4%)	1.4 (6.0%)	2.5 (10.8%)

Olsen, J., et al. 1983. "Tobacco Use, Alcohol Consumption and Infertility." *International Journal of Epidemiology* 12: 179-84.

Source: Primary sources, case-control study, Denmark, 1977-1979

Infertility Data:

This study evaluated two groups of couples from 1977 to 1979. The study group consisted of 1 069 infertile couples who attended an infertility clinic at Odense University Hospital and 4 305 fertile control couples who had a healthy infant born during the same period at the hospital.

Sociodemographic data were provided by 927 case and 3 728 control couples through a questionnaire. Control couples were defined as parents of a healthy child conceived within one year. Case couples were designated as having primary or secondary subfecundity on the basis of whether or not a live birth had ever been achieved prior to the time of seeking hospital treatment for a fecundity problem (presumably, subfecundity was defined as the inability to achieve conception within 12 months of regular unprotected intercourse). The relative risk of primary subfecundity for women smokers was 1.6%. The relative risk of secondary subfecundity for women smokers was 2.1%. The authors also examined the effect of alcohol consumption and the use of birth control pills on fertility with equivocal results.

Page, H. 1989. "Estimation of the Prevalence and Incidence of Infertility in a Population: A Pilot Study." *Fertility and Sterility* 51: 571-77.

Source: Primary sources, clinic-based data, United Kingdom

Infertility Data:
The author quotes Rachootin and Olsen (1982) as giving primary infertility rates of 15% and secondary infertility rates of 13% (lifetime rates). He cites Mosher and Pratt (1987) as stating that 8.5% of all couples aged 15-44 years experience infertility at one point in their lives. The study consisted of 250 females chosen at random from 2 500 female patients of a small (six physicians) group practice. Infertility was defined as 12 or more months of unprotected intercourse without conception. Data were obtained through a questionnaire that was returned by 201 (80%) of the participants involved in the study. The author differentiates between "incidence" and "prevalence":

> Incidence: "the number of women aged 20 to 44 years each year who reach the point at which they have been trying for 12 months unsuccessfully to conceive, divided by the number of married or cohabiting women aged 20 to 44 years."
> Prevalence: "the number of women aged 20 to 44 years who have been [trying to conceive] for more than 1 year, divided by the number of married or cohabiting women aged 20 to 44 years, in the population."

Of the 201 respondents, 165 (82%) were cohabiting and were considered the "population at risk." One hundred and fifty-three provided complete information (it was not clear whether this was 153 of the 201 respondents or 153 of the 165 who were cohabiting). Of these, 20 were not practising birth control and had not conceived for a period of 12 months or more, giving a prevalence of infertility of 13.1%. Primary infertility was found to be 5.9% and secondary infertility was 7.2%. The incidence of infertility (i.e., unprotected intercourse for exactly 12 months without a pregnancy) was calculated to be 1.31%. In addition to the 20 infertile women, among the 134 women who had a previous pregnancy, 120 provided information on previous pregnancies. Twenty-seven had experienced an episode of infertility: 13 women required between one and two years to conceive, 7 between two and three years, and the remaining 7 required more than three years to conceive. Thus 22% (27/134) of those who eventually conceived had experienced infertility.

Poston, D.L., Jr., and K.B. Kramer. 1983. "Voluntary and Involuntary Childlessness in the United States, 1955-1973." *Social Biology* 30: 290-306.

Source: Secondary sources, U.S. Bureau of the Census data, 1910-1981, national surveys, United States, 1955, 1960, 1965, 1970, and 1973

Infertility Data:

The authors use census data to demonstrate childlessness from 1910 to 1981 and then propose trends in voluntary versus involuntary childlessness. Percent childlessness from 1910 to 1981 among married women 15-44 years of age is as follows (data from the U.S. Bureau of the Census):

YEAR	PERCENTAGE	YEAR	PERCENTAGE
1910	19.2	1971	15.9
1940	24.1	1974	18.9
1950	22.8	1975	18.6
1952	20.7	1976	18.8
1957	15.9	1977	19.2
1960	15.0	1978	18.9
1962	14.4	1979	19.0
1965	14.2	1981	18.6
1970	16.4		

The article describes two theories for determining "involuntary childlessness" as the cognitive model and the behavioural model. Based upon the two theories, the authors establish three categories of childlessness for married non-pregnant wives: voluntary childlessness, temporary childlessness, and involuntary childlessness (infertile). Temporary childlessness applies to those women who are practising birth control and, therefore, do not know their true fertility status. The authors reviewed data from five studies on fertility carried out in the United States from 1955 to 1973: the Growth of American Families Study for 1955 and 1960, National Fertility Survey for 1965 and 1970, and the National Survey of Family Growth for 1973. Using data from the 1973 survey, the authors looked at the 9 797 women involved in the study and then excluded all non-white respondents (3 933) and those who were pregnant (350). Of the remaining 5 514 women, 903 were childless, 121 (13.4%) of whom indicated that they were involuntarily childless. An examination of the five studies was undertaken to determine trends (Table 1).

Table 1. Percentage of White Non-Pregnant Wives Who Are Involuntarily Childless

Year	All ages	Under age 30	Over age 30
1955	5.9	6.7	1.8
1960	6.4	3.3	4.2
1965	2.0	0.9	2.5
1970	1.8	0.7	2.7
1973	2.2	1.6	2.6

Note: The denominator is the total number of white non-pregnant wives.

The authors suggest that "increasing childlessness in society is voluntary and the increases are not due to increasing sterility and subfecundity stemming from involuntary factors."

Poston, D.L., Jr., and R.G. Rogers. 1988. "Development and Childlessness in the States and Territories of Brazil." *Social Biology* 35: 267-84.

Source: Secondary sources, Brazil, 1980 census data

Infertility Data:
Using 1980 census data from Brazil, the authors found a correlation between more developed regions and an increased incidence of childlessness, especially at younger ages (Table 1).

Table 1. Descriptive Statistics of Childlessness Rates: Twenty-Five States and Territories of Brazil, 1980

Age group	Mean	Standard deviation	Maximum value	Minimum value
15-19	0.414	0.036	0.471	0.321
20-24	0.185	0.036	0.278	0.105
25-29	0.102	0.019	0.156	0.079
30-34	0.066	0.012	0.096	0.045
35-39	0.055	0.012	0.082	0.029
40-44	0.061	0.012	0.090	0.038
45-49	0.067	0.016	0.106	0.046

The authors hypothesize that increased childlessness at younger ages is voluntary and more closely reflects current trends in "developed countries," where women are postponing childbearing.

Pratt, W.F., et al. 1985. "Infertility — United States, 1982." *Morbidity and Mortality Weekly Report* 34 (12 April): 197-99.

Source: Primary sources, national surveys, United States, 1965, 1976, and 1982

Infertility Data:
The author outlines the findings of the National Survey of Family Growth, 1982. He states that "more than one in eight couples were classified as infertile" and that "nearly one in five ever-married women of reproductive age reported they had sought professional consultation during their lifetimes to increase their chances of having children." The author estimates that health care costs associated with infertility are at least $200 million annually in the United States. The profile of infertile couples in the United States is as follows:

- they are older;
- they are more likely to be black;
- they have no previous children; and
- they are more likely to have less than a high school education.

The risk of infertility among women aged 35-44 years is double that of women aged 30-34.

Quebec. Comité de travail sur les nouvelles technologies de reproduction humaine. 1988. *Rapport du comité de travail sur les nouvelles technologies de reproduction humaine.* Quebec: Ministère de la Santé et des Services sociaux.

Source: Secondary sources, multinational data

Infertility Data:
　　Infertility is defined as the inability to conceive after 12 months of unprotected intercourse. This report quotes Rochon (1986), who, accepting a fecundability rate of 25% for each menstrual cycle, estimates an infertility rate of 12.6%. Therefore, 53.8% of these women will conceive in the second year, 28.3% in the third year, and 14% in the fourth year. Sterility is stated as being 3%. The report addresses a number of related issues, including causes and treatment of infertility.
　　Based upon the studies reviewed, infertility in couples was distributed as follows:

Male factor	33-40%
Female factor	45-60%
Both partners	20%

Rachootin, P., and J. Olsen. 1982. "Prevalence and Socioeconomic Correlates of Subfecundity and Spontaneous Abortion in Denmark." *International Journal of Epidemiology* 11: 245-49.

Source: Primary sources, national survey, Denmark, 1979

Infertility Data:
　　The authors "randomly identified" 1.4 women per thousand in Denmark between the ages of 25 and 45 years. The total sample involved 953 women, of which 74% (709 women) were interviewed, 18% refused to be interviewed, and 8% could not be contacted.

Definitions:
Primary subfecundity: failure to achieve a first pregnancy after engaging in sexual activity without contraception for at least one year.
Secondary subfecundity: failure to achieve a second or subsequent pregnancy within one year of cohabiting without contraception.
Primary infertility: failure to produce a first child.

Of the 709 women who were interviewed, 657 had attempted conception, 631 had achieved conception, and 542 had either achieved or attempted two conceptions.

Primary and secondary subfecundity rates based upon one or more years of failing to conceive were 16% and 17% respectively. Primary and secondary subfecundity rates based upon two or more years of failing to conceive were 10% and 12% respectively. Four percent of the women never produced a desired first child. Four percent of the women never produced a second or subsequent desired child.

Rajulton, F., T.R. Balakrishnan, and Z.R. Ravanera. 1990. "Measuring Infertility in Contracepting Populations." London: University of Western Ontario, Population Studies Centre.

Source: Primary sources, national survey, Canada, 1984

Infertility Data:
The authors quote Mosher (1985) when stating the proportion of sterile women has increased from 0.035 in 1965 to 0.106 in 1982 among women aged 20-24 years, but not for women in other age groups. They also quote Johnson et al. (1987) when stating that the incidence of involuntary childlessness in England was 3.2% for those women born in 1950 and 4.5% for those women born in 1935. The authors used the Canadian Fertility Survey of 1984 as the primary source for their figures. An examination of the records of 1 741 multiparous women revealed 156 women who were in a stable relationship, were not sterilized, had had no miscarriages, were not practising contraception, and were not currently pregnant, and another 42 women who exhibited "clear signs of infertility." Infertility, therefore, was calculated as 11.4%.

Rantala, M.-L., and A.I. Koskimies. 1986. "Infertility in Women Participating in a Screening Program for Cervical Cancer in Helsinki." *Acta Obstetricia et Gynecologica Scandinavica* 65: 823-25.

Source: Primary sources, national clinic based data, Finland, 1981-1982

Infertility Data:
A short literature review is included in which the authors quote Kistner (1979) when stating that the prevalence of infertility is approximately 15%. This study was conducted in Finland from 1981 to 1982. The study population included all of those females aged 30, 35, and 40 years

who attended an annual screening program for cancer by Pap smear. Approximately 60% of the total eligible population participates in this program. The study involved an interview and a questionnaire.

Definitions:

Primary infertility: inability to achieve a first pregnancy within one year of unprotected intercourse.

Secondary infertility: inability to achieve a second or subsequent pregnancy within one year of unprotected intercourse.

Actual infertility: failure to establish pregnancy at the time of the interview.

Total infertility: all females who had experienced either primary or secondary infertility in the past or at the time of the study.

Of 4 879 women interviewed, 149 were excluded because their questionnaires provided incomplete data and 528 were excluded because they were "not at risk for pregnancy." Thus, 4 202 (86%) women were included in the study.

Findings:

Actual infertility was found in 438 (10.4%) of the women (Table 1). It was also found that infertility increased significantly with age.

Table 1. Infertility Rates					
Age group	n	Actual primary infertility (1)	Actual secondary infertility (2)	Actual infertility (1) & (2)	Total infertility
30	2 530	127 (5.0%)	103 (4.1%)	230 (9.1%)	322 (12.7%)
35	1 098	61 (5.6%)	67 (6.1%)	128 (11.7%)	208 (18.9%)
40	574	23 (4.0%)	57 (9.9%)	80 (13.9%)	119 (20.7%)
Total	4 202	211 (5.0%)	227 (5.4%)	438 (10.4%)	649 (15.4%)

In this study, lifetime prevalence of infertility is 15.4% and point prevalence is 10.4%.

"Recent U.S. Fertility Patterns Continue: Birthrates Climb Among Older Women, Childlessness Rises." 1988. *Family Planning Perspectives* 20: 44-45.

Source: Primary sources, U.S. Bureau of the Census data, United States, 1986

Infertility Data:
    This article is based upon the U.S. Bureau of the Census' *Fertility of American Women: June 1986*. Fertility rate figures are given based upon age, occupation, income level, and race. The article states that one out of eight women 40-44 years of age is childless, one in six women 35-39 years of age is childless, and one in four women 30-34 years of age is childless. No mention is made as to whether these women are "voluntarily or involuntarily" childless. Childlessness is less common among foreign-born women than women born in the United States. Six percent of foreign-born women 18-34 years of age stated that they "expected to remain childless," whereas 10% of women born in the United States expected to be childless (once again, no comment was made regarding voluntary versus involuntary childlessness).

Spira, A. 1986. "Epidemiology of Human Reproduction." *Human Reproduction* 1: 111-15.

Source: Secondary sources, multinational data

Infertility Data:
    The author states that, based upon a worldwide study of fecundity, 3-5% of couples in industrialized countries have not had a child at the end of their reproductive life even though they desire one (no reference provided). Selected studies of couples seeking clinical treatment indicate that the causes of infertility are as follows:

    57% due to the female partner alone
    29% due to ovulation disorders
    16% due to tubal factors
    2% due to cervical factors
    3% due to uterine factors
    7% due to endometriosis
    4% due to multiple factors
    21% due to the male partner alone
    4% due to a combination of both partners
    18% due to unknown factors

    From Léridon's (1981) estimates, the author calculates that 4% of couples will be sterile and 15% of couples will be subfecund; therefore, 19% of couples will have trouble conceiving.
    Subfecund couples have a fecundability of approximately four to five times less than normal couples. Given that for normal couples fecundability is estimated as 25% per month, subfecund couples have a fecundability rate of approximately 5%. Therefore, the author estimates that after three years, 22% of subfecund couples will not have conceived

(15% × 22% = 3.0%). If one assumes that these couples (3%) plus the sterile couples (4%) will seek treatment, the author estimates that approximately 7% of all newly married couples will likely turn to more complex diagnostic measures.

Sundby, J. 1989. "Methodological Considerations in the Study of Frequency, Risk Factors and Outcome of Reduced Fertility." *Scandinavian Journal of Social Medicine* 17: 135-40.

Source: Secondary sources, data from various countries

Infertility Data:
    This article is essentially a literature review. Primary infertility is defined as "never been pregnant" and secondary infertility as "couples unable to get pregnant after one or more previous pregnancies." The time span used to define infertility varies from one to two years depending upon the researcher and the organization. The author quotes Østby and Noack (1981) as stating that "7% of married couples [in Norway] are childless at the end of their reproductive period (35-44 years)." Only 4% were considered to be childless due to infertility, the remaining 3% were "voluntarily childless." The author quotes Rantala and Koskimies (1986), who estimate that 15% of all women in Finland are infertile at some point in their lives and that at the age of 40 years, this figure increases to 20%. She quotes Hull et al. (1985) as stating that 17% of all couples in England seek help for either primary or secondary infertility at some time. The author quotes Johnson et al. (1987) as stating that 14.3% of women born in 1950 and 7.7% of women born in 1935 in England were childless. The article focusses on examining trends associated with infertility.

Swerdloff, R.S., et al. 1985. "Infertility in the Male." *Annals of Internal Medicine* 103: 906-19.

Source: Secondary sources, United States

Infertility Data:
    Infertility is attributed to a couple that is unable to conceive despite a reasonable frequency of unprotected coitus for more than one year; "reasonable frequency" is not defined. The prevalence of infertility is given as 15% of all U.S. couples. The authors attribute infertility to 33.3% abnormalities in the female partner, 33.3% abnormalities in the male partner, and 33.3% abnormalities in both partners.

The bulk of the article addresses various causes and treatment of male infertility.

Templeton, A., C. Fraser, and B. Thompson. 1991. "The Epidemiology of Infertility in Aberdeen." *British Medical Journal* 301: 148-52.

Source: Primary sources, retrospective study, regional survey, United Kingdom

Infertility Data:
In this study, a questionnaire was mailed to 1 024 females aged 46-50 years; 130 of these were subsequently excluded. Of the remaining 894 women, 766 (86%) responded. The authors defined infertility as the inability to conceive after 24 months or more of unprotected intercourse.

Findings:
Of the 766 respondents, 78.6% reported no difficulties in conceiving, 7.3% chose not to have children, and 14.1% experienced infertility (8.9% experiencing primary infertility, of which 5.4% eventually conceived, and 5.4% experiencing secondary infertility, of which 3% eventually conceived). Overall, 5.7% of the women were left with unresolved infertility problems.

Thonneau, P., and A. Spira. 1990. "Prevalence of Infertility: International Data and Problems of Measurement." *European Journal of Obstetrics & Gynecology and Reproductive Biology* 38: 43-52.

Source: Literature review, secondary data from multinational studies

Infertility Data:
This article reviews a number of national studies from Europe and North America and comments on the strengths and weaknesses of various study designs and population characteristics. The authors address multinational, national, regional, and health centre based studies.
The authors quote Léridon (1986) as giving a subfecundity rate of 14.7% and a sterility rate of 3.7%. They also quote Rachootin and Olsen (1982) as giving a primary subfecundity rate of 16%, a secondary subfecundity rate of 17%, and primary and secondary sterility rates of 4%. They quote Pratt et al. (1985) as giving a prevalence of infertility between 13% and 14% in 1965, 1976, and 1982. The authors also reviewed a number of regional studies: Rantala and Koskimies (1986) gave an overall infertility estimate of 11% for Danish women between 25 and 45 years of age; Hull et al. (1985) estimate an incidence of infertility of 17%, 59% of which were

cases of primary infertility in the Bristol area of the United Kingdom; and the Institut national de la Santé et de la Recherche médicale (INSERM) in France found a lifetime prevalence of consultations for infertility (primary and secondary) of 16.2% (Thonneau et al. 1989).

Veevers, J.E. 1972. "Factors in the Incidence of Childlessness in Canada: An Analysis of Census Data." *Social Biology* 19: 266-74.

Source: Primary sources, Canada, 1961 census data

Infertility Data:
The author states that "it is generally felt that 10% of all couples are definitely sterile." She considers childlessness to result from one of two factors: physiological factors or psychological factors (Table 1). Psychological factors are those that lead to infertility in the absence of physical causes (i.e., psychosomatic infertility). Conclusions were based upon a 20% fertility sample of the 1961 Canadian census and refer to women ever-married and aged 45 years or older.

Table 1. Estimate of the Incidence of Psychological Childlessness Among Urban Women Aged 45 Years and Older by Age at First Marriage

Age at first marriage	Percentage remaining childless	Estimated percentage who are physiologically childless*	Estimated percentage who are psychologically childless*
15-19	5.03	2.02	3.01
20-24	8.20	2.78	5.42
25-29	15.03	3.81	11.22
30-34	27.22	9.47	17.22
35-39	48.33	23.74	24.59
40-44	74.77	50.00	27.77
45+	85.61	79.14	6.47
Total	15.22	6.59	8.63

* Percentage childlessness in rural areas was associated with physiological childlessness; the rest [childlessness in urban areas] was interpreted as psychological childlessness.

Conclusions:
The general concept that the incidence of sterility in the population is 10% is much too high; it should, in fact, be closer to 5%. The incidence of voluntary childlessness is decreasing; psychological factors account for more than 50% of childlessness.

Westoff, C.F. 1986. "Fertility in the United States." *Science* 234: 554-59.

Source: Secondary sources, United States

Infertility Data:
This article focusses on declining fertility rates in the United States. This citation refers to infertility prevalence in general terms. The author states that "all told, one in three can be classified with some type of impaired fecundity, but half of this results from elective sterilization for contraceptive reasons" (no reference given). Involuntary subfecundity consists of 8% who are surgically sterile (for medical reasons) and another 8% who are unable to conceive (Mosher and Pratt 1985). On the basis of 1982 data, some 15% of women both want and appear unable to have a child or another child (Alan Guttmacher Institute 1985).

Bibliography

Adadevoh, B.K. 1974. *Subfertility and Infertility in Africa.* Idaban: Caxton Press.

Alan Guttmacher Institute. 1985. "Infertility Services in the United States: Need, Accessibility and Utilization." New York: Alan Guttmacher Institute.

Anderson, K. 1989. "Infertility: The Silent Crisis." *Canada's Mental Health* 37 (March): 9-12.

Aral, S.O., and W. Cates, Jr. 1983. "The Increasing Concern with Infertility: Why Now?" *JAMA* 250: 2327-31.

Armitage, B. 1986. "Infertility: A Self-Instructional Package." Ottawa: Health and Welfare Canada.

Baird, D.D., and A.J. Wilcox. 1985. "Cigarette Smoking Associated with Delayed Conception." *JAMA* 253: 2979-83.

Balakrishnan, T.R., K.J. Krótki, and E. Lapierre-Adamcyk. 1985. "Contraceptive Use in Canada, 1984." *Family Planning Perspectives* 17: 209-15.

Barrett, J.C. 1986. "The Estimation of Natural Sterility." *Genus* 42 (3-4): 23-31.

Behrman, S.J., and R.W. Kistner. 1975. *Progress in Infertility.* 2d ed. Boston: Little, Brown.

Belsey, M.A. 1976. "The Epidemiology of Infertility: A Review with Particular Reference to Sub-Saharan Africa." *Bulletin of the World Health Organization* 54: 319-41.

—. 1984. "Infertility: Prevalence, Etiology, and Natural History." In *Perinatal Epidemiology*, ed. M.B. Bracken. New York: Oxford University Press.

Bendvold, E. 1989. "Semen Quality in Norwegian Men Over a 20-Year Period." *International Journal of Fertility* 34: 401-404.

Bergström, S. 1990. "Genital Infections and Reproductive Health: Infertility and Morbidity of Mother and Child in Developing Countries." *Scandinavian Journal of Infectious Diseases* (Suppl. 69): 99-105.

Blank, R. 1985. "The Infertility Epidemic." *Futurist* 19: 177-80.

Bongaarts, J. 1982. "Infertility After Age 30: A False Alarm." *Family Planning Perspectives* 14: 75-78.

Boyd, R.L. 1989. "Racial Differences in Childlessness: A Centennial Review." *Sociological Perspectives* 32: 183-99.

Bryant, H. 1990. "The Infertility Dilemma: Reproductive Technologies and Prevention." Ottawa: Canadian Advisory Council on the Status of Women.

Burgwyn, D. 1981. *Marriage Without Children*. New York: Harper & Row.

Cates, W., T.M.M. Farley, and P.J. Rowe. 1985. "Worldwide Patterns of Infertility: Is Africa Different?" *Lancet* (14 September): 596-98.

Clark, R.L., and B. Keefe. 1989. "Infertility: Imaging of the Female." *Urologic Radiology* 11: 233-37.

Dubin, L., and R.D. Amelar. 1980. "A Plea for a More Scientific Approach in the Treatment of Male Infertility." *Fertility and Sterility* 34: 74-75.

Ducot, B., and A. Spira. 1988. "Utilisation de la notion de fécondabilité dans le pronostic de l'infécondité." *Journal de Gynécologie obstétrique et Biologie de la Reproduction* 17: 461-66.

Ebomoyi, E., and O.O. Adetoro. 1990. "Socio-Biological Factors Influencing Infertility in a Rural Nigerian Community." *International Journal of Gynecology and Obstetrics* 33: 41-47.

Estrada, A., et al. 1972. *Resultados Generales: Encuesta Nacional de Fecundidad*. Publication No. 1. Bogota: Associacion Colombiana de Facultades de Medicina, Division de Medicina Social y Poblacion.

Fédération des centres d'étude et de conservation des œufs et du sperme humains, D. Schwartz, and M.J. Mayaux. 1982. "Female Fecundity as a Function of Age." *New England Journal of Medicine* 306: 404-406.

Greenhall, E., and M. Vessey. 1990. "The Prevalence of Subfertility: A Review of the Current Confusion and a Report of Two New Studies." *Fertility and Sterility* 54: 978-83.

Gunaratne, M. 1979. "The Epidemiology of Infertility: A Selected Clinic Study." *Ceylon Medical Journal* 24: 36-42.

Hirsch, M.B., and W.D. Mosher. 1987. "Characteristics of Infertile Women in the United States and Their Use of Infertility Services." *Fertility and Sterility* 47: 618-25.

Högberg, U., and S. Åkerman. 1990. "Reproductive Pattern Among Women in 19th Century Sweden." *Journal of Biosocial Science* 22: 13-18.

Howe, G., et al. 1985. "Effects of Age, Cigarette Smoking, and Other Factors on Fertility: Findings in a Large Prospective Study." *British Medical Journal* 290: 1697-1700.

Hull, M.G.R., et al. 1985. "Population Study of Causes, Treatment, and Outcome of Infertility." *British Medical Journal* 291: 1693-97.

Johnson, G., et al. 1987. "Infertile or Childless by Choice? A Multipractice Survey of Women Aged 35 and 50." *British Medical Journal* 294: 804-806.

Kistner, R.W. 1979. "Endometriosis and Infertility." *Clinical Obstetrics and Gynecology* 22: 101-19.

Korean Institute for Family Planning. 1971. *Fertility-Abortion Survey*. Seoul.

Léridon, H. 1981. "La stérilité: méthodes de mesure et modèles du démographe." In *Facteurs de la fertilité humaine*, ed. A. Spira and P. Jouannet. *Les Colloques de l'INSERM* 103: 475-86.

—. 1986. "Stérilité et hypofertilité." In *Recherches récentes sur l'épidemiologie de la fertilité*. Paris: Masson.

Li, Y., et al. 1990. "Infertility in a Rural Area of Jiangsu Province: An Epidemiological Survey." *International Journal of Fertility* 35: 347-49.

Link, P.W., and C.A. Darling. 1986. "Couples Undergoing Treatment for Infertility: Dimensions of Life Satisfaction." *Journal of Sex and Marital Therapy* 12: 46-58.

Lodh, F. 1987. *Explaining Fertility Decline in the West (with Special Reference to Canada): A Critique of Research Results from Social Sciences*. Ottawa: Vanier Institute of the Family.

MacMahon, B., and T.F. Pugh. 1970. *Epidemiology: Principles and Methods*. Boston: Little, Brown.

Marchbanks, P.A., et al. 1989. "Research on Infertility: Definition Makes a Difference." *American Journal of Epidemiology* 130: 259-67.

Martin, T.E. 1989. "Infertility in a Large Royal Air Force General Practice." *Journal of the Royal Army Medical Corps* 135 (June): 68-75.

Menken, J., J. Trussell, and U. Larsen. 1976. "Age and Infertility." *Science* 233: 1389-94.

Modawi, O. 1976. *Infertility in Sub-Saharan Africa with Special Reference to the Sudan*. Khartoum: Ministry of Health.

Moghissi, K.S. 1979. "Current Concepts in Infertility." *Clinical Obstetrics and Gynecology* 22 (March): 9-10.

Mosher, W.D. 1982a. "Fertility and Family Planning in the 1970s: The National Survey of Family Growth." *Family Planning Perspectives* 14: 314-20.

—. 1982b. "Infertility Trends Among U.S. Couples: 1965-1976." *Family Planning Perspectives* 14: 22-27.

—. 1985. "Reproductive Impairments in the United States, 1965-1982." *Demography* 22: 415-30.

—. 1988. "Fecundity and Infertility in the United States." *American Journal of Public Health* 78: 181-82.

Mosher, W.D., and S.O. Aral. 1985. "Factors Related to Infertility in the United States, 1965-1976." *Sexually Transmitted Diseases* 12: 117-23.

Mosher, W.D., and W.F. Pratt. 1985. *Fecundity and Infertility in the United States, 1965-82.* Advance Data from Vital Health Statistics, No. 104. Hyattsville: U.S. Department of Health and Human Services.

—. 1987. *Fecundity, Infertility, and Reproductive Health in the United States, 1982.* Vital and Health Statistics: Data from the National Survey of Family Growth, Series 23, No. 14. Hyattsville: U.S. Department of Health and Human Services.

—. 1990. *Fecundity and Infertility in the United States, 1965-88.* Advance Data from Vital and Health Statistics of the National Center for Health Statistics, No. 192. Hyattsville: U.S. Department of Health and Human Services.

Olsen, J., et al. 1983. "Tobacco Use, Alcohol Consumption and Infertility." *International Journal of Epidemiology* 12: 179-84.

Østby, L., and T. Noack. 1981. *Fertility Among Norwegian Women, Results from the Fertility Survey 1977.* Oslo: Central Bureau of Statistics.

Page, H. 1989. "Estimation of the Prevalence and Incidence of Infertility in a Population: A Pilot Study." *Fertility and Sterility* 51: 571-77.

Poston, D.L., Jr., and K.B. Kramer. 1983. "Voluntary and Involuntary Childlessness in the United States, 1955-1973." *Social Biology* 30: 290-306.

Poston, D.L., Jr., and R.G. Rogers. 1988. "Development and Childlessness in the States and Territories of Brazil." *Social Biology* 35: 267-84.

Pratt, W.F., et al. 1985. "Infertility — United States, 1982." *Morbidity and Mortality Weekly Report* 34 (12 April): 197-99.

Quebec. Comité de travail sur les nouvelles technologies de reproduction humaine. 1988. *Rapport du comité de travail sur les nouvelles technologies de reproduction humaine.* Quebec: Ministère de la Santé et des Services sociaux.

Rachootin, P., and J. Olsen. 1982. "Prevalence and Socioeconomic Correlates of Subfecundity and Spontaneous Abortion in Denmark." *International Journal of Epidemiology* 11: 245-49.

Rajulton, F., T.R. Balakrishnan, and Z.R. Ravanera. 1990. "Measuring Infertility in Contracepting Populations." London: University of Western Ontario, Population Studies Centre.

Rantala, M.-L., and A.I. Koskimies. 1986. "Infertility in Women Participating in a Screening Program for Cervical Cancer in Helsinki." *Acta Obstetricia et Gynecologica Scandinavica* 65: 823-25.

"Recent U.S. Fertility Patterns Continue: Birthrates Climb Among Older Women, Childlessness Rises." 1988. *Family Planning Perspectives* 20: 44-45.

Ring, A., and R. Scragg. 1973. "A Demographic and Social Study of Fertility in Rural New Guinea." *Journal of Biosocial Science* 5: 89-121.

Rochon, M. 1986. *Stérilité et infertilité: deux concepts, deux réalités*. Études de santé 3. Quebec: Ministère de la Santé et des Services sociaux.

Spira, A. 1986. "Epidemiology of Human Reproduction." *Human Reproduction* 1: 111-15.

Sundby, J. 1989. "Methodological Considerations in the Study of Frequency, Risk Factors and Outcome of Reduced Fertility." *Scandinavian Journal of Social Medicine* 17: 135-40.

Swerdloff, R.S., et al. 1985. "Infertility in the Male." *Annals of Internal Medicine* 103: 906-19.

Templeton, A., C. Fraser, and B. Thompson. 1991. "The Epidemiology of Infertility in Aberdeen." *British Medical Journal* 301: 148-52.

Thonneau, P., and A. Spira. 1990. "Prevalence of Infertility: International Data and Problems of Measurement." *European Journal of Obstetrics & Gynecology and Reproductive Biology* 38: 43-52.

Thonneau, P., et al. 1989. "Prevalence and Main Causes of Infertility (France)." Paper presented at the 13th World Congress on Fertility and Sterility, Marrakech.

Tietze, C., A.F. Guttmacher, and F. Rubin. 1950. "Time Required for Conception in 1727 Planned Pregnancies." *Fertility and Sterility* 1: 338-46.

United States. Bureau of the Census. 1943. *U.S. Census of Population: 1940. Differential Fertility: 1940 and 1910. Fertility for States and Large Cities*. Washington, DC: Government Printing Office.

—. 1955. *U.S. Census of Population: 1950*. Vol. IV, Special Reports, Part 5, Chapter C. "Fertility." Washington, DC: Government Printing Office.

—. 1969. *Marriage, Fertility, and Childspacing: June 1965*. Current Population Reports, Series P-20, No. 186. Washington, DC: Government Printing Office.

—. 1974. *Fertility Histories and Birth Expectations of American Women: June 1971*. Current Population Reports, Series P-20, No. 263. Washington, DC: Government Printing Office.

—. 1976. *Fertility of American Women: June 1975*. Current Population Reports, Series P-20, No. 301. Washington, DC: Government Printing Office.

—. 1987. *Fertility of American Women: June 1986*. Current Population Reports, Series P-20, No. 421. Washington, DC: Government Printing Office.

Unruh, A.M., and P.J. McGrath. 1985. "The Psychology of Female Infertility: Toward a New Perspective." *Health Care for Women International* 6: 369-81.

Ussing, J., and B. Schmidt. 1972. *Nogle resultatet fra fertilitet-sundersogelsen*. Study No. 22. Copenhagen.

Veevers, J.E. 1972. "Factors in the Incidence of Childlessness in Canada: An Analysis of Census Data." *Social Biology* 19: 266-74.

Vessey, M.P., et al. 1978. "Fertility After Stopping Different Methods of Contraception." *British Medical Journal* (4 February): 265-67.

Westoff, C.F. 1986. "Fertility in the United States." *Science* 234: 554-59.

World Fertility Survey. 1977. *The Survey of Fertility in Thailand: Country Report.* Report No. 1. Bangkok: Institute of Population Studies, Bangkok Chulalongkorn University and Population Survey Division, National Statistical Office.

World Health Organization. 1975. *The Epidemiology of Infertility: Report of a WHO Scientific Group.* Technical Report Series No. 582. Geneva: WHO.

Contributors

T.R. Balakrishnan, Ph.D.

Kerry J. Daly, Ph.D., Department of Family Studies, University of Guelph.

Michael R.P. de la Roche, M.D., M.Sc.

Corinne S. Dulberg, Ph.D., M.P.H.

Rajulton Fernando, Ph.D.

Paul Maxim, Ph.D., Population Studies Centre, University of Western Ontario.

Wendy L. Mitchinson, Ph.D., Department of History, University of Waterloo.

Michael P. Sobol, Ph.D., Department of Psychology, University of Guelph.

Thomas Stephens, Ph.D., Thomas Stephens and Associates.

Mandate

(approved by Her Excellency the Governor General
on the 25th day of October, 1989)

The Committee of the Privy Council, on the recommendation of the Prime Minister, advise that a Commission do issue under Part I of the Inquiries Act and under the Great Seal of Canada appointing The Royal Commission on New Reproductive Technologies to inquire into and report on current and potential medical and scientific developments related to new reproductive technologies, considering in particular their social, ethical, health, research, legal and economic implications and the public interest, recommending what policies and safeguards should be applied, and examining in particular,

(a)   implications of new reproductive technologies for women's reproductive health and well-being;

(b)   the causes, treatment and prevention of male and female infertility;

(c)   reversals of sterilization procedures, artificial insemination, *in vitro* fertilization, embryo transfers, prenatal screening and diagnostic techniques, genetic manipulation and therapeutic interventions to correct genetic anomalies, sex selection techniques, embryo experimentation and fetal tissue transplants;

(d)   social and legal arrangements, such as surrogate childbearing, judicial interventions during gestation and birth, and "ownership" of ova, sperm, embryos and fetal tissue;

(e)   the status and rights of people using or contributing to reproductive services, such as access to procedures, "rights" to parenthood, informed consent, status of gamete donors and confidentiality, and the impact of these services on all concerned parties, particularly the children; and

(f)   the economic ramifications of these technologies, such as the commercial marketing of ova, sperm and embryos, the application of patent law, and the funding of research and procedures including infertility treatment.

The Research Volumes

Volume 1: New Reproductive Technologies: Ethical Aspects

Approaches to the Ethical Issues Raised by the
Royal Commission's Mandate — W. Kymlicka

Assisted Reproductive Technologies:
Informed Choice — F. Baylis

Medicalization and the New Reproductive
Technologies — M. Burgess/A. Frank/ S. Sherwin

Prenatal Diagnosis and Society — D.C. Wertz

Roles for Ethics Committees in Relation to
Guidelines for New Reproductive
Technologies: A Research Position Paper — J.B. Dossetor/J.L. Storch

Economic, Ethical, and Population Aspects of
New Reproductive Technologies in
Developing Countries: Implications for
Canada — P. Manga

Volume 2: Social Values and Attitudes Surrounding New Reproductive Technologies

An Overview of Findings in This Volume — RCNRT Staff

Social Values and Attitudes of Canadians
Toward New Reproductive Technologies — Decima Research

Social Values and Attitudes of Canadians
Toward New Reproductive Technologies:
Focus Group Findings — Decima Research

Key Findings from a National Survey Conducted
by the Angus Reid Group: Infertility,
Surrogacy, Fetal Tissue Research, and
Reproductive Technologies — M. de Groh

Volume 3: Overview of Legal Issues in New Reproductive Technologies

Volume 4: Legal and Ethical Issues in New Reproductive Technologies: Pregnancy and Parenthood

Volume 5: New Reproductive Technologies and the Science, Industry, Education, and Social Welfare Systems in Canada

Volume 6: The Prevalence of Infertility in Canada

Volume 7: Understanding Infertility: Risk Factors Affecting Fertility

Volume 8: Prevention of Infertility

Volume 9: Treatment of Infertility: Assisted Reproductive Technologies

Volume 10: Treatment of Infertility: Current Practices and Psychosocial Implications

Volume 11: New Reproductive Technologies and the Health Care System: The Case for Evidence-Based Medicine

Volume 12: Prenatal Diagnosis: Background and Impact on Individuals

Volume 13: Current Practice of Prenatal Diagnosis in Canada

Volume 14: Technologies of Sex Selection and Prenatal Diagnosis

Volume 15: Background and Current Practice of Fetal Tissue and Embryo Research in Canada

Commission Organization

Commissioners

Patricia Baird
Chairperson
Vancouver, British Columbia

Grace Jantzen
London, United Kingdom

Bartha Maria Knoppers
Montreal, Quebec

Susan E.M. McCutcheon
Toronto, Ontario

Suzanne Rozell Scorsone
Toronto, Ontario

Staff

John Sinclair
Executive Director

Mimsie Rodrigue
Executive Director (from July 1993)

Research & Evaluation

Sylvia Gold
Director

Nancy Miller Chénier
Deputy Director
Causes and Prevention of Infertility

Janet Hatcher Roberts
Deputy Director
Assisted Human Reproduction

F. Clarke Fraser
Deputy Director
Prenatal Diagnosis and Genetics

Burleigh Trevor Deutsch
Deputy Director
Embryo and Fetal Tissue Research

Consultations & Coordination

Dann M. Michols
Director

Mimsie Rodrigue
Deputy Director
Coordination

Anne Marie Smart
Deputy Director
Communications

Judith Nolté
Deputy Director
Analysis

Denise Cole
Deputy Director
Consultations

Mary Ann Allen
Director
Administration and Security

Gary Paradis
Deputy Director
Finance